FOCUS ON MEDICAL SPECIALTIES

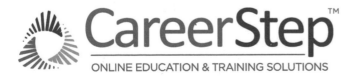

Career Step, LLC
Phone: 801.489.9393
Toll-Free: 800.246.7837
Fax: 801.491.6645
careerstep.com

This text companion contains a snapshot of the online program content converted to a printed format. Please note that the online training program is constantly changing and improving and is always the source of the most up-to-date information.

Product Number: HG-PR-11-009
Generation Date: March 13, 2015

TABLE OF CONTENTS

UNIT 1

Introduction

INTRODUCTION TO FOCUS ON MEDICAL SPECIALTIES

Learning Objectives

Medical Specialties Awareness – Students will be able to determine the correct use of specialty-specific information related to medical terminology, abbreviations, phrases, conditions, and treatments.

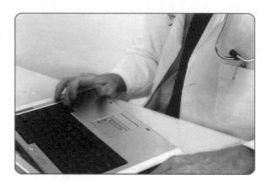

This Focus on Medical Specialties module is designed to provide full immersion in a variety of medical specialties—full immersion being attained by repeated exposure to specialty-specific terminology, abbreviations, medical phrases, conditions, assessment tools, and treatments. You may have been exposed to much of this information in various modules throughout this training program, but in this particular module we are pulling the information together for practical application by specialty.

All the reports in the "Focus," with examples from nearly every major medical specialty, are actual reports that were returned by actual transcription editors to actual medical facilities. They show you what medical transcription editing is: the language, the formats, the types of reports. They represent the results of the transcription editing process as they exist in the MTE workplace.

Traditional MTE training programs have used "sterile" as opposed to "live" transcription editing. That is, the reports—if they were actual reports to begin with—were scrubbed of inconsistencies, grammatical anomalies, and obvious mistakes. As a result, they did not represent the "real world" of medical transcription editing, and students who worked through them came out inadequately prepared for that world. Even reports by the best MTEs contain the acceptable variations, the typographical errors, the convoluted grammatical structures, and the occasional misspelled words that are an inevitable part of the workplace. Learning to identify such problems is a viable means for developing the questioning skill and judgment that the competent MTE or QA supervisor must have.

Keep in mind that in the workplace, turnaround times are usually short and unforgiving. As a working MTE, you may have one to four hours to return a stat report, and these days, in contrast to the past, most other reports must be edited and returned within twelve to twenty-four hours, depending on report type. Also keep in mind that most medical transcription editors are paid on production, so time spent trying to make every report perfect is simply not economical for the MTE, the MTE service, or the medical institution. For these reasons, there is tolerance in the workplace for imperfection. Most U.S. Government contracts, for example, which include military hospitals, Veterans Administration hospitals, and Public Health Service Hospitals, specify 98% accuracy. That works out—in their bid specifications—to about two errors per page. The reports in the medical specialties module are, using this criterion, close to 100% accurate. They do, however, represent "live" as opposed to "sterile" transcription editing, and you will find some imperfections and anomalies.

The upshot is that you are given an opportunity to begin to hone your editing, proofreading, and research skills.

That said, you should strive for 100% accuracy in Focus on Medical Specialties (often referred to as FOMS) reports and in your own transcription editing. It is often said that there is no shortage of medical transcription editors, but rather a shortage of quality medical transcription editors. We intend for you to be a top-quality MTE.

Since this material consists of reports sent to a number of different facilities, you will note variations in style and format. *Do not be overly concerned about this.* In addition, footnotes of explanation appear from time to time to indicate alternative ways of doing things, explain why certain things are done the way they are, and provide information on how to post notes for unintelligible dictation.

The Focus on Medical Specialties is comprehensive in scope, meaty in content, and is an excellent cross-section of 98% of what you will see as a medical transcription editor. Like anything else, it is only as valuable as the attention you give to it and the use you make of it.

THE BASIC FOUR

Most of the reports—a significant majority—in this module represent examples of what is commonly referred to in the MTE industry as the **Basic Four**. These reports represent work that was done for hospitals. You were introduced to the main medical report types in the Healthcare Documentation module of this training program, and you were given the general definitions and the headings most commonly used in these report types. To briefly review, the Basic Four are listed below.

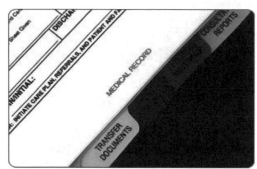

Admission History and Physical Exam

Often referred to as the **H&P**, this report type is dictated shortly after a patient is admitted. The reason for the admission is presented. History is elicited, both present and past. A review of systems is given, a physical exam is performed, and admission laboratory studies are done. A diagnosis/assessment is made, and a plan is outlined for the patient's treatment while in the hospital. The H&P contains all the information collected during this process.

As you work through the Focus on Medical Specialties, you will see that considerable variation in the details exists.

Operative Report

The **op report** is the narrative description of an operation performed on a patient while in the hospital. It generally includes at least the pre- and postoperative diagnosis, the indications for the procedure, the anesthesia given, the name of the surgeon and any assistants, the description of the actual procedure, estimated blood loss, and a description of complications (if any).

Discharge Summary or Narrative Summary

A **discharge summary** is required for any patient who is admitted to the hospital. It generally includes all of the information that appears in the Admission H&P and describes the patient's course of treatment in the hospital. It also includes any medications the patient is to take after discharge and reviews the instructions for post-hospital care and followup.

Consultation

A patient admitted to the hospital may be seen by physicians from various specialties who are called in (**consulted**) to examine and evaluate particular problems. A consulting physician examines, tests, and evaluates the patient and provides a report to the attending or primary care physician.

MAKING THE MOST OF FOMS

All the major specialties are covered in the Focus module. You have already learned how to build a medical record and the makeup of diagnostic reports, now it is time to apply what you have learned to the following specialties:

- Cardiology
- Gastroenterology
- Genitourinary
- Neurology
- Obstetrics/Gynecology
- Ophthalmology
- Orthopedics
- Otorhinolaryngology
- Pediatrics
- Surgery

If you use this text as intended, you will be prepared to perform the practicum modules of the program, ace the final exam, and move into the workplace. (However, just to sit down and simply read the reports would be a sure cure for insomnia!) The following are some suggestions on how to utilize this resource to your best advantage, both as part of the program and as a reference when you enter the workplace:

- **Do not skip any of the exercises**. First, they help keep you alert, and second, their purpose is to help you learn. They are a little different from the exercises in the other texts in that sometimes the answer key is the first place you will see the answer. You might, for example, see an abbreviation that is not expanded in the text. The exercise will ask you to expand that abbreviation, and the only way you can do that may be by looking at the answer key. That's okay. It is another way to learn.
- **Add new terminology to your hard copy or online word list**. You might want to make two lists on your computer as you work through the text: one general alphabetized list and one by specialty. This is up to you. *Choose the method that works best for you.* This exercise, while time consuming, helps fix the terminology in your mind. Remember, the more often you write the unfamiliar words down, the sooner they will become familiar. The terminology in Focus is especially valuable because it is all in context. You can generate word lists in MS Word, MS Excel (good, but expensive), or similar programs. Software such as the *Li'l Red Notebook* is also available and is designed especially for medical transcription editing. (Consult your *Resource Guide* or ask about such options on the Forum.)
- **Read with great concentration. Make sure that you understand every sentence—be certain that everything you read makes sense.** That's a big job, but if you do it, you will be miles ahead in your comprehension of medical reports. In an early editing of the text, for example, the word *repasteurization*, referring to the blood vessels in the leg, was found. The word has been corrected to *revascularization*. If you see a sentence like that one (and we hope you don't!) and ask yourself what it means, you will note the problem, figure out what it ought to be, and correct it, and that will be excellent training for finding errors in your own work. Remember, context is everything. We want you to be a *thinking* medical transcription editor. You are not expected to have the same knowledge as a physician, but MTEs often contribute to patient care by flagging inconsistencies. *If you can't figure out what it should be, and if there is no explanatory note, ask.*
- **Read some of the reports aloud or have someone read them to you.** That's the thing to do when you start to go to sleep! Start reading aloud. Get the sounds of medical language in your head.
- **Use the Focus on Medical Specialties as a reference.** Are you editing an orthopedic surgery report and find yourself stuck on a term or phrase or surgical instrument? Then refer to the Orthopedics unit of Focus and find a similar report. Maybe your answer will be there. What is the procedure for doing an MRI or CT scan? How do you format an x-ray examination? Look in the Radiology unit of Diagnostics Reports. Do the same thing when you take your final exam. You can use any of your resources for the final. As you are reviewing the dictation for the final, the first places to look would be in Diagnostics Reports and Focus. They show you formats, dosage notations, how procedures are done, all sorts of details, many of which are a problem for some who take the final exam—and the answers are right there! Then, when you get a job and have your first exposure to dictation, review the Diagnostics Reports and Focus modules. You will be way ahead.
- **Remember that your Career Step training program is a carefully designed "programmed learning" experience formulated to take you step by step to mastery of medical transcription editing.** All content and instruction is built on what you have learned before, and you are expected to comprehend the material in each increment before you move onward and upward. Because of this structure, each module is a valuable cross-reference to all of the others. So as you work through FOMS, refer back to the Anatomy, Pathophysiology, and Disease Processes and other modules, including the tests and the exercises, as often as needed. In the Focus on Medical Specialties, everything you have learned up to this point comes together so that you can really see how it works—all of the terminology, formats, principles. Apply these same principles when you approach the practicum portion of the training program, and they should help you master that as well.
- **Figure out your own ways to make an effective tool of the Focus on Medical Specialties.** Then let us know what you found so we can pass the tips on to other students.

In summary, it is our hope and intention that you will use FOMS as a learning tool to:

- Familiarize yourself with what edited reports look like in the real world.
- Enhance your research skills.
- Challenge your editing skills.
- Become aware of a variety of acceptable formats.
- Deepen your comprehension of the medical field.

All of these are important steps in the process of becoming a well-rounded MTE.

TIPS FOR SUCCESS IN FOMS

These are important! Read them. Understanding acceptable variation and stylistic nuances will help you get the most out of these FOMS units, and make you a better MTE in general.

Clinic Notes

There are no clinic notes to speak of in this text; your Clinic Notes modules will give you lots of experience with those. Some additional report types are not represented in this text—primarily psychology reports of one kind or another or VA reports, such as Compensation and Pension reports. The reason for this is that the information in those reports is usually so patient specific—e.g., types of incidents, injuries, accidents, service histories, psychological profiles—that confidential material is nearly impossible to delete entirely. You will have adequate exposure to the relevant terminology in other places in the program, however.

Numbers

When these materials were first published, the general rule for rendering numbers in the text was to type out the word if the number was ten or less, and type the numeral if the number was more than ten (i.e., seven and 17). This has been the classic rule for formal writing for a very long time, and it is still the rule for most formal writing. However, in recent years the trend has changed to using the numeral instead of spelling out numbers. The general preference now is to use the numeral in medical reports whenever it appears, no matter how small the number (i.e., 7 and 17). Note that this is a general guideline, not a hard and fast rule. In these FOMS reports, you will see some variation in this usage. The exceptions to the general guideline are as follows:

1. When the word is required to increase clarity and avoid any ambiguity. "The patient was given two 250 mg tablets of the medication," for example, rather than "The patient was given 2 250 mg tablets of the medication."
2. When a sentence begins with a number.
3. When the numeral is used as a pronoun as in "The patient had one of those fancy canes."

Also related to the use of numbers/numerals is the changing usage of Roman versus Arabic notations.

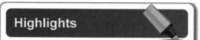

Highlights

You may choose to leave the reports as they appear, or you may strive to edit them to make all the numbers consistent.

Traditionally in medical transcription editing, types, classes, and grades were designated with Roman numerals: CIN-III Pap smear, II/VI systolic ejection murmur, type II diabetes. More and more, as time goes by, the usage is changing, with the Roman numerals being replaced by Arabic numerals. CIN-3 Pap smear, 2/6 systolic ejection murmur, type 2 diabetes. The changes are by no means universal, and in some cases (cranial nerves II-XII, grade IV chondromalacia), Roman numerals are still commonly used or even preferred. Again, in your program materials, both usages will appear—representing the preference of the MTEs who typed the reports and/or the institutions for which they were typed.

Dangerous Abbreviations

One other issue of style and format is the use of "dangerous abbreviations." You were introduced to some of these in the Foreign Terms unit of the Mastering Medical Language module. These, again, are a style issue. Some clients will prefer you adjust for dangerous abbreviations, which means you will change them to the more acceptable form. Other clients will prefer the "dangerous abbreviations" be edited as dictated. Because there is variation in how dangerous abbreviations are handled, it is important to have a firm grasp of what abbreviations are listed as dangerous. A list of dangerous abbreviations can be found online by searching *ISMP Dangerous Abbreviations*.

Possessive Eponyms

Dictators will often dictate possessive eponyms—they will say "Alzheimer's" or "Hodgkin's" or even "Babinski's sign." The current trend toward not using possessive eponyms would have you edit these as *Alzheimer disease*, *Hodgkin lymphoma*, and *Babinski sign*. Again, there is no steadfast general rule as to how this should be handled. While the trend may be moving away from including the *'s* (dropping the possessive form of eponym), some accounts or clients prefer the eponyms be edited as dictated. The reports in the FOMS module will vary with how possessive eponyms are handled (sometimes left as is and sometimes the possessive form is dropped). Without specific instruction on how to handle possessive eponyms, there is more than one correct way to edit the information.

None of these issues is of any dire significance to your learning process.

In fact, when you enter the MTE workplace, your client or employer will likely specify a preference. Until then, choose the style you are comfortable with and try to be consistent in its application. The same advice applies to any number of issues that are simply stylistic:

- capitalization
- punctuation
- hyphenation
- formatting
- numbering
- … and more!

Each specialty unit will begin with basic disease, diagnostics, and treatment information. This introduction will be followed by a specialty-specific language workshop and review. Sample reports with exercises will follow the language lessons, and each unit will end with a unit review test. The units will be full of exercises, sample reports, and even an audio file for comprehensive exposure to each specialty. Without further ado, we begin with Cardiology.

UNIT 2
Cardiology

CARDIOLOGY – INTRODUCTION

Cardiology is the branch of medicine that deals with the heart; pulmonology deals with the lungs; and vascular diseases and surgeries are related to the blood vessels. Cardiology and vascular surgery are often combined into one medical specialty—cardiovascular. Because the heart, lungs, and blood vessels are so closely related in function and disease, they are included in one unit.

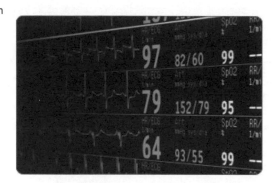

Some common diseases or conditions relating to the heart include:

- congestive heart failure
- rheumatic heart disease
- cardiomegaly
- cardiac dysrhythmias
- atherosclerotic coronary artery disease

Cardiology treatments and procedures include (but are not limited to):

- coronary artery bypass graft surgeries
- carotid endarterectomies
- percutaneous transluminal coronary angioplasties
- cardiac catheterization reports
- valve replacements
- pacemaker implantations
- coronary artery stent placements

Cardiology disorders are serious, and the patient generally requires hospitalization for both diagnosis and treatment.

PULMONOLOGY

Pulmonology is the branch of medicine that deals with diseases of the respiratory system. More specifically, pulmonary medicine deals with the causes, diagnosis, prevention, and treatment of diseases affecting the lungs.

While the primary functions of the respiratory system, with help from the circulatory system, are to provide a constant supply of oxygen to every cell in the body and remove gaseous waste from the body, the respiratory system is also responsible for important secondary functions as well. These include vocalization, assistance with abdominal compression which occurs during micturition (urination), defecation, parturition (childbirth), and the natural reflexes of coughing and sneezing, which assures the respiratory system is kept clean.

Pulmonology is generally considered a branch of Internal Medicine. Pulmonology is sometimes referred to as Chest Medicine or Respiratory Medicine.

Some common disease processes related to the lungs and the respiratory tract include (but are not limited to):

- acute respiratory distress syndrome (ARDS)
- asthma
- chronic obstructive pulmonary disease (COPD)
- cystic fibrosis
- interstitial lung disease
- pneumonia
- pneumothorax
- lung cancer
- pulmonary embolism
- pulmonary fibrosis
- sarcoidosis
- severe acute respiratory syndrome (SARS)

Pulmonology diagnoses are made through a variety of assessment methods, including (but again, not limited to):

medical history

- hereditary diseases
- exposure to toxins/infectious agents

physical exam

- visual inspection
- palpation
- percussion
- auscultation

laboratory tests

- spirometry
- bronchoscopy
- chest x-rays
- CT scanning
- nuclear scans
- PET scans

The treatment of pulmonology disease processes includes (but is in no way limited to):

surgical management

- bronchoscopies
- lobectomies
- thoracotomies
- medications (usually inhalation or oral)
- oxygen therapy
- chemotherapy

VASCULAR DISEASE/SURGERY

Finally, **vascular** diseases and surgeries are those related to the blood vessels.

Vascular diseases include conditions such as:

- aortoiliac disease
- carotid artery disease
- claudication
- cellulitis
- clotting disorders
- deep vein thrombosis and other thromboembolic diseases
- diabetic problems
- lymphedema
- varicose veins
- vessel lacerations

Vascular disease tests might include:

- angiogram
- ankle-brachial index (ABI)
- CT angiography
- duplex ultrasound
- MR angiogram

And finally, vascular treatments often include one or a combination of the following:

- amputation
- angioplasty stenting
- anticoagulation procedures
- carotid endarterectomy
- carotid stenting
- dialysis access
- diet/nutrition modifications
- endarterectomy
- exercise
- foot care
- thrombolytic therapy

In the medical workplace, you will have the opportunity to edit reports dictated by cardiologists, pulmonologists, thoracic surgeons, and vascular surgeons. While each specialty is distinct, a sampling of reports from these specialties will be presented together in this unit.

CARDIOLOGY LANGUAGE WORKSHOP

Although we have covered the components of cardiology language in the Abbreviations unit of the Mastering Medical Language module, in various units in Medical Word Building, and from a variety of angles in the Anatomy and Disease modules, it makes sense to do a more targeted review of cardiology terminology here before we dive into the cardiology FOMS reports.

Common Cardiology Root Words and Combining Forms

Root Word & Combining Form	Meaning	Example
aneurysm/o	widening	aneurysmoplasty
angi/o	vessel	angiorrhaphy
aort/o	aorta	aortostenosis
arteri/o	artery	arterial
arteriol/o	arteriole	arteriolitis
ather/o	fatty yellowish plaque	atherosclerosis
atri/o	atrium	atrioventricular
brachi/o	arm	brachiocephalic
cardi/o	heart	cardiomegaly
cholesterol/o	lipid	hypercholesterolemia
coron/o	heart	coronaritis
cyan/o	blue	cyanosis
hemangi/o	blood vessel	hemangioma
hemat/o	blood	hematochezia
my/o	muscle	myocardial
myx/o	mucus	myxoma
ox/o	oxygen	hypoxia
pericardi/o	pericardium	pericardiocentesis
phleb/o	vein	phlebotomy
sphygm/o	pulse	sphygmometer
thromb/o	blood clot	thrombolysis
valv/o	valve	valvotomy
valvul/o	valve	valvuloplasty
vas/o	vessel	vasospasm
vascul/o	vessel	vasculopathy
ven/o	vein	venous
ventricul/o	ventricle	ventriculotomy

Common Cardiology Prefixes

Prefix	Meaning	Example
brady-	slow	bradycardia
de-	from, away	defibrillate
dys-	bad, difficult	dysrhythmia
endo-	within	endocarditis
extra-	outside	extracardiac
hyper-	excessive, above normal	hypertension
hypo-	deficient, below normal	hypoplastic
inter-	among, between	interarterial
peri-	around	pericarditis
tachy-	rapid	tachycardia
tetra-	four	tetracrotic
trans-	across, through	transseptal
tri-	three	triangle

Common Cardiology Suffixes

Suffix	Meaning	Example
-constriction	sensation of pressure or tightening	vasoconstriction
-emia	blood	anemia
-gram	record, a writing	angiogram
-graph	instrument for recording	electrocardiograph
-graphy	a writing, recording, or description	echocardiography
-itis	inflammation	carditis
-lysis	destruction, loosening	cardiolysis
-megaly	large	cardiomegaly
-meter	instrument for measuring	thermometer (heat)
-osis	process, condition, state (abnormal)	cardiac cirrhosis
-plasty	surgical procedure	angioplasty
-sclerosis	hardening	arteriolosclerosis
-stenosis	a narrowing	arteriostenosis
-tomy	incision	cardiotomy

Common Cardiology Abbreviations

Abbreviation	Expansion
A-fib	atrial fibrillation
AV	atrioventricular
AVB	atrioventricular block
aVF	augmented voltage foot—unipolar limb lead on the left foot of EKG
AVM	arteriovenous malformation
AVN	atrioventricular node
aVR	augmented voltage right—unipolar limb lead on right arm of EKG
BVH	biventricular hypertrophy
CABG	coronary artery bypass graft/grafting
CV	cardiovascular
Defib	defibrillation
ECG/EKG	electrocardiogram (graphy)
EF	ejection fraction
IVC	inferior vena cava
LAD	left anterior descending
LBBB	left bundle branch block
LAO	left anterior oblique
LCA	left coronary artery (occasionally circumflex or carotid)
LICA	left internal carotid artery
LIMA	left internal mammary artery
LPA	left pulmonary artery
LV	left ventricle (ventricular)
LVH	left ventricular hypertrophy
MI	myocardial infarction
OMB	obtuse marginal branch
PTCA	percutaneous transluminal coronary angioplasty
PVC	premature ventricular contraction
RAD	right anterior descending
RBBB	right bundle branch block
RAO	right anterior oblique
RCA	right coronary artery (occasionally carotid)
SVC	superior vena cava
V-fib	ventricular fibrillation
V-tach	ventricular tachycardia

REVIEW: CARDIOLOGY LANGUAGE

TRUE/FALSE.
Mark the following true or false.

1. The combining form *coron/o* means vessel.

   ○ true

   ○ false

2. *Sphygm/o* is a combining form that means pulse.

   ○ true

   ○ false

3. The combining form *hemangi/o* means blood clot.

   ○ true

   ○ false

4. The suffix *-osis* means abnormal condition.

   ○ true

   ○ false

5. The abbreviation *SVC* stands for stenotic vena cava.

   ○ true

   ○ false

Multiple Choice.
Choose the best answer.

1. The patient underwent a 4-vessel CABG. *CABG* stands for (○ coronary, ○ carotid) artery bypass graft.

2. The term *tachycardia* means (○ slow, ○ rapid) heartbeat.

3. If a patient is cyanotic, this means that his or her lips or fingers may be (○ blue, ○ white).

4. If the physician dictates that the patient has RBBB, this means right (○ brachial, ○ bundle) branch block.

5. A patient who has arteriosclerosis has hardening of the (○ heart, ○ arteries).

Fill in the Blank.
Using the word(s) in the box, fill in the blanks.

1. A patient who has a blocked blood vessel around the heart may undergo a

   _____ transluminal coronary angioplasty.

2. The term for destruction of a blood clot is _____.

3. The left _____ mammary artery (LIMA) is often used for vessel grafting during CABG.

4. Cardiolysis involves _____ of adhesions between the heart and the sternal periosteum.

5. _____ is the term meaning elevated blood pressure.

percutaneous
internal
destruction
hypertension
thrombolysis

CARDIOLOGY REPORTS

Over the next few pages we will cover a variety of reports from the cardiology, pulmonology, and vascular surgery specialty areas. Pay special attention to the language, the medications, the surgical tools, the associated diagnoses and procedures, etc. in these reports. Up to this point in the training program you will have studied a great deal of background terminology and information—the following reports and associated exercises will give you not only an opportunity to learn new terms, but also to give your knowledge a specialty-focused practical application. Again, the sample reports found in these specialty units are actual cases taken from transcription editing databases. These reports are exactly what you can expect to be seeing and typing in your career as a medical transcription editor.

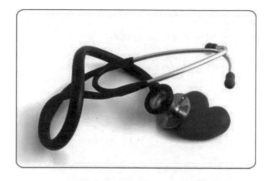

The patient confidentiality information has been washed from these files and made up names, places, and dates have been put in their place. Look closely, you may recognize some of the places and doctor names from TV and movies.

CARDIOLOGY REPORT 1 – DISCHARGE SUMMARY

PRIMARY DIAGNOSES

1. Severe right-sided heart failure.
2. Rheumatic heart disease.
3. Anemia.

HISTORY OF PRESENT ILLNESS: This is a 62-year-old male well known to me, who was readmitted for recurring anemia and congestive heart failure. Historically, he had been admitted first for this problem in the fall of 1999[1] and then most recently in 2002, when he appeared anemic and fatigued and short of breath and was found to have worsening rheumatic heart disease and right-sided heart failure. At that time, he was transfused and was doing well, and the plan was for him to follow up in cardiac clinic in the spring of 2000 and to be evaluated at that time for possible mitral valve replacement. Over the next 3 weeks, he apparently was very fatigued, not able to do much at home or at work, and had started to feel dizzy. This was reported over radio medical traffic, and I had him come to the hospital for evaluation.

PHYSICAL EXAMINATION: When he was first seen in the emergency room here, he was pale, slightly dyspneic at rest, and otherwise in no acute distress. Vitals: Pulse 120, afebrile, blood pressure 106/40, weight 132 pounds, which is 1 pound less than 1 month ago. Neck: Marked JVD and hepatojugular reflux as before, and again JVD even when standing. Cardiovascular exam revealed tachycardia with summation gallop and possible new aortic insufficiency murmur which was also listened to by Dr. Smith who agreed. He still had his very obvious mitral regurgitation. Lungs: Fine basilar rales.[2] Abdomen: Nontender. Liver may be a couple of fingerbreadths[3] below his costal margin, but did not percuss large. He did not have any edema. Most significantly and different from last month was that his legs demonstrated widespread purpura bilaterally from the midthigh down. Fundi did not reveal any hemorrhage or rough spots. He had no splinter hemorrhages in his extremities.

LABORATORY DATA: Hemoglobin 8; it was 10 one[4] month ago after transfusion. Chest x-ray revealed a silhouette of 19 cm, which was no change from a month ago.

HOSPITAL COURSE: He had multiple labs drawn, and then he was admitted for a transfusion and a consultation. We also at this time thought about evaluating his vasculitis, which he appeared to have. Over the next several days he received 4 blood transfusions with his hemoglobin raised to 10.5 with no evidence of ongoing blood loss. On admission, he had a reticulocyte count performed, which was 4.0%, but then corrected for his anemia it would be 2.8%, which was still slightly elevated. This is indicative of maybe a slight hemolysis. His direct and indirect Coombs was negative. His PT and PTT were within normal limits. His urine showed the usual 3+ blood, 3+ protein. His initial LDH was 1204. This was quite a marked increase from the previous month. His LDH then climbed to 1700 a couple of days later, and his clinical exam remained unchanged. Consultation was made with Dr. Smith in the hopes of getting a cardiac echo performed. At that time Dr. Smith said that they did have a new machine which had Doppler flow capability, and so the patient was transferred to their hospital for 1 day. There he received cardiac echo[5] with Doppler flow studies which demonstrated his usual severe mitral regurgitation. He did have some mild aortic insufficiency. However, this time, different from the fall time, he had marked tricuspid regurgitation with estimated pulmonary artery pressures of 25-27 and marked central venous pressures. Based on the fact that he does not have chronic lung disease, nor does he have left ventricular dysfunction, it is believed that he was exhibiting evidence of secondary pulmonary hypertension with subsequent right heart failure and tricuspid regurgitation. At the time of his ultrasound, it was found also that his liver was seen to be markedly engorged and enlarged. This was confirmed on their ultrasound of a homogeneous nature with no infiltrative pattern. The patient was transferred back to our facility for continued diuresis in the hopes that he might be transferred soon to County General Hospital to get cardiac valve replacement. On return to our facility, I did reexamine his liver, and much different from admission, his liver was huge and filling up most of his abdomen, down to his pelvic brim, across to his umbilicus, and over to the gastric area. It was tender to percussion. He also at this time had about 1+ peripheral edema, but he had been up on his feet a lot on this day. His purpura was fading, and his blood count was stable.

His rectal exam was negative for guaiac.[6] After the patient was back here for a couple of days, we got a report from the lab that he had 2 positive blood cultures from the dozen or so that had been done looking for SBE.[7] The 2 blood cultures were defined as growing strict anaerobes and of a pleomorphic, maybe gram-negative,[8] nature. Due to this and after consultation with a local internist, who then talked with an infectious disease specialist, we decided that he could be suffering from "culture-negative SBE" due to the HACEK[9] grouping of gram-negative pleomorphic anaerobic bacteria. We then checked the BUN and creatinine which were 29 and 1.0, and then started him on intravenous ampicillin and gentamicin. Dr. Smith was then informed of this, and we decided that it would be best, should he decompensate, that he be transferred back to County General Hospital in the hopes that they will be able to transfer him for urgent cardiac surgery. He was subsequently transferred back to County General on antibiotics for possible SBE. I should note that on Dr. Smith's repeat ultrasound of his heart, he did think that the patient had a large thickened area on his aortic valve, but apparently this was evident in the fall but not as clearly delineated. Dr. Smith also felt that the tricuspid regurgitation is probably from secondary pulmonary hypertension and right heart failure and most likely the purpuric lesions on his legs are due to his very high CV pressures and capillary fragility and leakage. He was transferred back in stable condition, and we await report from them as to his prognosis and decision making regarding cardiac surgery.

Footnotes:

1. 1.This "date" and all patient confidentiality information in this report are made up.
2. 2.This is pronounced "rals, rawls, or rails."
3. 3.A fingerbreadth is the length of breadth of a finger used as a linear measure. Although a dictator will sometimes dictate "fingersbreadth," the correct plural form of fingerbreadth is fingerbreadths.
4. 4.Note that the word *one* is spelled out. Note that the word *10* is typed numerically. ("...been 10 1 month ago" would be confusing.) It is generally preferred to not use adjacent numerals.
5. 5.The term *echo* is short or slang for echocardiogram. Some clients will require you expand any slang.
6. 6.If you are unsure how this or any other words are pronounced, use the pronunciation guide included with this training program.
7. 7.SBE = subacute bacterial endocarditis.
8. 8.A Gram stain is used to identify types of bacteria. When the results of a Gram stain are being stated, use a lowercase *g* (gram-negative or gram-positive).
9. 9.Look up the abbreviation *HACEK* in your medical dictionary, an abbreviations word book, or even the online Acronym Finder (http://www.acronymfinder.com).

SPELLING.

Determine if the following words are spelled correctly. If the spelling is correct, leave the word as it has already been entered. If the spelling is incorrect, provide the correct spelling.

1. reumatic _____

2. dyspneic _____

3. regurgitation _____

4. reticulocyte _____

5. Coombes _____

Fill in the Blank.

The following abbreviations and/or terms are used in the previous reports. Fill in the appropriate blank with either the abbreviation or its expansion.

1. CHF_____

2. JVD_____

3. blood pressure_____

4. hepatojugular reflux_____

5. CVP_____

6. SBE_____

7. blood urea nitrogen_____

CARDIOLOGY REPORT 2 – DISCHARGE SUMMARY

HISTORY OF PRESENT ILLNESS: The patient is a 63-year-old white female with no previous cardiac history, who awoke on the morning of admission with severe retrosternal chest pain. She was taken by ambulance to the emergency room where she received 4 mg of morphine IV and nitroglycerin sublingually times 2[1] with no relief of symptoms. The EKG showed acute myocardial infarction changes. The patient denied any previous chest pain, shortness of breath, orthopnea, or dyspnea on exertion, PND, or pedal edema.

SOCIAL HISTORY: Smoking: 50 pack-years. Alcohol: 3 to 4 drinks per night.

FAMILY HISTORY: Positive for breast cancer and colon cancer in her mother and father, respectively.

PAST MEDICAL HISTORY: Atherosclerotic peripheral vascular disease. Hyperlipidemia.

PAST SURGICAL HISTORY: Thyroidectomy in 2002, cholecystectomy in 2006.

ALLERGIES: No known drug allergies.[2]

PHYSICAL EXAMINATION: Pulse 72, blood pressure 150/92, temperature afebrile, respiratory rate 24, not labored. In general, the patient was an obese white female in moderate distress. HEENT exam was unremarkable except for arcus senilis bilaterally. Neck: Supple without lymphadenopathy. Lungs: Clear to auscultation and percussion bilaterally. Breasts: Fibrotic consistency without a discrete mass. Cardiovascular exam: Regular rate and rhythm with a normal S1 and a normal S2, positive S4, grade 1/6[3] ejection murmur at the left upper sternal border, no elevated JVD or carotid bruits. Pulses good symmetrically throughout. Abdomen: Positive normoactive bowel sounds, obese, no hepatosplenomegaly, nondistended, nontender. GU: Guaiac negative. Neurological exam: Nonfocal. Skin: Warm and dry.

LABORATORY AND X-RAY DATA: EKG: Normal sinus rhythm, 78 beats per minute. Marked ST elevation in leads I, aVL and V2 through V6 with Q-waves in V2 through V6. Chest x-ray: Normal heart size and silhouette with no effusions and no increased pulmonary vascularity.

HOSPITAL COURSE: The patient was admitted to the CCU[4] for staff evaluation by the cardiology service. It was apparent that she was having an acute anterolateral myocardial infarction manifested by EKG changes and chest pain. The patient was treated with thrombolytic therapy on admission with immediate reversal of her EKG changes. Cardiac catheterization was performed which showed a wedge pressure of 22, LVEDP[5] of 26, cardiac output of 4.7, LV-gram showed a large area of anterior apical dyskinesis and septal akinesis, 1-vessel coronary artery disease with an 80% mid-LAD stenosis and a large diagonal and 70% stenosis of a large diagonal at the takeoff. The patient was advised of the risks and benefits of PTCA[6] using the double-wire, single-balloon technique of her LAD and diagonal lesion. She underwent PTCA.

DISCHARGE DIAGNOSES

1. Acute anterolateral myocardial infarction by enzymes and electrocardiogram changes.
2. Atherosclerotic coronary artery disease, status post cardiac catheterization showing 1-vessel disease of the left anterior descending and large diagonal.
3. Status post percutaneous transluminal coronary angioplasty of the left anterior descending and large diagonal.
4. Hyperlipidemia.

Highlights

MURMURS

- **grade 1** – Lowest intensity, difficult to hear even by expert listeners
- **grade 2** – Low intensity, but usually audible by all listeners
- **grade 3** – Medium intensity, easy to hear even by inexperienced listeners, but without a palpable thrill
- **grade 4** – Medium intensity with a palpable thrill
- **grade 5** – Loud intensity with a palpable thrill. Audible even with the stethoscope placed on the chest with the edge of the diaphragm
- **grade 6** – Loudest intensity with a palpable thrill. Audible even with the stethoscope raised above the chest

PROCEDURES

1. Thrombolytic therapy.
2. Cardiac catheterization.
3. PTCA of an LAD and diagonal lesion.

DISCHARGE MEDICATIONS

1. Coumadin 5 mg p.o. q.d.[7]
2. Enalapril 2.5 mg p.o. q.d.
3. Cardizem SR 90 mg b.i.d.
4. Mevacor 20 mg q.d.
5. Lopressor 20 mg b.i.d.
6. Nitroglycerin sublingual p.r.n. q. 5 minutes times 3 for chest pain.

DISPOSITION AND FOLLOWUP: The patient will follow up in 1 month in the cardiology clinic. The patient will follow up in the anticoagulation clinic for 3 months.

Footnotes:

1. 1.This is also acceptably edited as x2 and x 2. When the word *times* is dictated for the number of times a thing can be done, the letter *x* can be used.
2. 2.Sometimes you will see this in all caps: NO KNOWN DRUG ALLERGIES, and other times a dictator will simply say "NKDA."
3. 3.Although some clients prefer murmurs be edited using Roman numerals, typically they are edited using Arabic numerals.
4. 4.CCU = Coronary Care Unit.
5. 5.Left ventricular end diastolic pressure.
6. 6.Percutaneous transluminal coronary angioplasty.
7. 7.The abbreviation *q.d.* is on the ISMP Dangerous Abbreviations list. Some clients may require it be expanded to "every day."

SPELLING.

Determine if the following words are spelled correctly. If the spelling is correct, leave the word as it has already been entered. If the spelling is incorrect, provide the correct spelling.

1. nitrogliceryn _____

2. sublingual _____

3. Coomadin _____

4. enalaprille _____

5. Cardizem _____

6. Mevacore _____

7. Lopressure _____

Fill in the Blank.

The following abbreviations and/or terms are used in the previous reports. Fill in the appropriate blank with either the abbreviation or its expansion.

1. auscultation and percussion_____

2. left ventricular end diastolic pressure_____

3. coronary care unit_____

4. PTCA_____

5. left anterior descending_____

6. PND_____

7. myocardial infarction_____

8. genitourinary_____

9. EKG_____

10. twice a day_____

CARDIOLOGY REPORT 3 – OPERATIVE NOTE

PREOPERATIVE DIAGNOSIS: 2-vessel coronary artery disease with 90% proximal left anterior descending stenosis and unstable angina.

POSTOPERATIVE DIAGNOSIS: Same.[1]

DRAINS: Two #36 chest tubes; a #10 Jackson-Pratt drain.

MATERIAL TO LAB: Portion of saphenous vein.

OPERATION PERFORMED: Coronary artery bypass grafting times 3 with left internal mammary artery to diagonal bypass and autogenous saphenous vein aortocoronary bypass graft to left anterior descending and obtuse marginal coronary artery.

FINDINGS: Diffuse coronary artery disease. The left anterior descending vessel was intramyocardial in its midportion and inaccessible for bypass. Therefore, the bypass was done to the distal one third[2] of the vessel utilizing a saphenous vein graft. The vessel in this region was free of disease and 1.6 mm in diameter. The diagonal coronary artery was 1.6 mm and free of disease. The obtuse marginal was 1.5 mm and free of disease. Satisfactory flow was noted in all grafts. The saphenous vein quality and internal mammary artery quality were good.

INTRAOPERATIVE COMPLICATIONS: None.

DESCRIPTION OF OPERATION: With the patient supine, under satisfactory general endotracheal anesthesia, and after the insertion of Swan-Ganz catheter and radial artery monitoring catheter, the chest, abdomen, and lower extremities were prepped with povidone and draped in a sterile manner. An incision was made overlying the course of the saphenous vein in the right lower leg. The vein was exposed at the ankle and cannulated with a small plastic vein cannula. The vein was gently distended with solution. The vein was then harvested from its bed. Branches were ligated with 3-0 silk and hemoclip application. After harvesting, the vein was examined and found to be satisfactory for use as a bypass conduit. The vein was marked for alignment and set aside for later use. The incision was closed using 2-0 Vicryl in the deep layers and 3-0 Vicryl subcuticular skin closure. Additional skin closure with staples was employed.

A median sternotomy was then made. Bleeding was controlled by electrocoagulation. The left hemisternum was then elevated and the internal mammary artery region exposed. A pedicle containing the internal mammary artery and adjacent veins was constructed with the electrocautery. Branches of the internal mammary artery were controlled with hemoclip application. The pedicle was dissected distally to the region of the bifurcation of the internal mammary artery, near the diaphragm and proximally to the level of the subclavian vein. The pedicle was infiltrated with papaverine solution. The pericardium was then opened in the midline and a pericardial well was constructed with 2-0 silk sutures. Concentric pursestring sutures of 2-0 Ethibond were placed in the distal ascending aorta for aortic cannulation. A pursestring was placed about the right atrial appendage, and a second atrial pursestring was placed for the retrograde cannula. Heparin was administered. The aorta was cannulated through a small stab aortotomy, and the cannula selected was a Sarns 6.5-mm aortic perfusion cannula. The cannula was secured with the pursestring sutures and connected to the heart/lung bypass circuit. A 2-stage venous cannula was inserted into the right atrium through the right atrial appendage and secured. The retrograde cardioplegia cannula was inserted through a small atriotomy and guided into the coronary sinus. Cardiopulmonary bypass was initiated. A cardioplegia tack was inserted on the anterior wall of the ascending aorta. The coronary vessels were marked for bypass. The vessels were identified conforming to the pattern noted on coronary arteriography. The left anterior descending artery could not be located in its midportion and appeared to occupy an intramyocardial course. The artery was found in its distal one third emerging from the myocardium, and a bypass was constructed at this point. The internal mammary artery, however, would not reach this distance. Therefore, we elected to use the internal mammary artery for a bypass of the diagonal coronary artery. The crossclamp was applied, and warm induction cardioplegia was administered, followed by total body hypothermia and myocardial hypothermia with iced saline lavage. Cold antegrade and retrograde cardioplegia techniques were employed. The saphenous vein bypass graft was fashioned for the obtuse marginal vessel. A small arteriotomy was made, and the vessel explored. An anastomosis was constructed with 7-0 Prolene. Good flow in the graft was verified. The left anterior descending was exposed in its distal one third as it emerged from the myocardium. A small arteriotomy was made, and a saphenous-vein-to-coronary-artery anastomosis was constructed with 7-0 Prolene. Good flow in this graft was also verified. The diagonal branch was likewise exposed and a small arteriotomy performed.

The internal-mammary-artery-to-coronary-artery anastomosis[3] was constructed with 8-0 Prolene. Good flow was verified upon removing the occluding internal mammary artery clamp. The pedicle of the internal mammary artery was secured to the epicardium with 6-0 silk sutures. The crossclamp was removed and a partial occlusion clamp placed on the ascending aorta. Two punch aortotomies were performed. Aorta-to-saphenous-vein-graft anastomoses were constructed with continuous 5-0 Prolene. The vein grafts were vented for air as the partial occlusion clamp was removed. Pacing wires were affixed to the right atrium and right ventricular myocardium.

The patient was weaned from cardiopulmonary bypass without difficulty. Cannulae were removed and protamine was administered. Cannulation sites and all anastomotic sites were carefully inspected for hemostasis and found to be secure. Wound hemostasis was achieved with electrocautery. A size #36 right-angle chest tube was placed in the left pleural space, and a straight thoracic catheter was placed in the retrosternal space. A Jackson-Pratt drain was placed in the bed of the internal mammary artery. The sternum was reapproximated with #5 stainless steel wires. Subcutaneous tissues were reapproximated with 0 Vicryl, the skin with 3-0 Vicryl subcuticular. Sterile dressings were applied. The patient was returned to the surgical intensive care unit in stable condition.

The aortic crossclamp time was 55 minutes; total bypass time: 109 minutes.

Footnotes:

1. 1.Typically when a dictator says "same," the entire preoperative diagnosis is repeated under postoperative diagnosis. This client allows "same," to be edited—many do not.
2. 2.It would be acceptable to edit this as 1/3. Also, do not hyphenate fractions when they are written out as a noun (only when an adjective).
3. 3.Some facilities will expect you to hyphenate the anastomosis description, as shown here. Others may not require it. However, adding the hyphens makes the nature of the anastomosis immediately clear to the reader.

SPELLING.
Determine if the following words are spelled correctly. If the spelling is correct, leave the word as it has already been entered. If the spelling is incorrect, provide the correct spelling.

1. hemoclip _____

2. anastamosis _____

3. aortaotomies _____

4. levage _____

5. circut _____

6. cannulae _____

Matching.
Match the correct term to the definition. Enter only the letter in the space provided (no punctuation).

1. ____ In the direction of normal movement.

2. ____ The clotting of tissue using high-frequency electric current.

3. ____ A drain used to pull excess fluid from the body by constant suction.

4. ____ Moving backward or against the usual direction of flow.

5. ____ Insertion of tube into hollow body organ.

6. ____ Procedure of stopping the flow of blood.

A. Jackson-Pratt

B. antegrade

C. electrocoagulation

D. retrograde

E. hemostasis

F. cannulation

CARDIOLOGY REPORT 4 – DISCHARGE SUMMARY

HISTORY OF PRESENT ILLNESS: The patient is a 77-year-old white male with a 10-year history of peripheral vascular disease who is status post multiple right and left lower extremity angioplasties. These were performed in 1982, 1983, 1984, and 1988. He underwent an aortobifemoral bypass in 1985. In addition he underwent a right femoral-popliteal bypass in 1986 with embolectomies in 1987 and 1989. He presented to the general surgery clinic with complaints of left lower extremity pain at rest that was of recent onset. The pain was primarily in the anteromedial thigh and calf. The patient has a significant smoking history but indicates that he discontinued cigarettes 2 to 3 years ago. Pulse volume recordings were taken in the clinic which noted an ABI of 0.33 on the left and greater than 1 on the right. The PVRs indicated that there was probably occlusion at the femoral artery. The patient was admitted for emergent angiography evaluation for angioplasty versus emergency surgery.

PAST MEDICAL HISTORY[1]

1. See HPI.
2. RSD.
3. Tobacco abuse.

PAST SURGICAL HISTORY: See HPI.

MEDICATIONS ON ADMISSION: Coumadin 7.5 mg p.o. q.d., Persantine 75 mg p.o. t.i.d., Tylox p.r.n., iron 325 mg p.o. q.d., calcium 1 p.o. b.i.d., lorazepam 30 mg p.o. q.h.s.[2] p.r.n., Benadryl 50 p.r.n. for hives.

ALLERGIES: TEGRETOL AND TRICYCLICS.

SOCIAL HISTORY: See HPI.

REVIEW OF SYSTEMS: Noncontributory.

PHYSICAL EXAMINATION: Vital signs are stable. He is afebrile. In general, he is alert and oriented times 3, in no apparent distress. HEENT are within normal limits. The neck is supple and nontender without adenopathy, no JVD, no thyromegaly. Heart: Normal S1 and S2, no gallops and no murmurs. Abdomen: There is a well-healed midline scar, normoactive bowel sounds, nontender and nondistended. There are no masses. Vascular exam: His pulses in the upper extremities are equal and symmetrical bilaterally. He only has a dopplerable left femoral pulse with a noted bruit, unable to obtain pulses in the popliteal or dorsalis pedis, with a very weak dopplerable pulse in the left posterior tibial. His right lower extremity pulses are all easily palpable. His neurological exam is nonfocal. The rectal exam is heme negative, good sphincter tone and no masses.

HOSPITAL COURSE: The patient was admitted to Seattle Grace and taken to the angiography suite for an emergency angiography. At angiography, they noted a complete thrombosis of the left AFB graft, with SMA to IMA to superior hemorrhoidal to femoral circumflex to the left SFA collateral pathways. He had diffuse left superficial femoral artery disease. His stratification was intact on the left. He was started on urokinase infusion after being given a 250,000 unit bolus. This was continued from Thursday through Sunday with additional angiographies performed. On Monday he underwent an angioplasty of the superficial femoral artery. This was successful with improvement of ABIs. He indicated that he no longer had chest pain and he had return of a palpable pulse. His case was reviewed by the vascular staff, and after examining the angiograms it was decided that the patient would need a left profundoplasty with a Gore-Tex patch, secondary to a stricture in the profunda femoris artery. This was performed on Wednesday, which was tolerated well. Postoperative ABIs were greater than 1. The remainder of the patient's postoperative course was unremarkable, with the patient restarted on Coumadin, and his PTT at the time of discharge within therapeutic levels. The patient was discharged to home, ambulating without assistance and tolerating a regular diet.

AFB – aortofemoral bypass
RSD – reflex sympathetic dystrophy
ABI – ankle-brachial index
PVR – pulse volume recording (also pulmonary vascular resistance)
SMA – superior mesenteric artery
IMA – inferior mesenteric artery
SFA – superficial femoral artery

FINAL DIAGNOSES

1. Aortofemoral bypass graft occlusion.
2. Profunda femoris artery stenosis.
3. Left superficial femoral artery stenosis.
4. History of atherosclerotic peripheral vascular disease.

PROCEDURES

1. Angiography with urokinase thrombolytic therapy.
2. Left SFA angioplasty, [DATE].

DISCHARGE MEDICATIONS

1. See admission medications.
2. Percocet 1-2 tablets p.o. q.4-6h.[3] p.r.n. for pain.
3. Persantine 75 mg p.o. t.i.d.
4. Coumadin 5 mg p.o. to alternate with 7.5 mg p.o. q.d.

DISPOSITION AND FOLLOWUP: The patient is to follow up with Seattle Grace, and he is to hand deliver his consult on the day of discharge. He is to return to the general surgery clinic on Monday at 1300 hours for routine followup.[4] He is to return to the emergency room or call the general surgery clinic if he notes an increase in pain in his left lower extremity. His activities are otherwise as tolerated. He is to maintain his diet. He should not drive for the next 1 week.

Footnotes:

1. 1."See HPI" means see history of present illness.
2. 2.The abbreviation *q.h.s.* and *q.d* are on the ISMP list of dangerous abbreviations. Some clients might prefer q.h.s. be expanded to "nightly" or "at bedtime," just as q.d. is sometimes required to be expanded to "daily." This is a "style issue."
3. 3.When mixing Latin and English dosing abbreviations, such as q.4 h. or q.2 hours, do not put a space after the q period, but do put one after the numeral so it is more easily read.
4. 4.You may notice that the first sentence in this paragraph used *follow up* as 2 words and it is being used here as 1 word. The distinction is this: when *followup* is an adjective or a noun, it is one word (followup appointment). When someone is going to follow up (verb), it is two words. *Followup* is never hyphenated.

SPELLING.

Determine if the following words are spelled correctly. If the spelling is correct, leave the word as it has already been entered. If the spelling is incorrect, provide the correct spelling.

1. lorazepam _____

2. Benadryl _____

3. Tegretal _____

4. trisyclics _____

5. urokinase _____

6. Percoset _____

Fill in the Blank.

The following abbreviations and/or terms are used in the previous reports. Fill in the appropriate blank with either the abbreviation or its expansion.

1. PTT_____

2. AFB_____

3. reflex sympathetic dystrophy_____

4. SMA_____

5. head, eyes, ears, nose, and throat_____

6. IMA_____

7. b.i.d._____

8. JVD_____

9. HPI_____

10. pulse volume recording_____

CARDIOLOGY REPORT 5 – OPERATIVE NOTE

PREOPERATIVE DIAGNOSIS: Right upper lobe/right middle lobe mass.

MATERIAL TO LAB: Multiple nodes, lung nodule and tissue.

OPERATION PERFORMED: Cervical mediastinal exploration and possible right posterolateral thoracotomy, pneumonotomy, and right upper/middle lobectomy.

DRAINS: A #36-French right-angle and #40-French chest tube.

INDICATIONS: This patient is a 71-year-old Caucasian man, with a 20+ pack-year history of smoking (quit 30 years ago) who on routine physical exam was found to have a right middle lobe/upper lobe mass. The patient underwent a CT scan which confirmed the mass, which was superior to the right hilum. There was, however, minimal hilar adenopathy. As the patient is elderly, a decision was made to proceed with a cervical mediastinal exploration. If the cervical mediastinal exploration is negative for carcinoma, we will proceed with a right posterolateral thoracotomy/pneumonotomy for diagnosis, and if positive for cancer, proceed with a right upper versus middle or bilobectomy.

DESCRIPTION OF PROCEDURE: The patient was given Ancef 1 g[1] intravenous piggyback on call to the operating room. General anesthesia was administered through an endotracheal tube. The patient was then sterilely prepped and draped in the usual fashion. A horizontal incision was made approximately 2 fingersbreadth above the sternal notch. This incision was extended through the platysma muscle down to the strap muscles. The strap muscles were then split vertically. The pretracheal fascia was grasped and then opened sharply. Then, using finger dissection, the pretracheal fascia was bluntly retracted, and then a mediastinoscope was placed into the opening. It was noted that the patient had right pretracheal and subcarinal masses, which were biopsied. Frozen section returned negative for carcinoma. A decision was made at that time to close the mediastinoscopy incision and then proceed with a right posterolateral thoracotomy. The pretracheal fascia and the strap muscles were reapproximated using 3-0 Vicryl suture in a running fashion, and the platysma was closed using a 3-0 Vicryl suture in a running fashion. The skin was closed using a 3-0 Vicryl suture in a subcuticular fashion and was reinforced with tincture of benzoin and Steri-Strips.

The patient was then placed right side up, left side down in the left lateral decubitus position and then sterilely prepped and draped in the usual standard fashion. A standard posterolateral thoracotomy incision was then made over the seventh rib. This incision was extended down to the fascia of the latissimus dorsi muscle. The auscultatory triangle was palpated posteriorly; then the latissimus dorsi muscle was cut at its most caudal insertion. Similarly, the serratus anterior was cut at its fascial attachments caudally. The wound was further extended posteriorly. The paraspinous muscles were separated from the rib and intercostal muscles; then the ribs were palpated and the 6th rib[2] was marked. The periosteum over the sixth rib cephalad was then separated from the intercostal muscle using electrocauterization. Then, using Alexander and Matson elevators, the periosteum was further removed both anteriorly and posteriorly. The pleura was visualized and then opened sharply. Prior to this, the lungs were deflated. Attention was directed posteriorly where the fifth and sixth ribs were cut using a Bethune cutter, and a 1-cm segment of the fifth and sixth rib was removed to prevent a rub. Then, 2 Wilson retractors were placed in the field, and the right chest was opened. Palpation of the lung demonstrated a mass in the right middle lobe involving the right upper lobe. A Tru-Cut needle biopsy was performed, which was sent to pathology and returned positive for carcinoma.

A decision was then made to perform a right upper and middle lobectomy. The major fissure was split, and the pulmonary artery was visualized. The branches leading to the upper and middle lobes were then secured and triply ligated[3] and then cut between the sutures. Similarly, the superior pulmonary vein was visualized, isolated, and secured with suture ligatures, 2-0 silk ties, and a 2-0 suture ligature. Then, the superior pulmonary vein was cut. Attention was turned to the right middle lobe bronchus and the right upper bronchus, which were visualized and isolated and then were separated from the mainstem bronchus and the bronchus intermedius via a TA-30 stapling device. Once the bronchus was cut, the remaining attachments were removed as well as the upper and middle lobes of the lung. In performing the dissection, multiple nodes were taken along with the specimen. It was noted that there was a hard mass over the right phrenic nerve on the pleura. This mass was excised, sparing the phrenic nerve, and sent off as specimen. The wound was checked for hemostasis. The bronchus was then reinforced with a pleural patch with 4-0 Prolene suture. The inferior pulmonary ligament was then cut, and the lung was allowed to expand to its fullest extent. A #36-French right-angle chest tube was placed in the posterior sulcus, as well as a #40-French straight chest tube, which was placed in the apex of the lung field. These chest tubes were secured using #1 Ethibond suture and then hooked to suction.

The wound was then irrigated with approximately 3 liters of sterile water. There was no evidence of gross bleeding. The lung was allowed to reexpand. The ribs were then reapproximated using eight #1 PDS sutures in an interrupted fashion. The intercostal muscle was then reattached to the periosteum using a 0 Vicryl suture. The serratus anterior was then reattached to its fascial attachments anteriorly, and the paraspinal muscles were reattached to the intercostal muscles posteriorly. The latissimus muscle and fascia were then closed using 2 running 0 Vicryl sutures. The subcuticular tissue was closed using a running 3-0 Vicryl suture. The skin was then closed using a running 3-0 Vicryl suture in a subcuticular fashion. The skin was further reinforced with staples. Dressing sponges were then used and tape covered the dressing sponges. The chest tubes were further secured using tape. The patient was then placed back in the supine position and extubated without complication and taken to the recovery room in good condition.

INSTRUMENT/SPONGE COUNT: Verified.

COMPLICATIONS: The procedure was performed without complication.

FLUIDS: Lactated Ringer's 1000 cc, Isolyte 1000, Hespan 500 cc, normal saline 100 cc.

ESTIMATED BLOOD LOSS: 200 cc.

URINE OUTPUT: 1240 cc.

Footnotes:

1. 1.The measurement gram can be acceptably notated as gram, g, or gm. When abbreviated, it is generally preferred to use g.
2. 2.While this could acceptably be edited as sixth, ordinals are generally edited 1st, 2nd, 3rd, etc. (Note, it is rarely okay to use formatted ordinals— those with *th* as superscript.)
3. 3.To ligate or place a ligature means binding something with a surgical thread. Triply ligate would be to tie three ligatures around something to bind it.

SPELLING.
Determine if the following words are spelled correctly. If the spelling is correct, leave the word as it has already been entered. If the spelling is incorrect, provide the correct spelling.

1. Anseff _____

2. benzoine _____

3. paraspinus _____

4. Matsen _____

5. Bethune _____

6. Isolyte _____

7. Hespan _____

Fill in the Blank.
The following abbreviations and/or terms are used in the previous reports. Fill in the appropriate blank with either the abbreviation or its expansion.

1.CA _____

2.LR _____

3.endotracheal _____

4.CT _____

5.RUL _____

CARDIOLOGY REPORT 6 – DISCHARGE SUMMARY

CHIEF COMPLAINT: Right lung mass times 2.

HISTORY OF PRESENT ILLNESS: This patient is a 57-year-old Caucasian man, with a 2- to 3-year history[1] of malaise and recent dyspnea on exertion after shoveling for 10 minutes. The patient also notes a recent history of hemoptysis. The patient was evaluated by Pulmonary Service.[2] A chest x-ray performed demonstrated a right apex and right hilar mass, and a CT scan confirmed. In addition, the patient was noted to have anterior tracheal lymph nodes. A bronchoscopy was nondiagnostic. A peripheral biopsy as well was nondiagnostic. The patient is admitted now to undergo a CME and possible further surgery. The patient has a 150+ pack-year history of smoking and notes a positive PPD in the past. He denies weight loss, good appetite. A preoperative FEV1 was 2.6 liters, preoperative ABG 7.42, 38, and 58%.

PAST MEDICAL HISTORY: Hypertriglyceridemia, non-insulin-dependent diabetes mellitus, DJD, BPH, hypertension, and a history of polio.

PAST SURGICAL HISTORY: T&A, appendectomy, and tendon transfer.

CURRENT MEDICATIONS

1. Lopid 600 mg p.o. b.i.d.
2. Atenolol 50 mg 1 q.d.
3. Glipizide 15 mg q.a.m. and 10 mg q.p.m.

SOCIAL HISTORY: The patient notes having a 150+ pack-year history of smoking; he quit in 2006. He notes occasional alcohol use. The patient is a retired OR perfusionist.[3]

ALLERGIES: The patient has no known drug allergies.

REVIEW OF SYSTEMS: Noncontributory except as mentioned in the HPI.

PHYSICAL EXAMINATION: The patient is afebrile. Vital signs are stable. He is in no acute distress, oriented times 3. HEENT: Unremarkable. The patient has both upper and lower dentures. There is no evidence of any carotid bruits. The patient has a palpable right cervical lymph node. Cor: Regular rate and rhythm. The lungs are clear to auscultation. The abdomen is soft and nontender. No evidence of hernia bilaterally. GU exam: A previous exam demonstrates an enlarged prostate of approximately 25 g. Extremities: Left-greater-than-right varicosities. The patient has palpable dorsalis pedis pulses posteriorly. No posterior pulse is palpable.

ADMISSION LABORATORY DATA: PT, PTT, UA, CBC, electrolytes were within normal limits. Glucose was mildly elevated at 189, and the hematocrit was 40.5 on admission.

HOSPITAL COURSE: The patient was admitted to the cardiothoracic surgery service on Thursday. He was preoperatively counseled, and on Friday the patient underwent a cervical-mediastinal exploration. Findings at the time of surgery demonstrated right peritracheal, left peritracheal, and subcarinal masses which were biopsied. A frozen section returned no evidence of carcinoma, final pathology confirmed. The patient's postoperative course was unremarkable. On postoperative day 5, the patient was preoperatively counseled to undergo a right posterolateral thoracotomy with the thought of either performing a right pneumonectomy or a right middle lobe and right upper lobectomy, depending on the findings at the time of surgery. The patient underwent a right posterolateral thoracotomy and a radical mediastinal exploration. Findings at the time of surgery demonstrated primary lung cancer at the mediastinum which crossed the midline. As the patient was found to have an advanced cancer on frozen section, a decision was made not to resect the right lung or a portion of the right lung. His postoperative course was unremarkable. He was in the intensive care unit for 2 days. His hematocrit remained stable. His chest tubes were removed when the air leak stopped, which was postoperative day 4. His diet was advanced to where he could tolerate a regular diet. The final pathology returned consistent with moderate-to-poorly-differentiated squamous cell carcinoma, T2, N2, M0. The patient is now discharged to home. His staples have been removed. The patient is tolerating a regular diet and is afebrile.

FINAL DIAGNOSES

1. T2, N2, M0 squamous cell carcinoma, moderately to poorly differentiated.
2. History of non-insulin-dependent diabetes mellitus.
3. History of degenerative joint disease.
4. History of benign prostatic hypertrophy.
5. History of hypertension.
6. History of polio.

OPERATIONS

1. Cervical mediastinal exploration.
2. Radical mediastinal exploration.

DISCHARGE MEDICATIONS

1. Lopid 600 mg p.o. b.i.d.
2. Atenolol 50 mg q.d.
3. Glipizide 50 mg q.a.m. and 10 q.p.m.
4. Percocet, 30 dispensed, 1-2 q.4-6h. p.r.n. pain.
5. Colace 100 mg p.o. b.i.d.

DISPOSITION AND FOLLOWUP: The patient is to follow up with Urology for the BPH. He is to follow up with the nuclear medicine service for a bone scan; a consult was given to him. He has already been seen by Hematology/Oncology and Radiation Therapy. He is to follow up with the radiation therapy service next Friday, and to follow up with Hematology/Oncology next week.

Footnotes:

1. 1.This may look a little funny, but it is the correct way to hyphenate this information.
2. 2.This name is capitalized here because it is being referred to as an entity. Had the dictator said "the pulmonary service," it would have been edited without initial caps. That said, some clients prefer you always cap department or clinic names and some prefer you never cap them.
3. 3.An OR (operating room) perfusionist is a trained health professional who operates the heart-lung machine during cardiac surgery and other surgeries that require cardiopulmonary bypass.

SPELLING.
Determine if the following words are spelled correctly. If the spelling is correct, leave the word as it has already been entered. If the spelling is incorrect, provide the correct spelling.

1. hylar	_____	2. Caucasian	_____
3. mellitus	_____	4. trachial	_____
5. subcarinal	_____	6. sqamous	_____

Fill in the Blank.

The following abbreviations and/or terms are used in the previous reports. Fill in the appropriate blank with either the abbreviation or its expansion.

1. BPH_____

2. urinalysis_____

3. OR_____

4. ABG_____

5. noninsulin-dependent diabetes mellitus_____

6. complete blood count_____

CARDIOLOGY REPORT 7 – OPERATIVE NOTE

Medical Record

PREOPERATIVE DIAGNOSIS: Rule out Wegener granulomatosis versus Goodpasture disease.

OPERATION PERFORMED: Left thoracoscopic versus video-assisted open lung biopsy.

INDICATIONS: This patient is a 49-year-old man who noted shortness of breath and hemoptysis in March of last year. The patient at that time had URI symptoms and was treated with antibiotics. His cough and hemoptysis persisted. He was seen by the pulmonary service. Chest x-ray demonstrated pulmonary nodules. CT scan demonstrated necrotic cavitations bilaterally. The patient is now to undergo a thoracoscopic lung biopsy versus open lung biopsy of the left lung.

DESCRIPTION OF PROCEDURE: The patient was given Ancef 1 g IV piggyback. General anesthesia was administered through a double-lumen Robertshaw endotracheal tube.[1] The patient was then placed left side up, right side down, in the right lateral decubitus position. He was then sterilely prepped and draped in the usual fashion. Examination of the chest film and CT scan demonstrated a superficial mass located approximately 13-cm from the spine along the 7th rib. An incision was made at that point. This incision was extended through the latissimus dorsi muscle and through the intercostal muscles using electrocautery, removing the periosteum over the 7th rib. The pleura was then entered sharply. A fiberoptic TV camera was then placed into the left chest via an 11-mm trocar. It was noted that the patient had multiple large masses, in addition to small pulmonary nodules. A second port was made anterior along the 6th intercostal space. An 11-mm trocar port was placed. The camera was then placed through the anterior port, and the large mass in the left lower lobe was grasped with ring forceps and brought into the field. A Satinsky clamp was then used to further grasp the mass. Then using a 3-0 Vicryl suture on a taper needle, a horizontal mattress, then a baseball stitch, was used to oversew and secure a portion of lung tissue. The lung tissue was removed. A small portion was sent for AFB[2] and fungus. Multiple cultures were taken, and the specimen was sent for frozen section.

A similar procedure was performed on a large left upper lobe mass. The residual lung and the suture line were checked for an air leak to 30-cm of air pressure. There was no evidence of leak. The laparoscopic equipment was removed. A 36-French straight-angle chest tube was placed through the anterior port. The chest tube was secured with a 1-0 Ethibond suture. A 1-0 PDS suture was used to reapproximate the ribs. The intercostal muscle, as well as the muscle fascia, was closed using a running 1-0 Vicryl suture. The subcutaneous tissue was closed using a running 3-0 Vicryl suture. The skin was closed using a running 3-0 Vicryl suture on a cutting needle in a subcuticular fashion. The wound was further secured with tincture of benzoin and Steri-Strips and a bandage dressing. The bandages were then taped. The patient was placed back in the supine position and then extubated without difficulty. The patient was taken to the recovery room in good condition.

A tincture of benzoin is a pungent solution of benzoin resin in alcohol. It is often applied to skin before applying tape or other adhesive bandages. To some degree, it protects the skin from allergy to the adhesive in the tape or bandage, but mostly it makes the tape or bandages adhere much longer.

Complications: None. Estimated blood loss. Minimal. Fluids: 2000 cc of Isolyte.[3]

Footnotes:

1. 1.A good surgical word book, such as Tessier's *The Surgical Word Book*, is very helpful in verifying accurate spelling of surgical equipment.
2. 2.AFB here means acid-fast bacillus (in cardiology it can also mean aortofemoral bypass).
3. 3.This information is presented in paragraph format but could easily be edited in heading format with COMPLICATIONS, ESTIMATED BLOOD LOSS, and FLUIDS as their own headings.

SPELLING.
Determine if the following words are spelled correctly. If the spelling is correct, leave the word as it has already been entered. If the spelling is incorrect, provide the correct spelling.

1. Weggener _____   2. hemoptisis _____

3. cavitations _____   4. sterily _____

5. trocar _____   6. extubated _____

7. Satinzky _____

Matching.
Match the correct term to the definition.

1. ____ To remove a tube from a hollow organ or passageway.   A. supine

2. ____ A dense fibrous membrane covering the surface of   B. periosteum
bones.   C. intercostal

3. ____ Lying face upward.   D. extubate

4. ____ A convex needle that narrows to a point.   E. taper

5. ____ Between the ribs.

CARDIOLOGY REPORT 8 – DISCHARGE SUMMARY

FINAL DIAGNOSES[1]

1. Pneumonia with Klebsiella pneumoniae.
2. Anemia.
3. Anxiety.
4. Hypokalemia.
5. Syncope.
6. Dehydration.

OPERATIONS/PROCEDURES: Potassium replacement, IV fluids, IV antibiotics, telemetry, mental health consult.

CONDITION AT DISCHARGE: Improved.

HISTORY OF PRESENT ILLNESS: The patient is a 83-year-old female for whom there was little history available; the patient could not give much and speaks only Lithuanian. Her caregiver is not reliable. According to them, approximately 3 days prior to admission she fell in her bathroom, and she had fallen from bed about 10 days prior to that. She had required assistance with ambulation while at home because of some inability to walk, and her left side was hurting from being lifted. She was occasionally dizzy. She had been having emesis for 3 days prior to admission and was unable to walk since the beginning of May.

PAST MEDICAL HISTORY: She has depression which has been listed as being in remission and anxiety which has been treated with Xanax. She is status post upper GI bleed in 1999. She was diagnosed with peptic ulcer disease in 2001 and had a gastrotomy and biopsy and ligation of bleeders. She had another upper GI bleed in 2003. She has anemia secondary to her bleeds. She has a history of COPD. She is status post TB with a right upper lobe resection. She has glaucoma and bilateral cataracts. She has mild bilateral hearing loss.

Medications at the time of admission were unable to be elicited. She has no allergies. She lives with a homemaker who is not a relative and who feels as though she was tricked into becoming the live-in caregiver for the patient.

SURGERY: She is status post cholecystectomy, appendectomy, and bilateral hip prostheses. She has severe DJD. She is status post fracture of her right and left humeri, left fibula, left tibia, and left metacarpal.

PHYSICAL EXAMINATION: Performed on admission at 11:10. She had anisocoria with the right pupil 1-2 mm and with the left 2-3 mm; both were reactive. Heart was regular. Lungs had decreased breath sounds throughout. She had an O2 sat of 98. Abdomen was soft and nontender. Heme-negative stool. Extremities had no edema and good strength.

LABORATORY DATA: Chest x-ray showed old scarring and bilateral humeral head fractures. EKG showed normal sinus rhythm with a questionable old lateral wall MI. Her potassium was 2.8 on admission. Other labs were within normal limits, except for a sputum Gram stain which showed 3+ gram-positive cocci in pairs which grew out Klebsiella pneumoniae.

HOSPITAL COURSE: The patient was admitted and begun on penicillin. She was given potassium replacement and IV fluids. She was placed on a cardiac monitor which showed no ectopy or dysrhythmia.

She continued to improve during her stay, but there was a problem discharging her because her caregiver did not wish to take her home. She also had some problems sleeping and some anxiety over her caregiver not being present. She was begun on Xanax which helped her sleep and helped her deal with her days slightly better. She was discharged per wheelchair on Septra p.o. following the culture results from her sputum. She was also discharged on ranitidine b.i.d. because of her history of upper GI bleed. She was given Xanax 0.5 mg q.h.s. She was to follow up in 3 to 4 weeks.

Her caregiver brought her back on Friday because of concern over her anxiety and a question of an increased cough. On repeat exam, she had total normal labs and normal chest x-ray. It was elicited that the caregiver is stressed and does not wish to take care of the patient any longer. For that reason, nursing home placement procedures will be done via the hospital social worker.

FINAL DIAGNOSES

1. Pneumonia, no organism isolated.
2. Ventricular septal defect.
3. Dehydration.

OPERATIONS/PROCEDURES: Antibiotics, IV fluids, blood cultures.

CONDITION AT DISCHARGE: Improved.

Footnotes:

1. 1.While "diagnoses" seems like the better fit here, since there is more than one listed, the term "diagnosis" is not necessarily wrong as it can refer to a group of diagnoses. Without specific instruction on which is preferred, it would be acceptable to edit this as singular or plural.

SPELLING.

Determine if the following words are spelled correctly. If the spelling is correct, leave the word as it has already been entered. If the spelling is incorrect, provide the correct spelling.

1. Clebseilla _____

2. Zanax _____

3. anisocoria _____

4. ranitedine _____

5. cefuroxime _____

Fill in the Blank.

The following abbreviations and/or terms are used in the previous reports. Fill in the appropriate blank with either the abbreviation or its expansion.

1. tuberculosis _____
2. PUD _____
3. myocardial infarction _____
4. COPD _____
5. ventricular septal defect _____
6. GI _____
7. H&H _____

CARDIOLOGY REPORT 9 – DISCHARGE SUMMARY

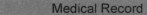

HISTORY OF PRESENT ILLNESS: The patient is a 68-year-old white male who presented with complaint of bilateral feet being cold and painful for approximately the past year, his left foot being more greatly affected. Within the last several weeks, the patient has noted 2 purplish spots on his left foot, primarily his great and second[1] toes. These spots are tender to palpation, making walking difficult at times. He has no claudication symptoms. He has had no prior surgeries or significant injuries to either of his lower extremities with the exception of a fracture of the left fourth metatarsophalangeal joint as a child.

PAST MEDICAL HISTORY: Significant for some degenerative joint disease of the neck, mild chronic obstructive pulmonary disease, congenital deafness of the right ear, hypertension, dysrhythmias. He had no prior knowledge of atherosclerotic disease. The patient smoked 2-3 packs of cigarettes per day for approximately 41 years, having quit in 2002. Prior surgeries included strangulated right inguinal hernia and sinus surgery.

ADMISSION MEDICATIONS

1. Digoxin 0.125 p.o. q.d.
2. Dipyridamole 75 mg t.i.d.
3. Enalapril 5 mg q.d.
4. Indocin 75 mg t.i.d.

Allergies: CODEINE.

PHYSICAL EXAMINATION: On admission, the patient was found to be 6 feet 6 inches tall,[2] weighing 190 pounds, with a normal temperature and a regular pulse at 72, and a blood pressure of 170/90. HEENT exam was remarkable for a right hypoplastic pinna without visible external auditory canal. Pupils equally round and reactive to light and accommodation. Extraocular movements intact. Positive arcus senilis. Upper and lower dentures in place. The neck was supple and nontender with mild-to-moderate decreased range of motion globally, secondary to his degenerative disc disease. There was no thyroid irregularity and no carotid bruits. The back was unremarkable. The chest was clear to auscultation bilaterally. The heart was regular rate and rhythm with a constant split S1, S2. The abdomen was benign. Genitourinary exam: Normal uncircumcised male with normal descended testes. Rectal exam: Positive nontender external hemorrhoids, normal tone, guaiac-negative brown stool, nontender prostate with an approximately 0.5-cm left inferior lobe apical nodule. Extremities: Lower extremities were unremarkable for deformity. He had bilaterally 2+ palpable dorsalis pedis and posterior tibial pulses. He had bilateral palpable popliteal pulses. There were bilateral femoral harsh bruits. He had 2 approximately 1 cm purplish areas on the plantar aspects of both the left first and second toes; these areas were tender to palpation. There was no clubbing, cyanosis, or edema of either lower extremity. Ankle-brachial indices were greater than 1 on both right and left.

HOSPITAL COURSE: The patient was admitted for a workup of his suspected atherosclerotic peripheral vascular disease and embolic phenomenon to the left lower extremity. Prior to his angiogram, the patient underwent evaluation by the cardiology service. He underwent a standard echocardiogram showing normal left ventricular size and function and normal valvular function. There was no cardiac source of embolus or thrombus identified. Cardiology felt that, with his history of supraventricular tachycardia on digoxin for approximately 1 year, the patient should undergo 24-hour Holter monitoring on return to his home base. During his hospitalization, he also underwent formal pulmonary function tests which indicated an FVC of 91% and an FEV1 of 70.7% with an FEV1/FVC ratio of 58.9. He was originally scheduled for angiogram on Tuesday, which was postponed due to equipment difficulties. His arteriogram on Wednesday revealed diffuse infrarenal atherosclerotic disease with focal stenosis, approximately 60% to 70% in the left external iliac artery. Successful angioplasty of this lesion was immediately performed with good result. Postprocedure runoff was brisk, and there was no evidence of flap or dissection. The patient returned from the procedure without complications. He was discharged to home on Friday in good condition.

PROCEDURES

1. Echocardiogram.
2. Pulmonary function tests.
3. Abdominal ultrasound.
4. Angiogram of bilateral lower extremities and abdominal aorta.
5. Angioplasty of left external iliac.

LABORATORY: Digoxin level was found to be less than 0.2. PSA 0.8. Chem-7[3] normal except for mildly elevated BUN of 23. Urine and complete blood count were within normal limits.

DISPOSITION: The patient was discharged to home via private vehicle on Friday. He is to follow up in the vascular clinic in 3 months or p.r.n. return of lower extremity symptoms. He is to follow up locally with his cardiologist to schedule a 24-hour Holter monitor and to return with these results in 3 months. The patient is to follow up locally for workup of his prostate nodule.

DIET/ACTIVITY: Diet can be regular. Activity ad lib with slow increase to normal activity over the next several weeks.

Footnotes:

1. 1.As stated previously, ordinals are generally preferred, but writing out *second* is just as acceptable as using *2nd*.
2. 2.Of note, it is generally preferred to not use "and" for feet and inches.
3. 3.The lab test chem-7 is more commonly referred to as a BMP (basic metabolic profile). It was also previously referred to as an SMA-7.

SPELLING.

Determine if the following words are spelled correctly. If the spelling is correct, leave the word as it has already been entered. If the spelling is incorrect, provide the correct spelling.

1. Pediazole _____

2. erythromyacin _____

3. Metaprelle _____

4. candidiasis _____

5. Eucerin _____

6. dipyridamal _____

7. Indocin _____

8. Valsalva _____

Fill in the Blank.

The following abbreviations and/or terms are used in the previous reports. Fill in the appropriate blank with either the abbreviation or its expansion.

1. range of motion_____

2. PERRLA_____

3. ankle-brachial index_____

4. DJD_____

5. PFT_____

UNIT 3
Gastroenterology

GASTROENTEROLOGY – INTRODUCTION

Gastroenterology is the study of the digestive system: the esophagus, the stomach, and the intestines and their diseases, often referred to in the short form as "GI," meaning *gastrointestinal*. GI complaints are very common reasons for going to the doctor or being admitted to the hospital, and any acute-care hospital account will require MTE proficiency in producing GI reports according to client specifications.

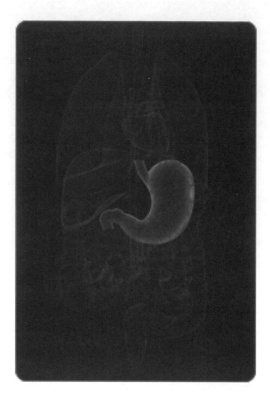

Common GI complaints include but are not limited to:

- peptic ulcer disease
- hiatal hernia
- diverticulitis or diverticulosis
- cholecystitis and cholelithiasis
- colonic polyps
- GERD – gastroesophageal reflux disease (heartburn)
- IBS – irritable bowel syndrome
- Crohn disease
- chest or abdominal pain
- abnormal LFTs (liver function tests)
- appendicitis
- GI malignancies

Examples of diagnostic and surgical procedures for gastrointestinal problems include (but again are not limited to):

- colonoscopy
- endoscopy
- Nissen fundoplication
- cholecystectomy
- gastrectomy
- laparotomy
- splenectomy
- colectomy with accompanying colostomy apparatus
- flexible sigmoidoscopy
- gastric stapling and anastomosis
- Whipple procedure (pancreatoduodenectomy)
- esophagogastroduodenoscopy
- Billroth operations

Some GI procedures are performed by gastroenterologists, others by general surgeons.

GASTROENTEROLOGY LANGUAGE WORKSHOP

It makes great sense to review common GI terminology before jumping into the reports in this Gastroenterology FOMS unit. The following is meant to be a review of terminology you have already been exposed to in the Abbreviations unit of the Mastering Medical Terminology module.

Common Gastroenterology Root Words and Combining Forms

Root Word & Combining Form	Meaning	Example
abdomin/o	abdomen	abdominal
adip/o	fat	adipose
aer/o	air	aerobic
append(ic)/o	appendix	appendicitis
bil/i	bile	biliary
cec/o	cecum	cecal
chol/e	bile	cholecystectomy
cholecyst/o	gallbladder	cholecystitis
col/o	colon	colonoscopy
enter/o	intestine	enterocolitis
esophag/o	esophagus	esophageal
fibr/o	fiber	fibroma
gastr/o	stomach	gastrectomy
ile/o	ileum	ileocecal
jejun/o	jejunum	jejunostomy
lapar/o	flank/abdominal wall	laparoscope
lith/o	stone	lithotomy
onc/o	bulk/tumor	oncology
ventr/o	ventral/belly side	ventral

Common Gastroenterology Prefixes

Prefix	Meaning	Example
dia-	through, between, across	dialysis
dys-	difficult/abnormal	dysphagia
en-/endo-/em-/eso-	inside	encapsulated
intra-	within/inside of	intra-abdominal
multi-/poly-	many/excessive	multinodular/polyhydramnios
para-	near, beside, abnormal	parahepatic

Common Gastroenterology Suffixes

Suffix	Meaning	Example
-ase	enzyme	amylase
-cele	hernia	cystocele
-ectomy	excision or removal	appendectomy
-emesis	vomiting	hematemesis
-emia	blood	anemia
-itis	inflammation	pancreatitis
-ium	membrane	hypogastrium
-oid	resembling	adenoid
-oma	tumor	hepatoma
-ostomy	creation of an opening	colostomy
-rrhage/-rrhagia	excessive flow	hemorrhage
-tripsy	pulverization	lithotripsy
-trophy	nourishment	hypertrophy

Common Gastroenterology Abbreviations

Abbreviation	Expansion
EGD	esophagogastroduodenoscopy
EGF	epidermal growth factor
EGJ	esophagogastric junction
ERCP	endoscopic retrograde cholangiopancreatography
GERD	gastroesophageal reflux disease
GIA	gastrointestinal anastomosis
HJR	hepatojugular reflux
PEG	percutaneous endoscopic gastrostomy

REVIEW: GASTROENTEROLOGY LANGUAGE

Multiple Choice.
Choose the best answer.

1. (⊙ Cholecystectomy, ○ Cholecystomy) means removal of the gallbladder.

2. A (○ rectocele, ○ vagocele) is a hernia of the rectum.

3. (○ Lithotripsy, ○ Lithotomy) means pulverization of stones.

4. The term *gastritis* means inflammation of the (○ liver, ○ stomach).

5. HJR stands for (○ hepatojugular, ○ hepatojejunal) reflux.

Fill in the Blank.
Using the word(s) in the box, enter the appropriate term in the space provided.

1. _____ means incision of the abdominal wall.

2. _____ is the study of cancers or tumors.

3. GERD stands for _____ reflux disease.

4. A _____ is an operation to remove a stone.

5. Surgery performed to remove the appendix is called _____ .

oncology
gastroesophageal
appendectomy
laparotomy
lithotomy

TRUE/FALSE.
Mark the following true or false.

1. *PEG* stands for percutaneous endothelial gastrotomy.

    ○ true

    ○ false

2. A hepatoma is a tumor of the liver.

    ○ true

    ○ false

3. Gastrectomy is removal of the pancreas.

    ○ true

    ○ false

4. Inspection of the colon with a scope is called colonoscopy.

    ○ true

    ○ false

5. Inflammation of the appendix is called appendicitis.

    ○ true

    ○ false

GASTROENTEROLOGY REPORTS

Stomach complaints are common and can be related to a number of problems. Any hospital, whether small or large, will do a substantial amount of gastrointestinal procedures and have many admissions for stomach problems. Therefore, for a hospital MTE or a transcription editor doing work on a hospital contract, a working knowledge of the various report types will be essential.

The following are examples of common GI reports, including discharge summaries and procedure notes. Make sure you understand the terminology in each report before moving on to the next. The reports in this unit will give you broad exposure to what you can expect to be exposed to in the working environment and in the practical components of the training program.

GASTROENTEROLOGY REPORT 1 – OPERATIVE NOTE

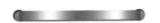

INDICATIONS: The patient is a 59-year-old white male who presents for elective total colectomy with creation of a J-pouch.[1] This procedure is to be done for sporadic adenomatosis coli which was identified several months ago. He presents for a total colectomy because of the increased risk of development of adenocarcinoma. Patient is otherwise a healthy male.

DESCRIPTION OF PROCEDURE: Having obtained informed consent, the patient was taken to the operating room and placed in a dorsal low lithotomy position, after having undergone general endotracheal anesthesia. Dura-Prep was used on the abdomen, and a standard Betadine scrub was used for the perineal prep. The patient was then draped for simultaneous peritoneal and abdominal surgical approaches. A midline incision was created, extending from above the umbilicus down to the pubic tubercle. This incision was then carried down to the median raphe using Bovie electrocautery. Hemostasis was achieved. The peritoneum was then elevated and sharply incised, taking care not to damage underlying bowel. Once the abdominal cavity was opened, it was explored both visually and with palpation. Liver and spleen appeared normal. The abdominal cavity appeared pristine, and several intraluminal masses were noted throughout the colon. First the antimesenteric border of the ascending colon was freed using electrocautery. The ascending colon mesentery was then taken down in a standard fashion using Kelly clamps and 0 silk ties for hemostasis. A short section of the mesentery was then dissected away from the terminal ileum allowing introduction of an Endo GIA 60 and subsequent transection of the terminal ileum from the cecum. The appendix and cecum were normal in appearance. Next, attention was turned to the transverse colon which was freed from the omentum using Kelly clamps and 0 silk ties. Electrocautery was also used for hemostasis. The mesentery was then removed from the transverse colon in a similar fashion to the way it was taken from the ascending colon. Next, attention was turned to the descending portion of the colon which was released on its antimesentery border by electrocautery along the white line of Toldt. The splenic flexure was carefully reduced using sharp and electrocautery technique. The splenic capsule was left intact. The descending colonic mesentery was then carefully dissected away using Kelly clamps and 0 silk ties. This dissection was carried down into the pelvis. Hemostasis of the omentum and mesentery was achieved. At this time, the case was turned over to Dr. Richards[2] for creation of the J-pouch and eventual closure of the abdomen. That portion of the operation will be dictated separately. Complications for this portion of the operation were none. EBL will be included in the other portion of the dictation at the end of the case. Fluids also will be part of the final operative dictation by Dr. Richards.

Footnotes:

1. 1.A J-pouch is an artificial internal bowel reservoir created after removal of the entire colon; it is also known as an ileoanal reservoir.
2. 2.Remember, all references to people, places, and time in these FOMS reports are made up in an effort to protect patient identity.

SPELLING.
Determine if the following words are spelled correctly. If the spelling is correct, leave the word as it has already been entered. If the spelling is incorrect, provide the correct spelling.

1. Kelley _____

2. electricautery _____

3. descending _____

4. terminal _____

5. antimesinteric _____

6. spleen _____

Matching.
Match the correct term to the definition.

1. ____ A fold of peritoneum supporting the viscera.

2. ____ A small projection at the anterior extremity of the crest of the pubis.

3. ____ Surgical removal of the colon or part of the colon.

4. ____ Lateral reflection of posterior parietal pleura of abdomen.

5. ____ The smooth membrane lining the cavity of the abdomen.

6. ____ Malignant tumor originating in glandular epithelium.

A. white line of Toldt

B. omentum

C. colectomy

D. adenocarcinoma

E. peritoneum

F. pubic tubercle

GASTROENTEROLOGY REPORT 2 – DISCHARGE SUMMARY

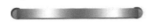

Medical Record

ADMITTING DIAGNOSIS: Dilantin ingestion, spastic diplegia.

HISTORY OF PRESENT ILLNESS: This is a 6-year-old male who took an unknown amount of Dilantin at approximately 9:30 on the morning of admission, which was unwitnessed. Sister has a seizure disorder and is on Dilantin for this. Mom subsequently heard, after she gave sister her dose, that the brothers were talking about taking these medications. The history is very sketchy from the mother. The mother has difficulty hearing. The patient went to school, and when he came home around 4 p.m.,[1] he was noted to be drowsy and not walking well. He was given ipecac at 5:45 p.m. and vomited. There was a bottle of 50 mg tabs, 420 of them dispensed with only 293 tablets. Of note, the 3-year-old brother was also admitted because he also took the medications. Normally, this patient walks on his toes and does not talk a lot. He has some evidence of developmental delay.

PAST MEDICAL HISTORY: The patient has spastic diplegia, cause unknown. He has been tried in an ankle-foot orthosis for walking, without much luck. He was seen in orthopedics clinic in January, but they did not recommend surgery at that time. He has delayed motor developments. He started walking at age 2, but he was seen by Dr. Romney at age 4, who felt that his speech was normal at that time. He also has a diagnosis of cerebral palsy from Dr. David. He was born by normal spontaneous vaginal delivery with Apgars of 9 and 10. Past surgical history is negative. He has never had any allergies. He lives with his 2 siblings and his parents. He is not on any medications at this time.

PHYSICAL EXAMINATION: On admission, exam revealed a 6-year-old male who was alert, in no apparent distress. He was initially vomiting, but later during history and physical was eating potato chips and lying on a gurney. HEENT: Normocephalic. Pupils were equally reactive to light. There was some horizontal nystagmus noted. Tympanic membranes were noted to be gray and mobile. Nose was without discharge. Throat was without erythema. Uvula and tongue were in the midline without fasciculations. Neck was supple. Heart: Regular rate and rhythm, no murmurs.[2] Lungs revealed occasional rhonchi, but no retractions. Chest was without retractions and symmetric. Abdomen was soft, bowel sounds present. There was no hepatosplenomegaly, no masses. The abdomen was not tender. Extremities revealed that the hands and ankles were plantar flexed with somewhat increased tone. The patient was grabbing things and moving all extremities equally. Deep tendon reflexes revealed 1+ in the upper extremities and 2+ in the lower extremities. It was difficult to get ankle reflexes. Genitalia revealed downgoing testes, male.

LABORATORY DATA: Chest x-ray on admission was normal and Dilantin level initially was 42.6. Electrolytes revealed sodium 145, potassium 3.5, chloride 109, CO_2 of 23, and glucose 92.

HOSPITAL COURSE: Assessment on admission was Dilantin ingestion with spastic diplegia and developmental delay. Poison control was called on admission, and they recommended observation for CNS depression and cardiac toxicity, although cardiac toxicity was noted to be extremely rare from oral Dilantin overdose. They also said that liver toxicity was more common with chronic overdose, not acute overdose. The patient was watched over the next couple of days and levels gradually decreased, although yesterday he was given some GoLYTELY to decrease transit time through the gut, and this morning the Dilantin level was down to 11.0,[3] which is low therapeutic range. The patient was active and alert, running around this morning, playful. No neurologic signs, and heart had regular rate and rhythm. He was sent home. Mom was again given instructions by me to place the medicines either under lock and key or up out of the reach of the children. She will follow up with the health aide should the boy show any signs of shortness of breath, chest pain, headaches, or drowsiness.

DISCHARGE DIAGNOSES

1. Dilantin ingestion.
2. Spastic diplegia.

Footnotes:

1. 1.It would be acceptable to edit this as 4:00 pm, but typically the :00 is dropped on the hour time notations.
2. 2.Notice how sometimes a subheading in PE is given and a colon is used and other times it is written in paragraph format. Some accounts will prefer (or even require) all PE subheadings are followed by a colon and the information has initial cap. Others prefer you edit all PE information in paragraph format without subheadings. In this report, the transcription editing was mixed (some headings some sentence format). This is probably verbatim.
3. 3.Oftentimes the trailing zero on a whole number is dropped so as not to confuse something like 11 with 110. In this case, the number was likely edited as dictated.

Multiple Choice.
Choose the best answer.

1. Palpation revealed no (○ hepatosplenamegaly, ○ hepatosplenomegaly).
2. At birth his (○ Appars, ○ Apgars) were 9 and 10.
3. The patient will follow up with a home health (○ aide, ○ aid).
4. The patient's sister suffers from (○ sezures, ○ seizures).
5. Initially the patient was (○ vomiting, ○ vomitting).

Fill in the Blank.
The following abbreviations and/or terms are used in the previous reports. Fill in the appropriate blank with either the abbreviation or its expansion.

1. TM_____
2. deep tendon reflexes_____
3. HPI_____
4. HEENT_____
5. central nervous system_____

GASTROENTEROLOGY REPORT 3 – OPERATIVE NOTE

PREOPERATIVE DIAGNOSIS: Imperforate anus.

OPERATION PERFORMED: Colostomy revision with end transverse colostomy in right lower quadrant and mucous fistula in left lower quadrant.

INDICATIONS: This is a two-and-a-half-year-old[1] male with history of duodenal atresia and loop colostomy at birth for imperforate anus. He has recently had problems with his colostomy. The parents of the child now note pain with his bowel movements and straining. Physical exam revealed narrowing of his colostomy and unable to pass finger below the fascia. He therefore now presents for planned revision of his colostomy.

DESCRIPTION OF PROCEDURE: He was administered a general endotracheal anesthesia in the supine position. The abdomen was prepped and draped in the usual sterile fashion. The colostomy was occluded with a figure-of-eight silk suture. The colostomy was then circumscribed with the electrocautery in order to completely free this loop colostomy up. The fascia was divided until the abdomen was freely entered. Some adhesions were encountered within the abdomen, which were taken down in sharp fashion. Upon palpating the course of the colon, it was felt that this colostomy was not a sigmoid but was more likely a loop transverse colostomy. There was a long segment of mucous fistula[2] on the distal segment of the loop, which contained a lot of inspissated mucus-type contents. It was felt in order to completely decompress this segment, since the distal segment was somewhat larger actually than the proximal segment, that a separate mucous fistula and colostomy site would be more favorable by dividing this loop. Therefore the loop was divided and the mesentery was cleared back from a small segment in order to bring these 2 ends up through the abdominal wall for planned stoma. A separate skin incision was made in the right lower quadrant in the transverse plane. A cruciate-type incision was made on the anterior and posterior rectus sheaths, and the proximal colostomy was then brought up through this incision and secured through the skin in 4 quadrants with interrupted Vicryl sutures. The colostomy was further secured to the skin with interrupted Vicryl between these quadrant stitches. The mucous fistula was also secured at the present colostomy site in a similar fashion. Stomal appliances were then placed onto the stomas. He was then awakened from general endotracheal anesthesia, extubated, and returned to the recovery room awake, alert, and in stable condition.

Footnotes:

1. 1.This is one way to notate this age, but another would be 2-1/2-year-old. This is what we call acceptable variation—more than one way to do something correctly (or is that 1 way?).
2. 2.Note this is not mucus fistula, but a mucous fistula. When the word *mucus* is being used as an adjective, it is *mucous*. Later in this same sentence the dictator says "mucus-type." This is the noun form (you always use the noun form with *-type*). Don't let this trip you up in the practicum.

SPELLING.
Determine if the following words are spelled correctly. If the spelling is correct, leave the word as it has already been entered. If the spelling is incorrect, provide the correct spelling.

1. imperferate _____

2. atresia _____

3. inspisated _____

4. fistula _____

5. proxemal _____

Matching.
Match the correct term to the definition.

1. ____ Opening established in the abdominal wall by
colostomy, ileostomy, or a similar operation.

2. ____ A fibrous band of scar tissue that binds together
normally separate anatomical structures.

3. ____ Extending across.

4. ____ Situated farthest from point of attachment or origin.

5. ____ A double layer of peritoneum attached to the abdominal
wall.

6. ____ Within the trachea.

A. transverse

B. stoma

C. distal

D. endotracheal

E. adhesion

F. mesentery

GASTROENTEROLOGY REPORT 4 – PROCEDURE NOTE

PREOPERATIVE DIAGNOSIS: Reflux esophagitis.

SURGEON: Dr. Monroe.

OPERATION PERFORMED: Endoscopy.

INDICATIONS: Reflux esophagitis resistant to H2 blockers.

HISTORY: Patient has had reflux esophagitis which has failed treatment with cimetidine and ranitidine. He has been on omeprazole for 2 weeks prior to current visit, although it was prescribed 1 month ago. He says the symptoms are much improved on this treatment, and he has no side effects of the medication. Risks were explained, and consent was signed. Of note, the patient has had an increase in his weight over the last month and is also on ferrous sulfate therapy. Examination prior to procedure was within normal limits.

DESCRIPTION OF OPERATION: The scope was passed into the duodenum at 85 cm and then was withdrawn slowly. The duodenum was entirely normal with a normal pylorus and antrum. The stomach mucosa was normal, although there were thickened gastric folds throughout. Three[1] biopsies were taken in the area of the cardia. The scope was able to be retroflexed, and this area was visualized and was normal. On withdrawing the scope into the esophagus, there was a sliding, moderately-sized hiatal hernia, but the mucosa in that space looked normal. The lower esophageal sphincter seemed somewhat decreased in pressure and remained open most of the time it was visualized. The esophageal mucosa appeared normal, but several biopsies were taken. The patient tolerated the procedure extremely well.

He is to continue on omeprazole 20 mg p.o. q.d. for a total of 6 weeks. Although there is no good indication that going back to H2 blockers will "maintain" his remission, because omeprazole is not approved for longterm use, this will probably be a prudent decision. It is possible that medication can be provided to increase his lower esophageal sphincter pressure as well, and this may help. If H2 blocker is unable to keep him symptom free, it may be worthwhile trying intermittent omeprazole therapy. The above will be discussed with Dr. Henry at Springfield General Hospital,[2] and the patient will follow up with him in 2-3 weeks. Only medications given at the time of procedure are midazolam 1 mg IV, Cetacaine spray and viscous Lidocaine, both topically.

Footnotes:

1. 1.A numeral is not used here because it is typically preferred to not begin a sentence with a numeral.
2. 2.The names (places and dates), obviously, are fictional substitutions in order to wash any patient confidentiality information from these reports. Do you recognize these names?

SPELLING.
Determine if the following words are spelled correctly. If the spelling is correct, leave the word as it has already been entered. If the spelling is incorrect, provide the correct spelling.

1. duedenum _____

2. reflux _____

3. pilorus _____

4. sphincter _____

5. midazolam _____

Matching.
Match the trade name to the generic form.

1. ____ Tagamet

2. ____ Zantac

3. ____ Prilosec

4. ____ Versed

5. ____ Lidocaine

A. ranitidine

B. cimetidine

C. lidocaine

D. midazolam

E. omeprazole

GASTROENTEROLOGY REPORT 5 – DISCHARGE SUMMARY

FINAL DIAGNOSES

1. Upper gastrointestinal bleed.[1]
2. Blood loss anemia.
3. Iron deficiency anemia.
4. History of uric acid stones.

PROCEDURES: Blood transfusion times 2 units.

HISTORY OF PRESENT ILLNESS: The patient presents with 1 month of stomach pain increased with eating and intermittent black bowel movements for 1 month. He notes these symptoms are better when he takes Mylanta. They have been worse over the last few days, and his appetite has been very poor. He does not use cigarettes or alcohol. He quit chewing tobacco approximately 1 week prior to admission. His hemoglobin was noted to be 5.5.

PAST MEDICAL HISTORY: Current medications are Naprosyn, allopurinol, and nitrofurantoin. He has a history of undocumented uric acid stones with urinary retention and urinary tract infection in 1999. He had an upper GI bleed of unknown cause in 2001. He has DJD of his back that has been treated with Naprosyn and physical therapy for years. He had a sigmoid polyp removed in 2003. He had Haemophilus influenzae in 2005. He has a past history of hypertension that resolved, and he has not been on medicines for many years for this problem.

PHYSICAL EXAMINATION: Alert male with pulse 120, respiratory rate 28, blood pressure 150/74. He initially in the emergency room was in considerable pain but apparently this resolved rapidly with IV cimetidine. Weight 159 pounds; typical weights are 162 to 174 pounds. Physical exam was basically normal except for guaiac positive stools.

LABORATORY DATA: Hemoglobin 5.6, hematocrit 18, MCV 68 with MCHC of 31 and MCH 21. Liver enzymes and clotting times were normal.

ASSESSMENT: Upper gastrointestinal bleed, ulcerative versus gastritis, iron deficiency and acute blood loss anemia.

HOSPITAL COURSE: The patient was transfused with 2 units of packed red blood cells and placed on cimetidine. His hemoglobin on Tuesday was up to 8.1, and the patient was feeling markedly stronger at that time. There was no further bleeding or abdominal pain while in the hospital. He was therefore discharged to home on Thursday.

DISCHARGE MEDICATIONS: Cimetidine 800 mg p.o. q.h.s. for 6 weeks, allopurinol 300 mg p.o. q.h.s., nitrofurantoin 50 mg p.o. q.h.s., and ferrous sulfate 5 grains 1 p.o. twice a day for 2 months.

FOLLOWUP: The patient was told to stop his Naprosyn. He was given an appointment for an upper GI for Monday and to be seen at that time.

Footnotes:

1. 1.It is likely the author dictated "GI bleed," but it is generally preferred abbreviations be expanded under the diagnosis and assessment headings. (This is an assumption, since we don't have the audio available for this file.)

SPELLING.
Determine if the following words are spelled correctly. If the spelling is correct, leave the word as it has already been entered. If the spelling is incorrect, provide the correct spelling.

1. Milanta _____

2. Nitrophutantoin _____

3. deficency _____

4. Haemophilus _____

5. guaiuc _____

Fill in the Blank.
The following abbreviations and/or terms are used in the previous reports. Fill in the appropriate blank with either the abbreviation or its expansion.

1. DJD_____

2. urinary tract infection_____

3. GI_____

4. ER_____

5. physical therapy_____

6. intravenous_____

GASTROENTEROLOGY REPORT 6 – OPERATIVE NOTE

PREOPERATIVE DIAGNOSIS: Zenker diverticulum.

POSTOPERATIVE DIAGNOSIS: Zenker diverticulum.[1]

DRAINS: 7-mm Blake drain.

MATERIAL TO LAB: Excised Zenker diverticulum.

OPERATION PERFORMED: Cricopharyngeal myotomy with esophageal diverticulectomy.

ESTIMATED BLOOD LOSS: 50 cc.

INDICATIONS: This is a relatively healthy 48-year-old male who relates a several month history of intermittent difficulty swallowing and worsening halitosis. Preoperative evaluation included an upper gastrointestinal series, which demonstrated a moderately large Zenker diverticulum with a wide base. He presents now for elective excision of this diverticulum and cricopharyngeal myotomy.[2]

DESCRIPTION OF PROCEDURE: The patient was taken to the operating room where general anesthesia was attained. His neck was prepped and draped in the usual sterile fashion. A scalpel was used to make an incision paralleling the anterior border of the left sternocleidomastoid muscle. The electrocautery was used to perform dissection down through the platysma muscle layer and then along the anterior border of the sternocleidomastoid muscle until the carotid sheath was reached. The carotid sheath with its contents was retracted laterally and careful dissection begun medially, next to the esophagus. Care was taken to identify and preserve the recurrent laryngeal nerve running in the tracheoesophageal groove. With dissection, the cricopharyngeus muscle became evident, as did the moderately large esophageal diverticulum arising just superior to the cricopharyngeus muscle. The cricopharyngeus was elevated from the esophagus using a right angle clamp, and divided with the electrocautery. The diverticulum was dissected free for its entire length. Anesthesia then passed a #40 French bougie esophageal dilator to prevent constriction of the esophagus with excision of the diverticulum. The base of the diverticulum was then stapled across using a TA 30 stapler. The diverticulum was excised and sent to Pathology as a specimen. The mucosal borders of the excised diverticulum site were bovied. The neck was then irrigated and checked for hemostasis. A 7-mm Blake drain was placed in the operative site and exited through a separate stab incision. Closure consisted of a running 3-0 Vicryl suture, reapproximating the platysma muscle layer. The skin was closed with staples. A dressing of Xeroform gauze and 4 x 8 sponges was placed. The patient was then awakened and extubated in the operating room and taken to the Surgical Intensive Care Unit for recovery. He did demonstrate a normal voice upon extubation. Estimated blood loss was 50 cc. There were no apparent complications.

Footnotes:

1. [1] Author likely said "same" here, but as is typically preferred, it was expanded out to repeat the preop diagnosis.
2. [2] Note the last sentence is an odd sounding construction, but it is one that is commonly dictated. "He is now for..." or even "He presents for..."

SPELLING.
Determine if the following words are spelled correctly. If the spelling is correct, leave the word as it has already been entered. If the spelling is incorrect, provide the correct spelling.

1. Zenker _____
2. crisopharingeal _____
3. halitosis _____
4. platysma _____
5. boogie _____
6. disection _____
7. esophagus _____
8. Xeraform _____

Multiple Choice.
Classify the following terms as either anatomical or equipment.

1. Blake
   - ○ anatomical
   - ○ equipment

2. cricopharyngeus
   - ○ anatomical
   - ○ equipment

3. sternocleidomastoid
   - ○ anatomical
   - ○ equipment

4. Xeroform
   - ○ anatomical
   - ○ equipment

5. platysma
   - ○ anatomical
   - ○ equipment

6. diverticulum
   - ○ anatomical
   - ○ equipment

7. bougie
   - ○ anatomical
   - ○ equipment

8. dilator
   - ○ anatomical
   - ○ equipment

GASTROENTEROLOGY REPORT 7 – OPERATIVE NOTE

DRAINS: Suprapubic 24-French Malecot catheter, Foley, left lower quadrant 10 Blake drain, left lower quadrant colostomy bag.[1]

INDICATIONS: The patient is a 61-year-old white male who presented with a history of several months of persistent bladder infection and a 2-week history of nocturia. He was admitted to the medicine service for workup of these problems. On attempted colonoscopy he was found to have a large fungating[2] mass in his distal sigmoid colon. During the night prior to operation, he developed a total bowel obstruction and was taken emergently to exploratory laparotomy with diverting colostomy for relief of the obstruction and to identify the nature of his colon mass and to repair a probable enterocystic fistula.

DESCRIPTION OF PROCEDURE: After obtaining informed consent the patient was taken to the operating room and placed in the supine position. Under general endotracheal anesthesia the patient was prepped and draped in the usual sterile fashion. A midline incision was made just above the umbilicus to a point near the pubis. This was carried down in a sharp and blunt fashion to the peritoneum, making sure to maintain meticulous hemostasis. The peritoneum was lifted up and entered sharply, taking care not to damage underlying bowel. The abdomen was then explored both visually and by palpation. Liver and spleen appeared normal. The small bowel appeared normal. The small bowel mesentery and omentum appeared normal without any evidence of enlarged lymph nodes. The sigmoid colon was found to have a large hard mass, which was adherent to the posterior and lateral walls. The sigmoid colon was mobilized along the white line of Toldt to approximately the mid descending colon. The Bovie electrocautery was used to separate the sigmoid colon from the posterior bladder wall. No obvious fistula was identified. The distal segment of sigmoid colon beyond the mass was then freed using sharp and blunt dissection. The GIA stapler was then used to transect the sigmoid colon, both proximal and distal to the mass, leaving a 5-10 cm margin on both ends. The specimen was then handed off and opened in the operating room. Examination showed a large cancerous appearing lesion within the segment removed, which was foul smelling and lobulated. Attention was then turned to the bladder wall, which appeared to be integrated and abnormal. Since this was suspicious for extension of the tumor mass, a piece was sent for frozen section. At this point the operation was turned over to the urology team, which had been standing by, for the ultimate partial resection of the urinary bladder. This portion of the case will be dictated separately. After partial resection of the bladder by the urology team, which included 3-layer closure and placement of a suprapubic catheter, the general surgery team once again resumed control of the operation. The sigmoid colon was brought up through the left lower quadrant abdominal wall, through the rectus abdominis muscle. The Bovie electrocautery was used to make a circular skin incision, and then a cruciate shaped incision was created in the rectus fascia and rectus abdominis musculature to facilitate passage of the sigmoid colon for maturing of colostomy. Then 4-0 silk sutures were then used to attach the colonic mucosa to the prerectus fascia. During the course of pulling the sigmoid colon through the abdominal wall defect, an incidental enterotomy occurred at the staple line. Because of the great pressure that the proximal colon and small bowel were under due to the original obstruction, there was gross spillage of bowel contents into the area of the colostomy site. A GIA 60 was then used to restaple[3] the distal portion of the sigmoid colon to prevent leakage of more bowel contents. Attention was then turned back to the original midline incision. The abdominal cavity was irrigated with copious amounts of saline antibiotic solution. The mesentery along the descending colon was closed with a 3-0 Vicryl running stitch to prevent future herniation of small bowel. Hemostasis was noted to have been achieved prior to the closure. A Blake drain was then laid in the cavity just superior to the bladder and brought out through the left lower quadrant abdominal wall. The midline incision was then closed using running 0 Prolene stitches. The subcutaneous tissues were irrigated copiously and the skin was closed with staples. Attention was then turned back to the maturing of the colostomy. This was done in the usual fashion using 3-0 Vicryl sutures. The colonic mucosa appeared vital at the end of the case, and a colostomy bag was placed. During the maturing of the colostomy the bowel continued to spontaneously decompress large amounts of gas and fecal material. The suprapubic and Blake drains were sewn in place using 2-0 silk. The patient was then awakened from general anesthetic, having tolerated the procedure well. He was taken to the Surgical Intensive Care Unit in stable condition.

COMPLICATIONS: Incidental enterotomy of the proximal sigmoid stump prior to maturing of the colostomy.

ESTIMATED BLOOD LOSS: 1300 cc.

FLUIDS: 1000 cc normal saline, 500 cc Hespan, and 5000 cc Isolyte.

Footnotes:

1. 1.Lists like this are easier read when they are presented in list format. Some clients prefer lists only be edited when dictated specifically as a list. It is always important to stick with account instructions regarding stylistic issues.
2. 2.Just what is a fungating mass? Glad you asked. *Fungating* means a mass or lesion which is marked by ulcerations (breaks on the skin or surface of an organ) and necrosis (death of living tissue) and that usually has a bad smell.
3. 3.Although some words like *re-cover* (cover again) and *re-create* (create again) need a hyphen for clarification (*recover* without the hyphen would mean regain and recreate would be play) *Restaple* is clearly to staple again and needs no hyphen.

Matching.
Match the correct term to the definition.

1. ____ Excessive urination at night.

2. ____ A large quantity.

3. ____ Bulging of tissue through an opening in a membrane, muscle, or bone.

4. ____ Above the pubic bone.

5. ____ Marked by ulcerations and necrosis.

6. ____ Surgical removal of part of a structure or organ.

A. suprapubic

B. herniation

C. nocturia

D. resection

E. copious

F. fungating

Multiple Choice.
Choose the best answer.

1. The fungating mass was found in the patient's distal (○ sigmoid, ⌣ small) colon.

2. A Foley (⌣ catheter, ⌣ drain) was inserted.

3. The patient was taken for an emergent exploratory (⌣ appendectomy, ⌣ laparotomy).

4. The patient was taken to the (⌣ Critical Care Unit, ⌣ Surgical Intensive Care Unit).

5. Estimated blood loss was (⌣ 1300, ⌣ 1000) cc.

GASTROENTEROLOGY REPORT 8 – DISCHARGE SUMMARY

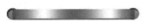

DISCHARGE DIAGNOSES

1. Partial small bowel obstruction, resolved.
2. Renal cell carcinoma, status post left nephrectomy.
3. Urinary tract infection, Escherichia coli.

ADMITTING HISTORY: This is a 72-year-old female who was discharged from Sacred Heart Hospital 1 week prior to admission following a left nephrectomy for a large left renal cell carcinoma. She did well postoperatively until the morning of admission when she developed diffuse crampy abdominal pain with vomiting, anorexia, and a sensation of some rectal pressure, but denied any bowel movement since the morning of admission.

PAST MEDICAL HISTORY: She was on no medication at the time of admission. Her past medical history was remarkable for an exploratory laparotomy in 1996 with adhesions found, a hysterectomy in 2001, and a left shoulder repair in 2003. There was a history of mild asthma, recurring E. coli urinary tract infections resistant to Septra, and hypertension, currently on no medications. She quit smoking 20 years prior to admission. SHE WAS ALLERGIC TO CODEINE WHICH CAUSED GI INTOLERANCE.[1] There was a past history of tuberculosis, treated in the 1950s. She lives at home with her husband. She had not yet resumed work since her surgery.

PHYSICAL EXAMINATION: She was an alert, cooperative female in mild distress. Her weight was 134 pounds, temperature 98, pulse 120, respiratory rate 20, and blood pressure 140/80. Head, eyes, ears, nose, throat exam was negative. Lung exam showed slightly decreased breath sounds at the left base with no wheezes, rales, or rhonchi. Heart rhythm was basically regular with occasional skipped beats, no murmur. Breast exam was normal. Abdomen showed a recent left abdominal surgical scar, healing well without evidence of infection. She had high-pitched bowel sounds and mild diffuse tenderness, especially in the center of the abdomen. However, the abdomen was soft without distention. Rectal exam showed guaiac negative stool. Extremities were normal. Her neurologic exam was normal.

LABORATORY AND X-RAY FINDINGS: X-rays showed a small effusion at the left base. Abdominal films showed a normal amount of gas with no air-fluid levels. Her laboratory studies showed a sodium of 143, potassium of 3.8, chloride of 97, bicarbonate of 30, BUN of 9, and white count of 11,900.

HOSPITAL COURSE: She was admitted with a diagnosis of partial small bowel obstruction. She was treated initially with IV fluids and kept n.p.o.[2] An NG tube was not placed, as she had no further vomiting after admission. By the second hospital day, she was complaining of feeling hungry, had improving bowel sounds, still some left upper quadrant and epigastric tenderness. Her laboratory studies remained normal. She was begun on clear liquids, as well as ambulation. Over the next several days, her diet was further advanced gradually, to a regular diet. She tolerated this reasonably well, although she did have one recurrent episode of fairly severe abdominal pain about 12 hours after starting her regular diet. She received a single injection of Demerol with relief of her symptoms. A repeat abdominal series at that time was unremarkable. By the following morning, she was again hungry, no nausea, and no further pain.

A urinalysis at the time of admission showed 3+ bacteria with 0-1 white cells and 2-4 red cells. A urine culture grew out E. coli, again resistant to amoxicillin and Septra. She was treated with IV Ancef initially. When she was eating normally, she was switched to oral Keflex. She tolerated this medication well.

She remained afebrile through her hospital stay. Her blood pressure remained well in the normal range. Respirations remained unlabored at 16-20. Her weight remained stable at about 131 pounds.

She did initially complain of left hip pain with symptoms somewhat suggestive of a radiculopathy involving the left buttocks and hip area. A plain film of her pelvis was obtained showing a normal appearing hip joint and no evidence of intrinsic bony disease, although there was one little area of sclerosis in the right hip, which was her asymptomatic side. She was given Motrin with good relief of pain. By the third hospital day, she had no further complaints of left hip or buttocks pain.

DISPOSITION: She was discharged on the eighth hospital day. Her discharge medications were Keflex 250 mg p.o. q.i.d. for 5 more days, Motrin 400 mg every 6 hours as needed for pain, and nitrofurantoin 100 mg 1 tablet daily for 3 months as prophylaxis against these frequently recurring UTIs, to start after she completed the course of Keflex. She will follow up with the next urology clinic. She is to follow up in the regular outpatient clinic in 3 weeks for a recheck. She will let us know at any point should she redevelop the abdominal pain, vomiting, fevers, or other new symptoms.

Footnotes:

1. 1.Some accounts will require any allergy information be presented in ALL CAPS. Still others require allergy information be separated from regular text and placed under an ALLERGY: heading and then edited in ALL CAPS. You will see it a number of acceptable ways.
2. 2.The abbreviation *n.p.o.* means literally "nil per os," or nothing per mouth. Some clients may require this be edited as NPO so as to make it stand out (as is also the case with DNR status).

Fill in the Blank.
The following abbreviations and/or terms are used in the previous reports. Fill in the appropriate blank with either the abbreviation or its expansion.

1. UTI_____
2. tuberculosis_____
3. GI_____
4. UA_____
5. blood urea nitrogen_____
6. nasogastric_____

TRUE/FALSE.
Mark the following true or false.

1. An admission urinalysis showed 0-1 white cells.

    ○ true

    ○ false

2. The patient was discharged on the ninth hospital day.

    ○ true

    ○ false

3. HEENT exam was negative.

    ○ true

    ○ false

4. The patient had no medical allergies.

    ○ true

    ○ false

5. The patient lives alone.

    ○ true

    ○ false

GASTROENTEROLOGY REPORT 9 – OPERATIVE NOTE

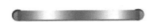

PREOPERATIVE DIAGNOSIS: Sigmoid obstructive mass.

DRAINS: #7 French Malecot suprapubic catheter.[1]

OPERATION PERFORMED: Exploratory laparotomy. Sigmoid colectomy with diverting colostomy. Partial cystectomy.

INDICATIONS: The patient is a 61-year-old white male with approximately a 3-week history of intermittent pneumaturia and frequent urinary tract infections times 3 months, admitted to the general surgery service with a large sigmoid mass that became obstructing acutely on the day of surgery. The patient was taken to the operating room, where an exploratory laparotomy was performed. At the time of surgery, an intraoperative consult to urology was made secondary to possible involvement of the bladder with colon cancer.[2]

DESCRIPTION OF PROCEDURE: See operative dictation by the general surgery service under separate dictation.

At the time of consultation, the dome of the bladder appeared to be thickened and hard from where the sigmoid colon had been removed and peeled off the exterior of the bladder. A cystotomy was made over the dome of the bladder, and the mucosa was found to be indurated and irregular. The affected area plus about 1-cm margins was resected, which involved a large portion of the dome and anterior portion of the bladder. This was sent to Pathology for frozen and permanent sections. In addition, the inflamed areas on the right posterior and left sides of the bladder were biopsied and sent for frozen section and found to be negative for carcinoma involvement. The ureters were visualized with clear urine efflux bilaterally. The mucosa was thus closed with 3-0 chromic suture in a running locking stitch. A #7 French Malecot suprapubic tube was inserted through the dome of the bladder and was brought out through the abdominal wall without difficulty. The musculature of the bladder was closed over the mucosa with 3-0 Vicryl interrupted sutures. Because the peritoneum was found to be quite thickened, the peritoneum was closed over the bladder with 3-0 Vicryl in a running fashion. After closing the cystotomy, the bladder was filled with saline; approximately 100-150 cc was instilled until the bladder was found to be quite taut. There was only mild seepage from the cystotomy. The suprapubic tube was secured in place, and the remainder of the surgery was turned to the general surgeons.

Footnotes:

1. 1.Some accounts do not allow the use of symbols such as #, &, and %. This account is not one of them, obviously, but it is good to note that some require these be expanded to *number, and,* and *percent.*
2. 2.Recognize this gentleman? He is the Operative Report patient from Gastroenterology Report 7.

Matching.
Match the correct term to the definition.

1. ____ The passage of gas or air from the urethra during or after urination.
2. ____ The process of flowing out.
3. ____ Pulled tight.
4. ____ Surgical incision into the abdominal wall.
5. ____ The muscular part of the body.

A. efflux
B. laparotomy
C. pneumaturia
D. musculature
E. taut

Multiple Choice.
Choose the best answer.

1. A (⚪ superpubic, ⚪ suprapubic) catheter was placed.

2. Patient has a history of (⚪ intermittent, ⚪ intermitent) UTIs.

3. Patient had urinary (⚪ track, ⚪ tract) infections times 3 months.

4. The (⚪ perineum, ⚪ peritoneum) was found to be thickened.

5. There was mild (⚪ seapage, ⚪ seepage) from the cystotomy.

UNIT 4
Genitourinary

GENITOURINARY – INTRODUCTION

Genitourinary is the branch of medicine that deals with the male and female urinary tracts, as well as the male genital and reproductive structures. This is often referred to simply as "GU."

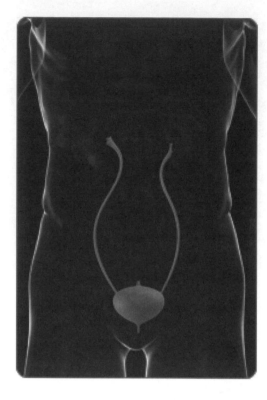

Many different problems are treated by urologists. Among these are:

- testicular torsions or other testicular problems
- hernias
- bladder incontinence
- urinary tract infections (UTIs)
- bladder, prostate, and rectal cancers
- inability to urinate
- impotence and other sexual dysfunctions
- bladder and urinary tract obstructions
- kidney stones
- various kidney diseases such as nephritis or nephrosis

Where appropriate, these problems are treated with such procedures and surgeries as:

- cystoscopies
- ureteroscopies
- orchiopexies
- resections of the prostate
- transurethral resection of the bladder or bladder tumor (TURB/TURBT)
- herniorrhaphies
- circumcisions
- stent placements
- catheter placements
- penile prostheses
- vasectomies
- kidney transplants

Hemorrhoids may also be diagnosed by urologists and either treated or excised as part of the medical management. The cross-disciplinary relationships between GI and GU are apparent when problems such as these are considered.

GENITOURINARY LANGUAGE WORKSHOP

Again, this list is in no way an exhaustive list of Genitourinary word-building word parts and abbreviations. It is meant merely to be a review of words commonly associated with the GU specialty—words you are likely to be exposed to in this FOMS unit, in the practicum modules of this training program, and as a successful working medical transcription editor.

Common Genitourinary Root Words and Combining Forms

Root Word & Combining Form	Meaning	Example
angi/o	vessel	angiotensin
balan/o	glans penis	balanitis
crypt/o	hide, conceal	cryptococcosis
cyst/o	cyst, bladder	cystocele
epididym/o	epididymis	epididymitis
genit/o	genitals	genitourinary
gonad/o	gonad	gonadectomy
granul/o	grain, particle	granulocyte
hom/o	common, same	homosexual
hydr/o	water, watery fluid	hydrocele
infer/o	lowermost, below	inferior
lapar/o	flank, abdominal wall	laparotomy
lith/o	stone	lithotripsy
muc/o	mucus	mucosectomy
my/o	muscle	myoblastoma
nephr/o	kidney	nephrolithiasis
orchi/o	testicle	orchiectomy
py/o	pus	pyogenic
pyel/o	trough, renal pelvis	pyelonephritis
semin/o	semen	seminal
spermat/o	seed	spermatocele
ur/o	urine	polyuria
ureter/o	ureter	ureterovesical
vas/o	vessel, vas deferens	vasodilation

Common Genitourinary Prefixes

Prefix	Meaning	Example
bi-/di-	two	bifid/dissect
de-	down from, removing	decompression
dys-	difficult, abnormal	dysenteric
epi-	above/on	epididymis
in-	not	incidental
multi-/poly-	many, excessive	multifocal/polyuria
mono-/uni-	one	monoclonal/unilateral
para-	near, beside, abnormal	paraesophageal
peri-	around, near	periurethral
supra-	above, over	suprapubic

Common Genitourinary Suffixes

Suffix	Meaning	Example
-centesis	procedure to aspirate fluid	paracentesis
-emia	blood	anemia
-lysis	loosening/breaking apart	clysis
-megaly	enlargement	pancreatomegaly
-rrhage/-rrhagia	excessive flow	ureterorrhagia
-rrhea	flow or discharge	diarrhea
-tripsy	surgical crushing	lithotripsy

Common Genitourinary Abbreviations

Abbreviation	Expansion
BPH	benign prostatic hypertrophy or hyperplasia
CAUTI	catheter-associated urinary tract infection
DVIU	direct-vision internal urethrotomy
UPJ	ureteropelvic junction
TURP	transurethral resection of prostate, transurethral prostatectomy
TURBT	transurethral resection of bladder tumor
TURB	transurethral resection of bladder tumor
UA	urinalysis
ESWL	extracorporeal shock wave lithotripsy
KUB	kidneys, ureters, bladder
VCUG	voiding cystourethrogram

REVIEW: GENITOURINARY LANGUAGE

TRUE/FALSE.
Mark the following true or false.

1. *Suprapubic* means behind the pubic area.

    ○ true

    ○ false

2. *Polyuria* means excessive urination.

    ○ true

    ○ false

3. *Vasectomy* is removal of all or part of the vas deferens.

    ○ true

    ○ false

4. *KUB* stands for kidneys, urethra, and bladder.

    ○ true

    ○ false

5. A cystoscope is a tubular instrument equipped with a light and used to examine the interior of the urinary bladder.

    ○ true

    ○ false

Fill in the Blank.
Using the word(s) in the box, enter the appropriate term in the space provided.

1. Transurethral _____ of the prostate, also known as TURP, is considered the most effective treatment for BPH.

2. _____ shockwave lithotripsy uses high-energy sound waves to destroy kidney stones.

3. A _____, literally meaning water hernia, is a pathological accumulation of serous fluid in a bodily cavity, especially in the scrotal pouch.

4. _____ means absence of urine formation.

5. Inflammation of the glans penis is called _____.

hydrocele
balanitis
anuresis
resection
extracorporeal

Multiple Choice.
Choose the best answer.

1. (○ Dysuria, ○ Dystonia) means difficulty urinating.

2. An incision made into the urethra is called a (○ urethrotomy ○ urethrectomy).

3. (○ Nephrolith, ○ Anorchism) means absence of testicles.

4. BPH is a non-malignant enlargement of the (○ prostrate, ○ prostate).

5. The uncontrolled or involuntary discharge of urine is known as (○ diuresis, ○ enuresis).

GENITOURINARY REPORTS

Although GU reports come in a variety of shapes and sizes, the terminology and anatomy for most urology reports are generally similar. Prostate cancer is one of the most common cancers and is treated by urologists. Additionally, urinary tract infections, hemorrhoids, and hernias are quite common. Thus, all hospitals have urology departments and as far as transcription editing is concerned, there are many urology reports to be typed in hospital settings. The terminology is relatively specialized, but mostly as it relates to the anatomy.

Remember to look up terms that are unfamiliar to you. A full understanding of the information in these reports will better prepare you for the practical component of this training program.

GENITOURINARY REPORT 1 – OPERATIVE NOTE

PREOPERATIVE DIAGNOSIS: Right testicular torsion.

POSTOPERATIVE DIAGNOSIS: Right testicular torsion.

MATERIAL TO LAB: Excised appendix epididymis, and excised appendix testis bilaterally.

OPERATION PERFORMED: Bilateral orchiopexy.

INDICATIONS: This is a 14-year-old male with a history of right testicular torsion this week, who was brought here for bilateral testicular orchiopexy.

[1]DESCRIPTION OF PROCEDURE: Consent was obtained. After subarachnoid block was induced, the patient was placed on the operating table in the supine position, prepped and draped in the usual sterile fashion. A transverse incision was made in the right hemiscrotum approximately 3 cm in length, and taken down using Bovie electrocautery through the tunica vaginalis. Examination of the testis found a normal testicle with a slightly anterior lie. The head of the epididymis was somewhat bullous,[2] perhaps consistent with recent torsion. The appendix epididymis and appendix testis were identified, picked up using a DeBakey forceps, and removed using electrocautery. The testis was then pexed[3] in place, using 4-0 Nurolon on the medial side to the median raphe to the lateral side and to the inferior pole. The wound was irrigated. The dartos muscle was closed using a running lock of 3-0 chromic. The skin was closed using interrupted horizontal mattress stitches of 4-0 chromic. The left hemiscrotum was then opened in a transverse fashion approximately 3 cm in length, taken down through the tunica vaginalis using Bovie electrocautery. The testis was examined. There was found to be a somewhat long mesorchium. The appendix epididymis and appendix testis were removed using electrocautery and sent for pathologic examination. The testis was then pexed in place from the tunica albuginea to the dartos muscle in the lateral and medial and inferior pole positions. The wound was irrigated. The dartos muscle was closed using a running lock of 3-0 chromic, and the skin was closed using interrupted horizontal mattress stitch of 4-0 chromic. The wound was cleaned with a wet and dry sponge. Xeroform gauze, fluffs and scrotal support were applied. The patient was then washed of the excess Betadine on his skin. He was transported to the recovery room via gurney in stable condition. There were no complications. The patient tolerated this procedure well.

Footnotes:

1. 1.This report is really chock full of good words: *orchiopexy, tunica vaginalis, epididymis, tunica albuginea, dartos,* etc. Make sure to look them up if you are unsure what they mean.
2. 2.Word differentiation—do you know the difference between *bullous* and *bolus*? Look it up!
3. 3.*Pexis* means fixation by tissue or surgical fixation by suture. Although the term *pexed* is not easily referenced in reputable resources, it is a word that is commonly used in GI and GU surgeries (and it will likely eventually find its way into those reputable resources).

SPELLING.
Determine if the following words are spelled correctly. If the spelling is correct, leave the word as it has already been entered. If the spelling is incorrect, provide the correct spelling.

1. torsion _____

2. epidydymis _____

3. orchiopexy _____

4. hemescrotum _____

5. toonica _____

6. vaginalis _____

7. DeBakey _____

8. raffe _____

9. meso-orchium _____

10. albuguinea _____

Matching.
Match the proper name to the common term it belongs with.

1. ____ Xeroform
2. ____ DeBakey
3. ____ Bovie
4. ____ Nurolon

A. forceps
B. suture
C. gauze
D. electrocautery

GENITOURINARY REPORT 2 – OPERATIVE NOTE

PREOPERATIVE DIAGNOSIS: Invasive transitional cell carcinoma of the bladder.

MATERIAL TO LAB[1]
1. Distal ureteral segment, negative for cancer by frozen section.
2. Bladder, prostate, and seminal vesicles.

OPERATION PERFORMED: Radical cystoprostatectomy, Bricker ileal conduit diversion.

DRAINS: Urethral Foley catheter as pelvic drain, Jackson-Pratt drain times 2, nasogastric tube, 8 French feeding tubes as ureteral stents.

ESTIMATED BLOOD LOSS: 1500 cc.

FLUIDS: 6000 cc crystalloid, 500 cc Hespan, 450 cc autologous blood.

COMPLICATIONS: None.

INDICATIONS: This is a 57-year-old white male found to have muscle invasive transitional cell carcinoma of the bladder by transurethral resection of a bladder tumor. During his staging workup for this tumor, he was found to have a 5 cm abdominal aortic aneurysm. After consultation with Dr. George of the vascular surgery service, it was decided that the aneurysm should be repaired first. This was accomplished on January 28, 2006.[2] It was planned that he should wait to allow time for epithelialization and incorporation of his aortic graft prior to radical cystoprostatectomy.

DESCRIPTION OF PROCEDURE: The patient was brought to the operating room and epidural anesthetic, arterial line, and general endotracheal anesthesia were performed by the anesthesia service. The patient was placed in the supine position with sacral roll and a rectal tube. The abdomen was prepped and draped in the usual manner. An incision was made through the prior midline incision, which had been for his abdominal aortic aneurysm repair. This was carried down through the scar and subcutaneous tissue with electrocautery. The monofilament sutures in the fascial layer were removed using a Kocher clamp. The rectus fascia was opened throughout the length of the incision. The peritoneum was entered sharply and opened throughout the extent of the incision. Care was taken to take down any adhesions of the bowel to the peritoneum sharply. The abdomen was explored. The liver was soft with no evidence of metastatic lesions. The kidneys and spleen were palpated and were normal. The abdominal aortic graft was well incorporated and had a strong pulsation. The urachus[3] was divided sharply between clamps and the ends ligated. Using the inferior limb of the urachus for traction the peritoneum was incised in an inverted V-shape along both sides of the bladder. This incision was carried laterally along the avascular line of Toldt on each side. Care was taken to avoid exposing the vascular graft at all times. The ureter was identified on each side coursing through the retroperitoneum. Dr. Bradford participated in the surgery at this point and assisted in dissecting the ureters as they coursed over the vascular graft. The ureters were dissected down to the level of the bladder. The obliterated umbilical arteries were doubly ligated and divided on each side. At the most distal aspect of the bladder the ureters were doubly clipped and divided. A segment of each distal ureter was sent for frozen section. There was no transitional cell carcinoma found in either ureter. The lateral vascular pedicles of the bladder were then dissected, and all vessels were ligated and divided as they passed close to the bladder wall. The main hypogastric arteries were not ligated in this case, out of concern that this would lead to devascularization of the rectum. The inferior mesenteric artery had been ligated during the abdominal aortic aneurysm repair. After dissection of the lateral vascular pedicles down to the level of the endopelvic fascia, the peritoneum was incised posteriorly at the reflection between the bladder and the rectum. The posterior vascular pedicles of the bladder were similarly dissected and all blood vessels divided. Next, the endopelvic fascia was divided on each side. The puboprostatic ligaments were divided sharply under direct vision. A Storey right angle clamp was passed between the dorsal venous complex and the urethra. The dorsal vein complex was doubly ligated. A chromic suture was used on the anterior surface of the prostate to ligate the distal branches of the dorsal vein complex. The dorsal vein complex was divided sharply. A 0 chromic suture ligature was used to suture ligate the stump of the dorsal vein complex. The urethra was dissected free, and a right angle clamp passed posterior to the urethra. This was used to place a vessel loop behind the urethra.

The anterior wall of the urethra was divided. Foley catheter was pulled up into the wound and clamped with a Kelly clamp and divided. The posterior wall of the urethra was divided as well. The rectourethralis fibers were dissected off the apex of the prostate sharply and a finger used to bluntly dissect posterior to the prostate. The lateral vascular supply of the prostate was dissected on each side using a right angle to free up the blood vessels, which were doubly clipped. The seminal vesicles were dissected free and a clip placed on the tip of each seminal vesicle. The remaining blood vessels posterior to the bladder neck were dissected and doubly ligated. The bladder, prostate, and seminal vesicles were sent as a single specimen. The pelvis was examined for hemostasis. There appeared to be no significant bleeding. A 20 French Foley catheter was passed transurethrally and the balloon inflated to 30 cc. This was placed on traction.

An appendectomy was performed, dividing the mesoappendix between clamps and ligating blood vessels. A running pursestring suture was used around the base of the appendix. The appendix was doubly crushed, ligated at its base, and divided. The stump of the appendix was cauterized with the edge of a knife blade. The stump of the appendix was inverted into the cecum and the pursestring suture tied down. A segment of ileum was then selected, beginning approximately 15 cm from the ileocecal junction. The operating light was shone through the mesentery of the ileum to select a segment with a good blood supply and leaving adequate blood supply to the remaining segment of ileum. An 18 cm segment of ileum was selected. The peritoneum overlying the mesentery was divided sharply on each end of the segment. The blood vessels of the mesentery were divided between clamps and ligated. A GIA stapler was used to divide the ileum at each end of the selected segment. An ileal ileostomy was created, excising a corner of each limb, bringing the antimesenteric borders together, and a silk suture was used to approximate the limbs of ileum. A GIA stapler was then introduced with one limb in each segment of ileum. The GIA stapler was fired, and this created a side-to-side anastomosis. A TIA stapler was fired across the open ends of the ileum. Silk sutures were used to imbricate the TIA staple line. One end of the ileal conduit segment was opened after isolating it from the remainder of the wound with sterile towels. This was flushed with copious amounts of antibiotic-containing saline solution. The ureters were then anastomosed to the proximal end of this ileal segment. A small enterotomy was made on either side of the ileum, and the left ureter was brought through the sigmoid mesocolon. This was done taking care to avoid bringing the ureter in approximation to the abdominal aortic graft. Feeding tubes were passed through the conduit with the tip brought out each enterotomy. These were passed up the ureters to stent the anastomosis on each side. A running 4-0 chromic suture was used to create the anastomosis, running one chromic up each side of the ureter. This was done for each ureter. The butt end of the ileal conduit had been reinforced with imbricating silk sutures. This butt end was tacked to the psoas tendon. The skin at the selected stoma site was clamped with a Kocher clamp and a knife used to create a round stoma, by cutting underneath the Kocher clamp. Electrocautery was used to go through the subcutaneous tissue and to score the rectus fascia in a cruciate pattern. A defect in the rectus muscle was created, taking care to ensure that two fingers could be passed through the stoma site. A Babcock clamp was passed through the fascia and rectus muscle into the abdomen and used to bring the distal end of the conduit through the stoma site. The four Vicryl sutures that had been placed in each corner of the cruciate fascial incision were used to affix the conduit to the fascia at the stoma site. 3-0 Vicryl sutures were then used to evert the nipple of the stoma, taking a suture through the dermis, skin, to the proximal muscular layer of the stoma, and then finally through the lip of the ileal segment. Then several sutures were used to complete the anastomosis of the ileum to the dermis. The result was an everted nipple with good blood supply and a pink color. Two Jackson-Pratt drains were then placed in the pelvis, one near the site of the cystectomy and another near the ileal conduit. The fascia was closed with two running 1-0 Maxon sutures. The skin was closed with staples. A stoma appliance was placed over the ileal conduit. A sterile dressing was applied. The patient was awakened, extubated, and brought to the recovery room in satisfactory condition.[4]

Footnotes:

1. [1]Note, there is no colon after the heading because there is a list. Colons are typically only used when the information follows it directly on the same line with no list. (This is a style issue and a client may want it done differently.)
2. [2]Again, as is the case with all FOMS reports, the names, dates, places have been changed to ensure patient confidentiality.
3. [3]The urachus is a cord or band of fibrous tissue extending from the bladder to the umbilicus.
4. [4]This report is long, but it is really full of good useful terms and information. Make sure to read through this report at least once. Reading it out loud will help you practice saying some of the words and help train your ear!

SPELLING.
Determine if the following words are spelled correctly. If the spelling is correct, leave the word as it has already been entered. If the spelling is incorrect, provide the correct spelling.

1. puboprostatic _____

2. psoas _____

3. devascilarization _____ 4. hemodialysis _____

5. cystoprostate ectomy _____ 6. Bricker _____

7. conduit _____ 8. Story _____

9. rectourethrelis _____ 10. Babcock _____

TRUE/FALSE.
Mark the following true or false.

1. The skin at the selected stoma site was clamped with a Babcock clamp.

   ○ true

   ○ false

2. The patient is a male.

   ○ true

   ○ false

3. No material was sent to the lab.

   ○ true

   ○ false

4. The patient received a spinal block.

   ○ true

   ○ false

5. This patient had an appendectomy performed.

   ○ true

   ○ false

GENITOURINARY REPORT 3 – DISCHARGE SUMMARY

CHIEF COMPLAINT: Acute urinary retention.

HISTORY OF PRESENT ILLNESS: The patient has a long history of significant bladder outlet obstructive symptoms. He did note increase from his usual baseline in urinary frequency just prior to going into acute urinary retention, but denies dysuria, gross hematuria, or change in his baseline urgency at that time. He had Foley catheter placed one week ago, and he is brought here for further evaluation. He was scheduled for TURP with cystoscopy under anesthesia based on his symptoms, but developed shaking chills over the weekend prior to admission with fevers to 101 and 102. He also had anorexia and some mild low back pain. He is admitted now with febrile urinary tract infection for evaluation of his bladder outlet obstructive symptoms.

PAST MEDICAL HISTORY: Remarkable for rheumatoid arthritis times 16 years, otherwise unremarkable. He had usual childhood illnesses.

PAST SURGICAL HISTORY: Appendectomy at age 14.

SOCIAL HISTORY: Approximately 1 beer per month. He stopped smoking 24 years prior to admission after approximately a 60-pack-year smoking history.[1]

MEDICATIONS: He is on Naprosyn which he took the last 7 days prior to admission for possible surgery.

ALLERGIES: He has no known drug allergies.

REVIEW OF SYSTEMS: Noncontributory, except as in chief complaint and history of present illness.

PHYSICAL EXAMINATION: Temperature 102, vital signs stable. HEENT: Unremarkable. Neck: Supple. Lungs: Clear without wheezing or rales. Heart: Regular rate and rhythm with 2/6 systolic ejection murmur, no rub or gallop. Abdomen: Benign. Normal circumcised male phallus with bilaterally descended testes. Foley catheter in place. Digital rectal exam deferred secondary to probable prostatitis. Does have some moderate right CVA tenderness and negative left CVA tenderness. Extremities: Full range of motion, no clubbing, cyanosis, or edema. Neuro: Physiologic.

LABORATORY DATA: Urinalysis at the time of admission positive for nitrites and is sent for culture.

HOSPITAL COURSE: The patient is admitted to the hospital for evaluation of his febrile urinary tract infection and bladder outlet obstruction. The patient was started on IV antibiotics, and Foley catheter remained in place. He was given IV hydration, and oral hydration was pushed. The patient responded quite well and was afebrile after being on antibiotics for 24 hours. After being afebrile for 24 hours he was transferred over to oral antibiotics, and he remained afebrile throughout the remainder of his hospital course. Six days after admission he had evaluation with a voiding trial. He had 550 cc of fluid instilled into the bladder, and he was able to void 500 cc out. It was felt that his acute urinary retention was an exacerbation more by prostatitis than of his benign prostatic hypertrophy. To evaluate this further he had cystoscopy performed in the urology clinic. This was remarkable for capacity of 500 cc, normal mucosa, 1+ trabeculations of the bladder wall, trigone normal, ureteral orifices of normal size, shape, and position with clear efflux bilaterally. His anterior urethra was open. Prostatic urethra was 1.5 cm, lateral lobe hyperplasia, but noncoapting lobes. Essentially his cystoscopy did not support intervention with surgery at this time. He was started on a trial of terazosin, and since he was noted to have symptomatic improvement on this medication with increased force of stream and no nocturia, as well as passing his voiding trial, it was decided to discontinue the Foley catheter. He is voiding well now at a current level of 2 mg p.o. q.h.s. and is ready for discharge to home. He will be managed on medical therapy.

DISCHARGE DIAGNOSES

1. Febrile urinary tract infection with prostatitis, causing acute urinary retention.
2. Mild-to-moderate benign prostatic hypertrophy with bladder outlet obstruction amenable to medical therapy.
3. Rheumatoid arthritis.

PROCEDURES

1. Cystoscopy.
2. Voiding trial.

DISPOSITION: Usual diet, activity ad lib. He should have evaluation in 3 months with a Uroflow study and a UA symptom score to evaluate the efficacy of his Hytrin therapy. This medicine can be increased to initially 4 mg q.h.s. times 1 week and then to a level of 5 mg p.o. q.h.s. if his symptoms are not optimized. If the patient at a later date has further problems, he should be reevaluated by Urology here.

Footnotes:

1. 1.Smoking history is frequently expressed in the amount of packs per day times the number of years the person has been smoking. So with this patient it could mean he smoked 1 pack per day for 60 years, or 5 packs per day for 12 years, or 6 packs per day for 10 years, or 2 packs per day for 30 years, etc. The above hyphen usage is the correct way to hyphenate this, although oftentimes people leave out the hyphen between pack and year.

SPELLING.
Determine if the following words are spelled correctly. If the spelling is correct, leave the word as it has already been entered. If the spelling is incorrect, provide the correct spelling.

1. hemeturia _____

2. phallus _____

3. nitrites _____

4. trebeculations _____

5. hyperplasea _____

Matching.
Match the correct term to the definition.

1. ____ Readily reacting to influences.

2. ____ Painful or difficult urination.

3. ____ Enlargement or overgrowth of an organ.

4. ____ A smooth triangular area on the inner surface of the bladder.

5. ____ As desired.

6. ____ Diminished appetite and/or aversion to food.

A. hypertrophy

B. amenable

C. ad lib

D. trigone

E. dysuria

F. anorexia

GENITOURINARY REPORT 4 – OPERATIVE NOTE

PREOPERATIVE DIAGNOSIS: Benign prostatic hypertrophy and bladder neck hypertrophy.

POSTOPERATIVE DIAGNOSIS: Benign prostatic hypertrophy and bladder neck hypertrophy.

DRAINS: 22 French Foley catheter.

MATERIAL TO LAB: 11 g of prostatic chips.

OPERATION PERFORMED: Transurethral resection of the prostate.

FLUIDS: 1350 cc of crystalloid.

ESTIMATED BLOOD LOSS: Less than 150 cc.

COMPLICATIONS: None.

DISPOSITION: To recovery room in stable condition.

INDICATIONS: The patient is a 68-year-old white male with severe bladder outlet obstructive symptoms with an AUA score of 34/35. [1] He did not have a urinary tract infection, but on cystoscopy was noted to have 4+ trabeculations, and his creatinine was elevated at 2.1. The patient was given a trial of medical therapy. He had minimal improvement on this and requested surgical intervention be done. He presents at this time for TURP and assessment of the bladder neck under anesthesia.

DESCRIPTION OF PROCEDURE: The patient was brought to the operating suite after preoperative preparation, evaluation, counseling and consent. After he had an excellent subarachnoid block placed,[2] he was placed in the lithotomy position and prepped and draped in the usual sterile fashion. His urethra was calibrated using Van Buren sounds to 28 French. We then elected to use a 26 French Bakelite sheath with Timberlake obturator, which was then placed into the bladder without difficulty. Using a 30 and 70 degree lens for cystoscopy under anesthesia, the patient was noted to have 4+ bladder trabeculations. Bilateral ureteral orifices were normal size, shape, and position, with clear efflux. The patient had a 2-cm prostatic urethra with an elevated bladder neck and coapting lateral lobes with the right side a larger size than the left side. With this finding it was felt that the patient would be best served by TURP, as well as including the bladder neck area within the TURP, to increase the patient's flow. Using the 30 degree lens with the Iglesias resectoscope, the patient's bladder neck was taken down from the 7 o'clock to the 4 o'clock position[3] after locating the bilateral ureteral orifices and resecting distal to these. This enabled the scope to move freely, and then the right lobe was taken down from the 11 o'clock position to the 7 o'clock position and down to the level of the verumontanum. Hemostasis was obtained on the right lobe and attention was turned to the patient's left lobe, which was taken down in the same manner from the 12:30[4] position to the 5 o'clock position. Once this was done and hemostasis was intact, the bladder neck and the prostatic floor were taken down to the level of the verumontanum. The area was checked for hemostasis, and electrocautery was used for this. The resectoscope was removed from the patient's bladder. Using Ellik evacuator, prostatic chips were removed from the bladder. The bladder was assessed for remaining chips, and there were no chips remaining within the bladder after Ellik evacuation. Further attention was given to hemostasis with electrocautery. With this in good order the bladder was left full. The cystoscopic equipment was removed, and a 22-French Foley catheter was placed into the bladder without difficulty. The catheter was placed on mild traction and the effluent of bladder irrigation was clear after 200 cc. The catheter was placed on mild traction and connected to a urine collection device. After the patient had tolerated this procedure well, he was taken from the lithotomy to the supine position, transferred to a gurney, and then to the recovery room in stable condition. Total resection time was 39 minutes.

Footnotes:

1. 1.AUA is the American Urological Association. If you do a little research on this symptom scale, you will see that 20–35 is rated as "severe." This poor gentleman has 34–35.
2. 2.With the pain this gentleman was in, it is fitting that his anesthetic block should be "excellent."
3. 3.When giving anatomical positions or locations, o'clock is used instead of :00. This is typically the only time o'clock is used.
4. 4.This is one of those gray areas or exceptions to the rule. Likely the dictator said "twelve-thirty" position, so it would be best noted as "12:30 position." It would sound odd as 12:30 o'clock.

SPELLING.
Determine if the following words are spelled correctly. If the spelling is correct, leave the word as it has already been entered. If the spelling is incorrect, provide the correct spelling.

1. prostratic _____

2. benign _____

3. transuretheral _____

4. verumontanum _____

5. guerny _____

Matching.
Match the proper name to the common term it belongs with.

1. ____ French Foley

2. ____ Bakelite

3. ____ Iglesias

4. ____ Van Buren

5. ____ Ellik

6. ____ Timberlake

A. sound

B. obturator

C. sheath

D. catheter

E. evacuator

F. resectoscope

GENITOURINARY REPORT 5 – PROCEDURE NOTE

[1]PREOPERATIVE DIAGNOSIS: History of paraphimosis.

OPERATION PERFORMED: Elective circumcision.

INDICATIONS: History of paraphimosis.

DESCRIPTION OF PROCEDURE: The patient was brought into the operating room and placed in the supine position. He was prepped and draped in the normal sterile manner. The patient's foreskin was retracted and the glans was prepped with Betadine. The coronal eminence was marked externally. The foreskin was then retracted, and another mark was made circumferentially 0.5 cm proximal to the eminence. The foreskin was removed by using a skin knife. Hemostasis was achieved by Bovie electrocautery. The skin edges were approximated using a 4-0 chromic suture placed in a running fashion. Local anesthetic was applied at this point using approximately 1 cc of Marcaine applied subcutaneously circumferentially proximal to the incision site using a 28 gauge needle. Pressure dressing was applied. The patient was extubated and brought to the recovery room in stable condition.

Footnotes:

1. 1.This is not your "run of the mill" newborn circumcision. Paraphimosis is a relatively uncommon condition in which the foreskin, once pulled back behind the glans penis, cannot be brought down to its original position. This condition can occur when the foreskin is retracted for a long period of time, like during catheterization or cystoscopy.

SPELLING.
Determine if the following words are spelled correctly. If the spelling is correct, leave the word as it has already been entered. If the spelling is incorrect, provide the correct spelling.

1. circuncision _____

2. paraphimosis _____

3. forskin _____

4. subcutaneously _____

5. eminance _____

TRUE/FALSE.

Mark the following true or false.

1. The patient was prepped and draped in the normal sterile manner.

   ○ true

   ○ false

2. Marcaine was applied using a 28-gauge needle.

   ○ true

   ○ false

3. The patient was brought to the Intensive Care Unit in stable condition.

   ○ true

   ○ false

4. No dressing was applied to the wound.

   ○ true

   ○ false

5. An elective circumcision was performed.

   ○ true

   ○ false

GENITOURINARY REPORT 6 – OPERATIVE NOTE

PREOPERATIVE DIAGNOSIS: Left varicocele.

POSTOPERATIVE DIAGNOSIS: Left varicocele.

OPERATION PERFORMED: Laparoscopic ligation of left internal spermatic vein.

EBL: Minimal.

FLUIDS: 1500 cc of Crystalloid.

COMPLICATIONS: None.

INDICATIONS: 71-year-old white male with left scrotal pain and finding of a left varicocele on physical examination. He was scheduled for laparoscopic ligation of the internal spermatic vein, with the understanding that a guarantee of pain relief could not be made.

DESCRIPTION OF OPERATION: The patient was brought to the operating room and general endotracheal anesthesia was induced by the anesthesia service. An orogastric tube was also placed. The arms were tucked. Tape was placed across the chest and a strap across the legs. The patient was placed in Trendelenburg.[1] The abdomen and perineum were prepped and draped in the usual manner. A Foley catheter was inserted on the field.[2] A 1-cm infraumbilical incision was made sharply and carried down through the subcutaneous tissue with electrocautery. The fascia was nicked with a #11 blade, and a Veress needle was inserted into the peritoneal cavity. A syringe of water was injected through the needle and was returned on aspiration. The column of water rapidly fell into the needle upon removal of the syringe. Insufflation was begun at a low insufflation rate. The initial pressure was 7 mm of mercury. The perineum was then insufflated on high pressure that would hold the pressure of 20 mm of mercury. There was 4-quadrant tympany. The Veress needle was removed, and a 10 mm port with trocar was inserted through the infraumbilical incision. The trocar was removed. A laparoscopic camera was placed. The fascia screw was screwed down. The abdomen was examined. There was no evidence of trauma from the needle or trocar insertion. Under direct vision, a 10-mm suprapubic port and a 5-mm left lower quadrant port were placed. The left spermatic vessels were identified as they entered the internal ring. Using sharp dissection of electrocautery, a peritoneal window was made lateral to the spermatic vessels. This incision was carried across the vessels just proximal to the internal ring. Blunt dissection was used to divide the spermatic vessels into two packets. The pulsation of the spermatic artery could be seen in the lateral packet. Adventitial tissue was cauterized and divided with the scissors. Two large veins were doubly clipped and divided. Turning to the lateral packet, two more veins were doubly clipped and divided. There was one remaining vein that was adherent to the artery. This was dissected free, clipped, but not divided.

Pulsation of the artery could be seen at the completion of this dissection. There was no significant hemorrhage from the site of dissection. Under direct vision, the suprapubic and left lower quadrant ports were removed, and no bleeding could be seen from the insertion sites. The fascial screw was then screwed and the infraumbilical port was withdrawn over the camera. Finally, the camera was drawn into the wound, examined for hemostasis as it was removed through the abdominal wall. There was no significant bleeding. The two 10-mm ports were closed with a vertical mattress suture of 2-0 Nurolon. The subcutaneous tissue was approximated with a vertical mattress 4-0 Vicryl suture at each site. Skin was closed with Steri-Strips. Bandages were applied. The patient was awakened. The Foley catheter was removed. The patient was extubated and brought to the recovery room in satisfactory condition.

Footnotes:

1. 1.The Trendelenburg position is when a person is flat on his back (supine) with his feet higher than his head (same thing when it is a "her").
2. 2.The field here refers to the surgical field.

SPELLING.
Determine if the following words are spelled correctly. If the spelling is correct, leave the word as it has already been entered. If the spelling is incorrect, provide the correct spelling.

1. varicocele _____   2. Trendelanberg _____

3. Veres _____   4. trochar _____

5. quadarant _____

Matching.
Match the correct term to the definition.

1. ____ Traversing alimentary tract from mouth to stomach.

2. ____ A hollow drum-like sound produced when a gas-
containing cavity is tapped sharply.

3. ____ The act of binding.

4. ____ To blow into any cavity or orifice of the body.

5. ____ The flat layers of fibrous tissue that separate different
layers of tissue.

A. ligation

B. orogastric

C. tympany

D. fascia

E. insufflate

GENITOURINARY REPORT 7 – DISCHARGE SUMMARY

CHIEF COMPLAINT: Rectal bleeding.[1]

HISTORY OF PRESENT ILLNESS: The patient is a 47-year-old male with a history of bright red blood per rectum[2] for several years. Three years prior to admission he had a tubulovillous polyp removed from just inside his anal verge. A followup endoscopy revealed no residual lesion. The patient was noted to have increasing blood over the last several months, and on GI endoscopy he had a recurrence of a large tubulovillous adenoma in the lower rectum. He was scheduled for transanal excision.

PHYSICAL EXAMINATION ON ADMISSION: Pulse 96, respirations 16, blood pressure 136/85. The head, eyes, ears, nose and throat examination was unremarkable. The neck was clear with a full range of motion. The lungs were clear to percussion and auscultation. The cardiovascular exam revealed a regular rhythm without murmurs. The abdomen was soft and nontender with active bowel sounds. A genitourinary exam was not performed. The rectal exam revealed a fleshy 3 x 2.5 cm[3] sessile polyp, nonfixed, on the left posterolateral wall.

LABORATORY DATA ON ADMISSION: A CBC and a urinalysis were performed which were within normal limits.

HOSPITAL COURSE: On March 11, 2004, the patient was taken to the operating room where a transanal excision of the villous adenoma was performed under subarachnoid block anesthesia. The patient's postoperative course was unremarkable. He was discharged.

DIAGNOSIS: Tubulovillous adenoma of the rectum, recurrent.

OPERATION PERFORMED: Transanal excision of tubular adenoma.

PATHOLOGY: Complete excision of tubulovillous adenoma with focal adenomatous change.

Footnotes:

1. 1.Often rectal bleeding (hemorrhoids, etc.) issues are seen by GU doctors. This is one of those cross-disciplinary conditions where GI and GU overlap.
2. 2.This phrase "bright red blood per rectum," is very commonly dictated under the past medical history and review of systems headings.
3. 3.Even when dictated as two and a half centimeters, it is generally preferred to not use fractions with metric units of measurement. This is a style issue and it would not necessarily be incorrect to edit 2-1/2 if dictated that way.

SPELLING.
Determine if the following words are spelled correctly. If the spelling is correct, leave the word as it has already been entered. If the spelling is incorrect, provide the correct spelling.

1. reocurrence _____   2. tubovillus _____

3. sessile _____   4. transanal _____

5. tubuler _____

TRUE/FALSE.
Mark the following true or false.

1. The patient had a tubulovillous polyp removed in 2001.

    ○ true

    ○ false

2. The patient was noted to have a 2/6 murmur on physical exam.

    ○ true

    ○ false

3. Rectal exam revealed a nonfixed sessile polyp.

    ○ true

    ○ false

4. The tubulovillous adenoma was completely excised.

    ○ true

    ○ false

5. The polyp was removed under general anesthesia.

    ○ true

    ○ false

GENITOURINARY REPORT 8 – OPERATIVE NOTE

PREOPERATIVE DIAGNOSIS: Grade III[1] right vesicoureteral reflux.

POSTOPERATIVE DIAGNOSIS: Grade III right vesicoureteral reflux.

DRAINS: Penrose drain, Foley catheter.

OPERATION PERFORMED: Right ureteral reimplantation.

EBL: 10 cc.

FLUIDS: 450 cc crystalloid.

COMPLICATIONS: None.

INDICATIONS: A 4-year-old white female with grade III vesicoureteral reflux, who had had breakthrough infections and evidence of decrease in renal function and renal size. Thus she was scheduled for right ureteral reimplant.

DESCRIPTION OF PROCEDURE: Patient was brought to the operating room, and general endotracheal anesthesia was induced by the anesthesia service. The patient was brought to the end of the table, the perineum prepped in the usual manner. Cystoscopy was performed with a 14 French diagnostic pediatric cystoscope. The ureteral orifices were identified. The right ureteral orifice was patulous. There was minimal trabeculation of the bladder. The bladder was filled to 200 cc, and the cystoscope was removed. The patient was returned to a supine position with the legs slightly frog-legged. The abdomen was prepped and draped in the usual manner. A low transverse incision was made sharply and carried down through the subcutaneous tissue with electrocautery. Magnifying loupes were used throughout the case. Scarpa's fascia was entered with the electrocautery. The rectus fascia was incised in the midline. Bellies of the rectus muscle were reflected laterally. The transversalis fascia was entered sharply, and the peritoneum was swept off the dome of the bladder. Two stay sutures of 3-0 Vicryl were placed in the bladder. The Denis Browne ring retractor was used. The bladder was entered with the electrocautery, and the cystotomy was extended inferiorly on the bladder, approximately 3 cm, to the bladder neck. Stay sutures were placed at the inferior aspect of the cystotomy as well. The dome of the bladder was packed with Ray-Tec sponges. The ureteral orifices were identified. The right ureteral orifice was cannulated with a 5 French feeding tube, and 0 Vicryl was passed through the ureteral orifice and through the feeding tube to hold it in place. With traction on the ureteral orifice, the Bovie was used to circumscribe the ureteral orifice. Electrocautery and sharp and blunt dissection were used to dissect the attachments of the ureter to the detrusor muscle. Then blunt dissection was used to sweep the peritoneum off the ureter. The ureter was brought into the bladder with sufficient length for reimplantation. The detrusor's hiatus was closed with a single 3-0 Vicryl suture. The tenotomy scissors were used to create a submucosal tunnel to a position of approximately 1 cm superior and 1 cm lateral to the left ureteral orifice. A right angle was passed underneath this and used to bring the ureter through the tunnel. The distal 1 cm of ureter was incised across two thirds[2] of its diameter. A 4-0 chromic was used to anchor the lateral aspect of the ureter to its new position at the new ureteral orifice, connecting ureteral mucosa to bladder mucosa. Six more sutures of 5-0 chromic were used to complete the ureteroneocystostomy. The ureter was cannulated with a 5 French feeding tube, and the tube easily passed up the ureter without obstruction. The remainder of the bladder mucosa was closed with 4-0 chromic. A Foley catheter had been passed transurethrally into the bladder, and its position was confirmed. The cystotomy was closed in two layers, with the second layer imbricated over the first with running 2-0 chromic sutures. A Penrose drain was then placed in the space of Retzius and brought through the rectus fascia and through a separate stab incision. The rectus fascia was closed with a running 1-0 PDS suture. Subcutaneous tissue was approximated with 3-0 Vicryl, and the end closed with a running 5-0 Vicryl suture. Steri-Strips were applied to the wound. An Op-Site dressing was placed with gauze over the Penrose drain. The patient was awakened, extubated and brought to the pediatric intensive care unit in satisfactory condition.

Footnotes:

1. 1.In general, grades are presented with Arabic numerals. This is not a steadfast rule, but a general trend. A client may prefer Roman numerals, as it appears this client does.
2. 2.It is generally preferred to spell out fractions when they are less than one and do not precede a noun.

SPELLING.

Determine if the following words are spelled correctly. If the spelling is correct, leave the word as it has already been entered. If the spelling is incorrect, provide the correct spelling.

1. Ray-Tech _____

2. mucosa _____

3. canulated _____

4. transversalis _____

5. endotrachial _____

Matching.

Match the correct term to the definition.

1. ____ Through the urethra.

2. ____ The general region between the anus and the genital area.

3. ____ Surgical cutting of a tendon.

4. ____ Deep subcutaneous tissue of the abdominal wall.

5. ____ Beneath the epidermis.

A. transurethral

B. tenotomy

C. subcutaneous

D. Scarpa's fascia

E. perineum

GENITOURINARY REPORT 9 – OPERATIVE NOTE

PREOPERATIVE DIAGNOSIS: Right ureteral stone.

POSTOPERATIVE DIAGNOSIS: Same.[1]

MATERIAL TO LAB: None, but stone fragments will be sent through the urology clinic for stone analysis.

OPERATION PERFORMED: Right ureteroscopy with stone manipulation and extraction.

DRAINS: #7-French 22- to 32-cm multilength ureteral stent, and #18-French Foley catheter.

POSITION: Lithotomy.

PREP: Standard.

FLUIDS: 1600 cc crystalloid.

EBL: Minimal.

BLOOD ADMINISTERED: None.

INDICATIONS: The patient is a 41-year-old white male who had right renal colic on one previous occasion and was found to have an obstructing right ureteral stone. The patient had prior attempt at vascular stone removal. However, this surgery was complicated by ureteral perforation, as the stone appeared to be lodged with the hemi-ureteral mucosa. The patient had a right double-J ureteral stent placed at that time. We have allowed approximately 1 month to pass before pursuing re-attempt at removing this symptomatic stone. The stone measurement is approximately 3 x 6 mm. The patient has been counseled regarding the options of his stone, which is in the proximal portion of the middle third ureter, options regarding ESWL versus open versus ureteroscopic stone manipulation. After patient had been given options, he elected that attempt at ureteroscopy be performed.

DESCRIPTION OF PROCEDURE: The patient was brought to the operating suite after preoperative preparation, evaluation, counseling, and consent. The patient did receive perioperative IV antibiotics, as he had an indwelling ureteral stent prior to his surgery. After his sterile prep and drape, and excellent epidural catheter, the patient was placed in the lithotomy position, and prepped and draped in the usual sterile fashion. The 21-French ACMI cystoscope was then used to enter the bladder, at which time a safety wire of 0.038 was advanced through the right renal pelvis under fluoroscopic guidance. At this time, the patient's right double-J ureteral stent was removed using alligator forceps, while leaving the safety wire in place. A right retrograde ureteral pyelogram was performed under fluoroscopy, and this did confirm the presence of a stone, as was taken by a KUB prior to the initiation of surgery in the middle ureter. At this point the ureteral orifice was assessed. It did not appear to need dilating, as the patient did have an indwelling double-J ureteral stent. The #11-French ureteroscope was intubated into the ureteral orifice with the assistance of the guide wire,[2] which was in place, and advanced to the level of the stone. This cystoscope is the cystoscope which is attachable to the transurethral ultrasound lithotripsy unit. With attempt of basketing under direct vision using a 3.5-French basket with both 3 and 4 wires, the stone could not be engaged, and it was felt this was possibly due to the size of the stone, or the fact that the stone was somewhat embedded into the ureteral mucosa. With this in mind, it was elected that ultrasound lithotripsy be performed to reduce the stone's burden and the size of the fragments, so these could be extracted using the basket or grasping forceps. Under direct vision, the ultrasound lithotripsy was performed and the stone broken up into a minimum of 4 major pieces with other fragments and gravel. At this time, the patient had the ultrasound lithotripsy probe removed, and the 3.5 basket was advanced under direct vision, in addition to the assist by fluoroscopic guidance. With some difficulty the stone fragments were engaged with a basket and removed, with the ureteroscope advanced back to the stone at the time. There was no significant proximal migration of the stone with these manipulations, and there was no evidence of ureteral perforation. On both fluoroscopic evaluation with contrast, as well as under direct vision, there appeared to be no remaining significant stone fragments left other than gravel and minimal fragments, which would pass spontaneously with time. With this in mind, it was elected to terminate the procedure, and again, the ureteroscope was removed. The 21-French ACMI cystoscope was placed into the bladder using 30-degree lens, and a 22- to 32-cm multilength #7-French ureteral catheter was placed with the assistance of fluoroscopic and direct vision guidance. The patient then had the cystoscope removed, and an #18-French Foley catheter placed. There was minimal bleeding. The patient tolerated the procedure well. There was no evidence of complications. The patient was then taken down from a lithotomy position into the supine position.

Epidural was removed. He was transferred to a gurney, and then to the recovery room in stable condition. It is planned that patient will have a retrograde ureteral pyelogram in approximately 2 weeks with removal of the stent at that time if everything appears patent without any significant edema.

Footnotes:

1. 1.Again, it is typically preferred the postoperative diagnosis be edited again instead of simply putting "same." Client account preferences will determine how this is done.
2. 2.This is also acceptably edited as one word—guidewire.

SPELLING.
Determine if the following words are spelled correctly. If the spelling is correct, leave the word as it has already been entered. If the spelling is incorrect, provide the correct spelling.

1. pylogram _____

2. lithotripsy _____

3. fluoroscopic _____

4. uretral _____

5. dialating _____

Matching.
Match the correct term to the definition.

1. ____ Procedure that uses sound waves delivered inside a water bath to pulverize kidney stones.

2. ____ A dye injected intravenously during X-ray studies.

3. ____ An instrument used to compress or grasp tissues.

4. ____ Excessive accumulation of serous fluid in tissue.

5. ____ The period of time from hospitalization for surgery to the time of discharge.

A. lithotripsy

B. edema

C. perioperative

D. forceps

E. contrast

UNIT 5
Neurology

NEUROLOGY – INTRODUCTION

Neurology is the branch of medicine that deals with the brain and central nervous system, diseases associated with them, and the procedures related to them. The **neurologist** or **neurosurgeon** is concerned with the function of nerves in the body, particularly in the spine. **Neurology** or **neurosurgery** reports often describe procedures performed on the spine, such as foraminotomy, laminectomy, or spinal disc surgery. Other neurosurgical procedures include spinal fusions and the repair of spinal cord fractures. Neurologists and neurosurgeons also diagnose and treat brain tumors and brain injuries. They also are concerned with such intracranial problems as pituitary adenomas and problems with the internal auditory canal.

While neurology addresses primarily the physiological aspects of brain function, **psychiatry** deals with the study, treatment, and prevention of mental disorders. These may have their origin in physiological anomalies, such as chemical imbalances or brain injuries, but they may also have no apparent organic basis. Instead, they may arise from environmental problems, childhood abuse, hereditary factors, social factors, addictive behaviors, cultural factors, and life stresses.

Neurological disorders affect the central nervous system (brain, brainstem, and cerebellum), the peripheral nervous system (peripheral nerves including cranial nerves), and/or the autonomic nervous system (nerves which control involuntary body functions). Neurologists also diagnose and treat some conditions in the musculoskeletal system.

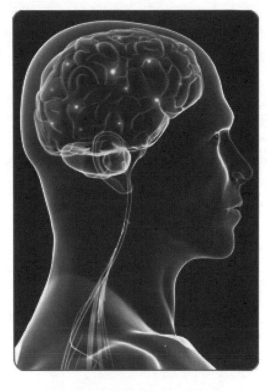

Neurologic conditions primarily include (but are not limited to):

- headache disorders
- epilepsy and seizure disorders
- neurodegenerative disorders
- cerebrovascular disease
- sleep disorders
- cerebral palsy
- neoplasms
- movement disorders
- demyelinating diseases
- spinal cord disorders
- traumatic injuries to the brain, spinal cord and peripheral nerves
- speech and language disorders

Evaluation of pathology includes analysis of laboratory data and utilization of other sophisticated techniques to study the neurological system. Common assessments include:

- electroencephalogram (EEG)
- x-rays
- imaging (MRI, CT)
- angiograms
- muscle/nerve testing, evoked potentials
- tomography
- ultrasound

Patient symptoms and pathologic problems are treated using pharmaceutical products, surgical repair, revision, plastic repair, nerve transfers and transplants.

Highlights

Overlapping Disciplines

- Psychiatry
- Internal Medicine
- Rehabilitation Medicine
- Infectious Disease
- General Practice
- Orthopedic Surgery
- Pulmonology
- Pediatrics
- Radiology

NEUROLOGY LANGUAGE WORKSHOP

Neurology terminology can be complex as it deals with the diagnosis and treatment of all categories of disease involving the brain and central, peripheral, and autonomic nervous systems. The following lists will provide a review of common Neurology language and should help get you primed and ready to jump into this Neurology FOMS unit.

Common Neurology Root Words and Combining Forms

Root Word & Combining Form	Meaning	Example
amygdal/o	almond shaped structure	amygdaloid
ankyl/o	crooked or fused	ankylosing
anter/o	anterior/before	anterolateral
arachn/o	spider	arachnoid
arthr/o	joint	arthroplasty
auricul/o	ear	auriculocranial
brachi/o	arm	brachiocephalic
caud/o	tail	caudolateral
cephal/o	head	cephalolateral
cerebr/o	relationship to cerebrum	cerebrocerebellar
cervic/o	neck	cervicothoracic
chemonucle/o	chemical/dissolution	chemonucleolysis
cistern/o	reservoir	cisternography
cost/o	rib	costovertebral
crani/o	cranium/skull	craniocervical
dextr/o	right	dextroscoliosis
disc/o	disc/disk	discogenic
dist/o	far/distant from origin	distoradial
dors/o/i	directed toward/on back	dorsiflexion
electr/o	electron	electrocorticography
encephal/o	brain	encephalography
epidur/o	upon or outside dura mater	epidurography
esthesi/o	feeling	esthesiologic, paresthesia
ethm/o	pertaining to ethmoid bone	ethmolacrimal
front/o	forehead/front	frontoradial
facet/o	facet	facetectomy
foramin/o	foramen, opening, passage	foraminotomy
infer/o	lowermost/below	inferoposterior
labyrinth/o	communicating cavities	labyrinthotomy
lamina and /o	thin flat plate/layer	laminectomy, laminagraph
later/o	side	lateromedial
lob/o	well-defined part of organ	lobation, lobotomy
lumb/o	lower back	lumbosacral
maxill/o	upper jaw	maxillectomy

medull /o	inmost part	medulloblastoma
mening/o	membrane	meningocele
muscul/o	muscle	musculotendinous
my/o	muscle	myometrium
myel/o	relationship to myelin	myeloclast
neur/o	relating to nerve	neurocentrum
occipit/o	pertaining to the occiput	occipitalization occipitomental
odyn/o	pain/distress	odynophagia
orbit	cavity of eyeball	orbitonasal
oste/o	pertaining to bone	osteoclasis
proxim/o	nearest point of origin	proximoradial
rhiz/o	relating to a root	rhizolysis
sequestrum/a	dead bone	sequestration
somat/o	body	somatoesthetic
spin/o	spinal column	spinogalvanization
spondyl/o	vertebra	spondylitis
tempor/o	temples	temporomandibular
thalam/o	brain division, ovoid mass	thalamotomy
ventricul/o	cavity	ventriculocisternostomy
vertebr/o	spinal bones	vertebrogenic

Common Neurology Prefixes

Prefix	Meaning	Example
ab-	away from	abduct
ad-	toward	adduct
bi-/di-	two	bilateral/diplegia
dia-	through, between	diastasis
epi-	above/on	epicondyle
extra-	outside	extradural
hemi-/semi-	half/partly	hemilaminectomy
hyper-	excessive, greater than normal	hypermobility
hypo-/sub-	beneath/below normal/under	hypodermic/subserosal
infra-	beneath	inframedullary
intra-	within	intraneural
multi-/poly-	many/excessive	multiaxial/polyneuritis
per-	through, by, or completely	perfusion
peri-	around/near	pericephalic
retro-	behind, backward	retroversion
trans-	across/through	translumbar

Common Neurology Suffixes

Suffix	Meaning	Example
-algia	pain	neuralgia
-ectomy	excision or removal	laminectomy
-edema	swelling	encephaloedema
-ia/-iasis	condition	psoriasis
-itis	inflammation	bursitis
-kinesia/-kinesis	movement/motion	hypokinesis
listhesis	slippage	spondylolisthesis
-lysis	loosening/freeing/breaking apart	neurolysis
-lytic	relating to destruction	meningolytic
-malacia	softening	encephalomalacia
-oid	resembling	sphenoid
-pathy	disease or abnormality	axonopathy
-penia	deficiency	osteopenia
-pexy	surgical fixation	neuropexy
-plasty	surgical repair	laminoplasty
-plegia	paralysis	paraplegia
-scopy	examination with an instrument	myoscopy
-stomy	forming an opening	temporostomy
-tome	an instrument for cutting	dermatome
-tomy	incision (cutting into)	craniotomy

Common Neurology Abbreviations

Abbreviation	Expansion
ANS	autonomic nervous system
AVM/AVMs	arteriovenous malformation/s
CNS	central nervous system
CP	cerebral palsy
CSF	cerebrospinal fluid
CT	computed tomography (scan)
CVA	cerebrovascular accident
CVD	cerebrovascular disease
EEG	electroencephalogram
EMG	electromyogram
HNP	herniated nucleus pulposus
LP	lumbar puncture
MRI	magnetic resonance imaging
MS	multiple sclerosis
PET	positron emission tomography
PNS	peripheral nervous system
R/O	rule out
RT	radiation therapy
SAH	subarachnoid hemorrhage
SNS	sympathetic nervous system
TIA	transient ischemic attack
TENS	transcutaneous electrical nerve stimulation

REVIEW: NEUROLOGY LANGUAGE

Fill in the Blank.
Using the word(s) in the box, enter the appropriate term in the space provided.

craniomalacia
neurotome
computed
encephalitis
emission
resonance
peripheral

1. A PET scan, or positron _____ tomography scan, is a nuclear medicine medical imaging technique that produces a three-dimensional image or map of functional processes in the body.

2. _____ means abnormal softness of the bones of the skull.

3. _____ tomography (CT) scan is an imaging method that uses x-rays to create cross-sectional pictures of the body.

4. Magnetic _____ imaging (MRI) is a safe, noninvasive test that creates detailed images of organs and tissues.

5. Inflammation of the brain, or _____ , is often caused by a virus.

6. The _____ nervous system (PNS) consists of neurons that carry information to and from the central nervous system.

7. A _____ is an instrument used in cutting or dissecting nerves.

Multiple Choice.
Choose the best answer.

1. (○ Arthroplasty, ○ Arthrogram) is surgery performed on a joint.

2. The term that literally means inflammation of communicating cavities is (○ labyrinthitis, ○ labyrinthosis).

3. (○ Myology, ○ Myopathy) means disease of muscle.

4. A (○ laminectomy, ○ laminotomy) is removal of lamina.

5. A transient (○ ischemic, ○ intracranial) attack is sometimes called a "mini-stroke," as symptoms generally last less than 24 hours.

TRUE/FALSE.
Mark the following true or false.

1. *Subdural* means above the dura.

    ○ true

    ○ false

2. *Neuralgia* literally means pain relating to the face.

    ○ true

    ○ false

3. *Paresthesia* is an abnormal sensation of the skin, such as numbness, tingling, pricking, burning, or creeping on the skin.

    ○ true

    ○ false

4. *Hemiplegia* means paralysis of one side of the body.

    ○ true

    ○ false

5. *Lumbar puncture* involves withdrawal of blood from the spinal cord.

    ○ true

    ○ false

NEUROLOGY REPORTS

Neurology is a vital part of a hospital's service; however, neurosurgery reports are not as common as general surgery or obstetrics and gynecology. The terminology associated with neurology is relatively uniform and, after doing only a few reports, relatively easy to pick up (especially if you have a comprehensive collection of online resources).

The websites provided below are full of specialty-related terminology. There are, of course, many other reputable, reliable online resources. In the process of doing research you will undoubtedly find many related sites. Bookmark the ones that work for you.

Neurology online resources:

- http://www.ninds.nih.gov/disorders/disorder_index.htm
- http://www.merck.com/mmpe/sec16.html

NEUROLOGY REPORT 1 – OPERATIVE NOTE

PREOPERATIVE DIAGNOSIS: C4-5 and C5-6 spondylosis.[1]

POSTOPERATIVE DIAGNOSIS: C4-5 and C5-6 spondylosis.

OPERATION PERFORMED: C4-5 and C5-6 anterior cervical diskectomy.[2]

COMPLICATIONS: None.

ESTIMATED BLOOD LOSS: 50 cc.

MONITORING: Intraoperative somatosensory blood potential monitoring.

INDICATIONS: This is a 61-year-old female with a progressive history of pain, paresthesias and stiffness in her upper extremities, and progressive gait dysfunction. On exam, she had signs and symptoms consistent with an early myelopathy. An MRI shows DJD at multiple levels with congenitally small canal with significant stenosis at C5-6, less so at C4-5. We have recommended anterior cervical diskectomy at both levels, and the patient agrees.

DESCRIPTION OF PROCEDURE: The patient was brought to the operating room, general endotracheal anesthesia induced, and placed in the supine position on the operating room table. She was induced into anesthesia through an awake intubation with no hyperextension. Neurologic exam was stable after intubation. At this stage, the patient's neck was prepped and draped in the usual sterile fashion for surgery. A horizontal linear incision was made in the right anterior neck and extended through the subcutaneous tissue. Self-retaining retractors were placed, and dissection was carried down to the platysma. The platysma was opened horizontally using Lincoln scissors. It was then undermined. At this stage, retractors were advanced, and a dissection plane was created between the tracheoesophageal region medially and the carotid/sternocleidomastoid region laterally, using sharp and blunt dissection. The prevertebral fascia was then opened using a sharp dissection, and the fascia was stripped off the anterior vertebral bodies using Kitners. At this stage, the correct level of operation was ascertained using intraoperative x-ray. The longus colli muscles were then dissected off the anterior face of the vertebral bodies using Bovie electrocautery and Key periosteal elevators. A self-retaining retractor system was placed behind the longus colli muscle. The C5-6 disk space was then entered using an 11 blade. The disk was then removed using various rongeurs and curets. Carter disk space spreaders were used to open up the disk space. As we approached the back of the disk space, there were obvious large osteophytes in the region running all the way across the disk space and into the neural foramina. These were removed using Kerrison rongeurs. There was a small rent[3] in the medial left posterior longitudinal ligament, and there was small-to-moderate sized free fragment of disk material through this rent. This was removed. The region was then explored using a nerve hook, and no further free disk material was found. The posterior longitudinal ligament was then opened all the way across the disk space using a Kerrison rongeur. The neural foramina were cleared out of encroaching bone using Kerrison rongeurs again. By the end of the disk and osteophyte removal, the entire disk space was clear of osteophytes, as were the neural foramina. The neural foramina were widely open. Hemostasis was achieved using thrombin-soaked Gelfoam. At this stage, a similar procedure was carried out at the C4-5 level. Interestingly, the disk was much more degenerated at this level, and the posterior osteophytes were considerably larger and bridging the disk space. By the end of disk and osteophyte removal at this level, a similar picture to the C5-6 level was obtained. There was good decompression of the osteophytes and the neural foramina. The wounds were then thoroughly irrigated with bacitracin solution, and closure was accomplished using interrupted 2-0 Vicryl sutures for the platysma and subcutaneous tissue and staples for the skin. The patient tolerated the procedure well. There were no complications. Estimated blood loss was 50 cc.

Footnotes:

1. 1.When transcription editing disk spaces, it is not required to repeat the letter (C4-5 doesn't have to be C4-C5.) However, it is preferred to repeat the letter before each numbered vertebrae or vertebral space in a list (C4-5 and C5-6, and not C4-5 and 5-6). Again, this is general style preference. It would not necessarily be incorrect to edit as C4-C5 or C4-5 and 5-6.
2. 2.Note spelling of disc/disk. Both are acceptable, but use should be consistent, especially within a report. Additionally, sometimes clients will have a preference. If they do, always use the form they prefer.
3. 3.As it is used here, *rent* refers to an opening or hole made by tearing something.

SPELLING.

Determine if the following words are spelled correctly. If the spelling is correct, leave the word as it has already been entered. If the spelling is incorrect, provide the correct spelling.

1. paresthesias _____

2. coli _____

3. myelopathy _____

4. osteophite _____

5. Thrombin _____

Matching.

Match the proper name to the common term that it belongs with.

1. ____ Kerrison

2. ____ Bovie

3. ____ Key

4. ____ Carter

5. ____ self-retaining

A. electrocautery

B. disk space spreader

C. rongeur

D. periosteal elevator

E. retractor

NEUROLOGY REPORT 2 – DISCHARGE SUMMARY

CHIEF COMPLAINT: Low back pain with radiation to the right lower extremity.

HISTORY OF PRESENT ILLNESS: The patient is a 66-year-old white male with a long history of low back pain since the late 1970s. [1] The patient states that about a year and a half ago the pain began radiating into the left lower extremity from the buttocks, posterior thigh, to the entire foot. The patient was treated with physical therapy including traction, ultrasound, heat, and exercises, with only temporary relief. A previous evaluation in 2000 revealed an L5-S1 herniated nucleus pulposus with foraminal encroachment. The patient is here for probable surgery. The patient also has a history of chronic diarrhea. A previous evaluation revealed increased LFTs of unknown etiology. Stool cultures were negative. A liver ultrasound and a liver-spleen scan showed hepatocellular disease without focal hepatic abnormality. The patient is readmitted for a probable liver biopsy.

PAST MEDICAL HISTORY: As per HPI, and a kidney stone in 1998.

PAST SURGICAL HISTORY: Pneumothorax in 1977 with a chest tube.

MEDICATIONS: Azulfidine 1 g p.o. b.i.d.

ALLERGIES: The patient has no known drug allergies.

SOCIAL HISTORY: The patient smokes a pipe and rarely drinks alcohol.

PHYSICAL EXAMINATION: The patient's general physical examination is within normal limits except for slight tenderness to palpation of his right lower quadrant, without masses. The liver is without enlargement. The back has positive straight leg raising[2] at 60 degrees, negative cross straight leg raising. Neurological: Cranial nerves II-XII are intact.[3] Strength is 5/5 in all 4 extremities. Sensory is grossly intact except decreased to pinprick, left S1. Reflexes are 2+ throughout except for an absent left ankle jerk. There is no clonus.[4]

HOSPITAL COURSE: This 66-year-old white male, with low back pain and left lower extremity pain, was admitted for evaluation of increased LFTs. The patient had a liver biopsy which showed a fatty liver with steatohepatitis.[5] GI recommended a dietary consult for hyperlipidemia. In addition the patient had a fasting lipid profile. The patient was cleared for general surgery after the liver biopsy. Thus, the patient was taken to the operating room where he underwent a left L5-S1 hemilaminectomy, diskectomy, and foraminotomy. The patient did well postoperatively with relief of his leg pain. The patient was thus discharged.

FINAL DIAGNOSES

1. Herniated nucleus pulposus.
2. Fatty liver.
3. Increased cholesterol.

OPERATION: L5-S1 diskectomy.

PROCEDURES

1. Liver biopsy
2. Dietary consult.

DISCHARGE MEDICATION: Percocet p.r.n.

DISPOSITION: Avoid nonsteroidal antiinflammatory[6] drugs and alcohol. The patient is to have a low-fat, low-cholesterol diet. The patient is to have no strenuous activity and walk for exercise. The patient should return to the neurosurgery clinic in 3 months.

Footnotes:

1. 1.When editing decades, it is generally preferred to add an *s* (no apostrophe). If it was dictated as "the '70s," then it would be edited with a preceding apostrophe.
2. 2.This can be straight-leg raising as well. Meaning is clear either way.
3. 3.The trend is to transcribe cranial nerves with Arabic numerals. However, some clients prefer Roman numerals for this. Without specific instruction, you can transcribe them either way.
4. 4.A form of movement marked by contractions and relaxations of a muscle.
5. 5.If you aren't sure what this means, look it up (http://www.onelook.com).
6. 6.This can be acceptably edited with a hyphen as anti-inflammatory.

SPELLING.

Determine if the following words are spelled correctly. If the spelling is correct, leave the word as it has already been entered. If the spelling is incorrect, provide the correct spelling.

1. encroachment _____

2. hepatocelular _____

3. Azulfidine _____

4. steatohepatitis _____

5. hemelaminectomy _____

6. foraminotomy _____

7. pulposous _____

Fill in the Blank.

The following abbreviations and/or terms are used in the previous reports. Fill in the appropriate blank with either the abbreviation or its expansion.

1. degenerative joint disease_____

2. NKDA_____

3. physical therapy_____

4. liver function test_____

5. GI_____

6. history of present illness_____

7. C-spine_____

8. b.i.d._____

NEUROLOGY REPORT 3 – OPERATIVE NOTE

PREOPERATIVE DIAGNOSIS: Cerebrospinal fluid leak, postoperative.

OPERATION PERFORMED: Suboccipital craniectomy and repair of cerebrospinal fluid leak.

COMPLICATIONS: None.

ESTIMATED BLOOD LOSS: 50 cc.

INDICATIONS: This is a 57-year-old male who recently underwent resection of an 8 nerve schwannoma[1] through a suboccipital route with drilling out of the internal auditory canal. The procedure went well. The patient made a very good recovery, but he, on the third postoperative day, exhibited CSF rhinorrhea.[2] An attempt to halt this process was made through a lumbar drain, but this was unsuccessful. The options were discussed with the patient who elected to undergo reexploration and repair of CSF leak.

DESCRIPTION OF PROCEDURE: Patient was brought to the operating room, induced in general endotracheal anesthesia, and placed in the supine position on the operating room table. All pressure points were well padded, and his head was held in the Mayfield head-holder with pins. His head was turned well to the left, and an incision was made through an old incision line in the right subocciput. Self-retaining retractors were placed, and dissection was carried down through the suboccipital musculature to the region of the previous craniectomy. Self-retaining retractors were advanced. At the site of the previous craniectomy, the mastoid region was thoroughly explored. There were no obvious areas of defect, but the area was again rewaxed with bone wax. The dura was then opened through the previous incision lines, and the remainder of the procedure was done under direct magnification with the microscope. The cerebellum was very lightly retracted superiorly and laterally, exposing the VII cranial nerve leading out into the well-drilled porus and canal. This region was explored thoroughly under the microscope, with the findings only of a simple area of very small roughened bone that may have represented a defect in cortical bone leading into small air cells. All areas of previously drilled bone were heavily waxed with bone wax. The whole region was then covered and stuffed with suboccipital muscle that was harvested from the patient. Thrombin-soaked Gelfoam was laid over the muscle. The wound was then thoroughly irrigated with bacitracin solution, and the dura was closed using interrupted 4-0 Nurolon sutures. Again the mastoid region was thoroughly explored, and there was no obvious area of CSF leakage. Again, the region was rewaxed. The wound was then thoroughly irrigated again with bacitracin solution and closed in multiple layers using interrupted 0 and 2-0 Vicryl sutures and 3-0 nylon for the skin. The wound was then dressed in a sterile fashion. The patient was awakened from anesthesia and returned to the recovery room in satisfactory condition. It should be noted that during the procedure the radial aspect of his left hand was noted to be quite cold. This may be a residual from the previous procedure, but it will be reviewed postoperatively.

Highlights

CRANIAL NERVES

1. Olfactory
2. Optic
3. Oculomotor
4. Trochlear
5. Trigeminal
6. Abducens
7. Facial
8. Vestibulocochlear
9. Glossopharyngeal
10. Vagus
11. Accessory
12. Hypoglossal

Footnotes:

1. [1]This is reference to a cranial nerve 8 schwannoma. Again, VIII or 8 is acceptable for cranial nerves.
2. [2]CSF is cerebrospinal fluid, rhino means nose, and -rrhea means flowing. You do the math.

SPELLING.
Determine if the following words are spelled correctly. If the spelling is correct, leave the word as it has already been entered. If the spelling is incorrect, provide the correct spelling.

1. dura _____

2. subociput _____

3. schwanomma _____   4. Mayfield _____

5. craniectomy _____

TRUE/FALSE.
Mark the following true or false.

1. The patient's estimated blood loss was none.

   ○ true

   ○ false

2. The patient's skin was closed with 3-0 Vicryl.

   ○ true

   ○ false

3. Cranial nerves can be edited using Arabic numerals or Roman numerals.

   ○ true

   ○ false

4. The wound was irrigated with thrombin.

   ○ true

   ○ false

5. The patient is 57 years old.

   ○ true

   ○ false

NEUROLOGY REPORT 4 – DISCHARGE SUMMARY

CHIEF COMPLAINT: Head injury.

HISTORY OF PRESENT ILLNESS: The patient is a 22-year-old white female. She reportedly was out drinking with friends last evening prior to admission and fell from the back of a truck traveling at 30 mph, onto her head with a loss of consciousness. The patient was brought to the ER at 0300[1] where her C-spine was reportedly clear. Due to combativeness alternating with lethargy, she was sent to an institution where a CT scan was done that showed a left temporal lobe contusion, blood in the sinuses, and pneumocephalus.[2] Her lacerations over her right scalp were cleaned and stapled, and the patient was transferred here. Upon arrival, the patient is awake with intermittent combativeness and lethargy. The patient is oriented to her name and age but not date, time or circumstances. She complains of abdominal, neck, and chest pain as well as the need for urination, though her Foley is in place. The patient is unable to name objects and has felt the inability to name parts of her body that hurt. The patient was also unable to recognize her parents in the hallway and is using abusive language in her attempt to urinate and be free of her restraints.

PAST MEDICAL HISTORY: Negative.

PAST SURGICAL HISTORY: Negative.

MEDICATIONS: Oral contraceptive pills.

The patient has no known drug allergies and does smoke tobacco.

PHYSICAL EXAMINATION: General: The patient is a well-developed, thin white female, combative, uncooperative, and oriented only to person, does not recognize her parents, intermittent lethargy. HEENT: The head has several small lacerations, staples are in place, and no active bleeding. The right TM has blood behind the membrane, no rupture, positive tenderness. No blood in the external canal. Pupils are equal and reactive. No papilledema. The left TM has a possible hemotympanum. Nose: Blood in the right nostril, no deformity or fluid leakage. Teeth: No trauma. Neck: Generalized tenderness. No point tenderness or deformity. Chest: Symmetric, no trauma or contusion. Lungs: Clear throughout. Cardiovascular: Regular rate and rhythm. Abdomen: Soft, nondistended, markedly decreased bowel sounds, diffuse tenderness, no guarding or rebound. GU: Normal external genitalia, no masses or blood in the vagina. Rectal: No masses, guaiac negative brown stool. Extremities: The right buttock has superficial abrasions and contusions. Cranial nerves 2-12 are intact. Motor: Normal tone and strength, no deficits. Sensory: Difficult to assess secondary to uncooperativeness. DTRs: Difficult to assess secondary to combativeness. Gait: Not assessed.

HOSPITAL COURSE: This 22-year-old, who fell out of the back of a truck with a closed head injury, was admitted for observation. The patient had a CT scan performed that showed a fracture of the sphenoid sinus, probably involving the clinoid process, with air in the cranium; the sphenoid sinus was filled with blood and air; a left temporal contrecoup contusion with small petechiae; and a possible small subdural. C-spine x-rays were performed that showed no evidence of soft tissue or bony lesions. A CT scan of the abdomen showed no abnormalities, though it was a substandard study secondary to movement. Pelvic and hip films were negative. The patient was observed in the SICU. A CT scan did show some hydrocephalus with a temporal lobe contusion. Thus a ventriculostomy was placed because of her intermittent lethargy. The patient continued to be followed in the SICU with a ventriculostomy and supportive care. The patient's neurological status remained stable. The patient remained mildly agitated and confused but had no focal abnormalities. An attempt was made to clamp the ventriculostomy.

The patient did not do well. Thus it was discussed with her parents to place a VP[3] shunt. The patient was taken to the operating room to place a VP shunt to control hydrocephalus. The patient continued to be followed in the unit until it was determined that she was stable. She was transferred to the neurosurgical ward on Friday. The patient continued to be more alert, although still somewhat confused. She was started in speech therapy, occupational therapy, and physical therapy. The patient continued to become more responsive and a little less confused. An MRI performed showed resolution of the posterior fossa hemorrhage, and the left temporal lobe contusion had resolved. She stated that she was doing well, no headaches. She said she scored 78% on a psych 101 course. The patient wants to return to work and exercise. Thus the patient had psychometrics performed to determine if she was fit for duty. In addition the patient had an EEG performed to see if her Dilantin could be tapered. The EEG was normal, and the patient was discharged with recommendations to taper her Dilantin.

FINAL DIAGNOSES

1. Severe closed head injury, resolving.
2. Basilar skull fracture.
3. Hydrocephalus.

OPERATIONS

1. Ventriculostomy placement.
2. Ventriculoperitoneal shunt placement.

PROCEDURES

1. Multiple CT scans and MRI scans.
2. Physical therapy.
3. Occupational therapy.
4. Speech therapy.
5. Neurological psychiatric testing.
6. Electroencephalogram.

DISPOSITION: The patient should taper her Dilantin to 200 mg q.h.s. for a week, 100 mg p.o. q.h.s. for a week, and then discontinue. The patient should follow up in the neurosurgery clinic in 3 months or sooner if she has difficulty concentrating or other problems.

Footnotes:

1. 1.Military time is a synonym for a 24-hour clock notation. The time starts at 0100 and goes through 2400. This time always takes 4 numerals and never uses a colon. This particular time would likely be dictated as oh-three-hundred hours.
2. 2.Word building! -pneumo means ___ and cephalus means ___ (fill in the blank).
3. 3.VP = ventriculoperitoneal.

SPELLING.
Determine if the following words are spelled correctly. If the spelling is correct, leave the word as it has already been entered. If the spelling is incorrect, provide the correct spelling.

1. pnuemocephalus _____

2. papiledema _____

3. hemotympanum _____

4. ventriculostomy _____

5. psychometrics _____

Fill in the Blank.

The following abbreviations and/or terms are used in the previous reports. Fill in the appropriate blank with either the abbreviation or its expansion.

1. ER_____

2. EEG_____

3. tympanic membrane_____

4. occupational therapy_____

5. VP_____

6. computed tomography_____

7. LOC_____

8. DTR_____

9. discontinue_____

NEUROLOGY REPORT 5 – OPERATIVE NOTE

PREOPERATIVE DIAGNOSIS: Metastatic spinal column tumor with cord compression.

OPERATION PERFORMED: T3-6 laminectomy and spinal cord decompression.

COMPLICATIONS: None.

ESTIMATED BLOOD LOSS: 2500 cc.

TRANSFUSION: Two units of packed red blood cells and two 6-packs of platelets.

INDICATIONS: This is a 71-year-old male with known prostatic carcinoma who presented with a rapid onset of paraparesis in his lower extremities. MRI disclosed severe epidural tumor with near total obliteration of the spinal cord in the T4-5 region. Because of the rapidity of the onset of the patient's deficit, it was felt that surgery would be the best option for rapid decompression of the spinal cord. The patient fully understands that the chances of neurologic recovery with his profound deficit is extremely limited.

DESCRIPTION OF PROCEDURE: The patient was brought to the operating room, induced in general endotracheal anesthesia, and placed in the prone position[1] on the operating room table. The patient's back was prepped and draped in the usual sterile fashion for surgery. The region of surgery was indicated by radiation therapy markings made just prior to surgery. A midline linear incision was made in the upper thoracic region and extended through the subcutaneous tissue. It should be noted that this patient had a platelet count of 56,000. Thus a 6-pack of platelets was begun right at the beginning of the procedure. The incision was carried through the subcutaneous tissue and self-retaining retractors were placed. Dissection was carried down to the deep fascia. The fascia was opened using Bovie electrocautery. Then a subperiosteal paraspinous muscle dissection was carried out bilaterally over T3-7 using Bovie electrocautery and Langenbeck periosteal elevator. It should be noted that the muscle bleeding here was heavy, but eventually controllable. At this stage the laminas of T3-6 were removed using Leksell and Kerrison rongeurs. In several areas the laminar bone was clearly abnormal and infiltrated with tumor. There was a large amount of epidural tumor tissue, especially lateral to the spinal cord. The cord could be seen clearly distorted by tumor. The laminectomies were extended laterally using Kerrison rongeurs, and much of the lateral tumor bulk was removed using pituitary rongeurs. Some tumor was sent off for pathologic evaluation. There was profuse bleeding from the tumor and the tumor infiltrated dome. Eventually we were able to define a more normal contour thecal sac above and below the region of the tumor. When this was accomplished, we thoroughly irrigated the wound and began trying to obtain hemostasis. This was obtained using bipolar electrocautery and multiple hemostatic agents, including Avitene, Gelfoam and Surgicel. Eventually the gutters of the resection were lined with Surgicel. By the end of the procedure, the spinal cord was well decompressed posteriorly and laterally, although there was clearly tumor coursing anteriorly and anterolaterally. The wound was then again thoroughly irrigated with bacitracin solution and closed in multiple layers using interrupted 0 and 2-0 Vicryl sutures. The skin was reapproximated using nylon, and it should be noted that a drain was placed just above the deep fascial layer. The wound was then dressed in a sterile fashion. The patient tolerated the procedure well, and there were no complications. Estimated blood loss was 2500 cc.

Footnotes:

1. 1.To review, the prone position is a position of the body lying face down.

SPELLING.
Determine if the following words are spelled correctly. If the spelling is correct, leave the word as it has already been entered. If the spelling is incorrect, provide the correct spelling.

1. chord _____

2. platlets _____

3. Surgicel _____

4. pituitary _____

5. hemestatic _____

Matching.
Match the correct term to the definition.

1. ____ Relieving pressure.

2. ____ Slight paralysis or weakness of both legs.

3. ____ Washing by stream of water or other fluid.

4. ____ Complete destruction of something.

5. ____ Permeating or penetrating into a substance, cell, or tissue.

A. paraparesis

B. infiltrated

C. obliteration

D. irrigated

E. decompression

NEUROLOGY REPORT 6 – DISCHARGE SUMMARY

CHIEF COMPLAINT: Right lower extremity pain.

HISTORY OF PRESENT ILLNESS: The patient is a 51-year-old white female with increasing numbness, pain, and weakness of the right lower extremity, extending from the right foot. This developed in early August without any history of trauma. The patient has been evaluated for right L5 radiculopathy, with weakness of dorsiflexion of the right foot. An MRI performed in August showed a large right central and paracentral L4-5 herniated disk extending superiorly and behind the L4 vertebral body, displacing the thecal sac to the left. The patient was started on dexamethasone with decreased symptoms. The patient is now admitted for surgery.

PAST MEDICAL HISTORY: Negative.

PAST SURGICAL HISTORY: D&C[1] in 1983. C-section x2 with a tubal ligation in 1985.

SOCIAL HISTORY: The patient has a 20-pack-year history of smoking. She does not drink alcohol.

MEDICATIONS: Dexamethasone 4 mg p.o. q.6 hours and Tagamet 300 mg p.o. q.i.d.

PHYSICAL EXAMINATION: The general physical examination is within normal limits. The gait is antalgic to the right with a foot drop. Reflexes are 2+ in both knees, 1+ in the right ankle, and 2+ in the left ankle. Motor: Right dorsiflexion is 3+/5; right extensor hallucis longus is 3+/5, otherwise 5/5.

HOSPITAL COURSE: This 51-year-old white female with a right L5 radiculopathy and a large herniated nucleus pulposus at L4-5 to the right, underwent a hemilaminectomy at L4-5 with excision of the disk. The patient did well postoperatively without complications, with relief of her right leg pain, and slight improvement in the strength in her right leg. The patient was thus discharged to home.

FINAL DIAGNOSIS

1. Right L5 radiculopathy.[2]

OPERATION

1. Right L4-5 hemilaminectomy and diskectomy.

PROCEDURES: None.

DISCHARGE MEDICATIONS

1. Tylenol No. 3 p.r.n. pain.
2. Colace 100 mg b.i.d.

DISPOSITION: Activity: No heavy lifting or housework, no strenuous activity. The patient may walk for exercise. The patient should follow up on the neurosurgery ward in 1 week for removal of staples, and follow up in the neurosurgery clinic in 1 month.

Footnotes:

1. 1.Some accounts or even platforms do not allow the use of symbols such as &, and might require this be expanded to "D and C" or even further to "dilatation and curettage."
2. 2.Typically, even when dictated as a list (dictator says "Diagnoses number one left L 5 radiculopathy"), it is preferred not to list a 1 without a 2. So this would just be edited after the heading. Again, this is a style issue. For a verbatim account, it would be okay to edit this as 1.

Multiple Choice.
Choose the correct spelling of the term.

1. In the condition of a soft, moist solid.
   - ○ pulpusus
   - ○ pulpousus
   - ○ pulposus
   - ○ pulpusous

2. A type of gait.
   - ○ antalgec
   - ○ antalgic
   - ○ entalgic
   - ○ antaligic

3. A corticosteroid drug.
   - ○ dexamethasone
   - ○ deximethasone
   - ○ dexamethisone
   - ○ deximethisone

4. Characterized by much energy.
   - ○ strinuous
   - ○ strenuis
   - ○ strenuoius
   - ○ strenuous

5. Removal of a portion of a vertebral lamina.
   - ○ hemilamenectomy
   - ○ hemilaminectomy
   - ○ hemelamenectomy
   - ○ hemelaminectomy

TRUE/FALSE.
Mark the following true or false.

1. The patient's surgery required no staples.

   ○ true

   ○ false

2. The patient's symptoms decreased after starting dexamethasone.

   ○ true

   ○ false

3. The patient's discharge activity level is no heavy lifting or walking.

   ○ true

   ○ false

4. The patient has had no previous surgeries.

   ○ true

   ○ false

5. The patient was discharged to a nursing home.

   ○ true

   ○ false

NEUROLOGY REPORT 7 – OPERATIVE NOTE

PREOPERATIVE DIAGNOSIS: Progressive left thoracolumbar[1] scoliosis.

POSTOPERATIVE DIAGNOSIS: Same.

OPERATION PERFORMED
1. Anterior spine fusion, T12-L4, with Zielke instrumentation and T10 rib autograft.
2. Posterior spine fusion, T12-L4, with Cotrel-Dubousset[2] instrumentation and right posterior iliac crest bone graft.

COMPLICATIONS: None.

INDICATIONS: The patient is a 53-year-old with progressive thoracolumbar scoliosis and pain.

DESCRIPTION OF PROCEDURE: The patient was taken to the operating suite where she was given a general endotracheal anesthetic without complication. She was then prepared by the anesthesia service with the appropriate lines. The patient was then positioned in a right side-down lateral decubitus position and held with bean bags. Her body was prepped and draped, and a left thoracoabdominal incision and exposure was provided. After exposure of the anterior spine, the position was confirmed with intraoperative radiographs. At this point, the T12-L1, L1-L2, L2-L3, and L3-L4 disks were incised and removed with a combination of rongeurs and curets. The endplates of all levels were curetted. After adequate decompression of the disk spaces and exposure of subchondral and cancellous bone in all vertebral bodies, the interspaces were then packed with Gelfoam. The patient's 10th rib was then morcellized[3] using a bone mill. At this point, the patient's vertebral bodies were then instrumented using Zielke instrumentation, beginning at the central vertebrae and extending cephalad and caudad. After the placement of the five appropriate-sized Zielke screws, a 3.25-mm rod was then placed between the screws, and nuts were used to lock the screws in place. During the tightening portion of the case, the spine was de-rotated with excellent correction of the spine. It should be noted that prior to application of the rod, all Gelfoam was removed. The endplates were decorticated using osteotomes, and the bone graft was packed in position. After tightening the rods, the spine appeared to have excellent alignment, and all bleeding was well controlled.

The case was then returned to the general surgery team who performed an anterior closure of the wound. After this was completed, and dressings were in place, the orthopedic team resumed care of the patient. AP and lateral radiographs were taken intraoperatively which showed excellent alignment of the spine in the coronal plane and some restoration of normal lumbar lordosis. With correction obtained, the decision was made to perform an instrumented posterior spine fusion for support from T12-L4. The patient was positioned prone on a 4-poster frame. All bony prominences were well padded. The patient's back was then prepped and draped in a sterile fashion. A midline longitudinal incision was then made from the area of the thoracolumbar junction down to approximately L4. Sharp dissection was carried out through the skin, and electrocautery dissection was carried down to the deep fascia. The spinous processes were outlined using electrocautery. Intraoperative radiographs were taken to confirm position. After this was done, the spine was exposed from T12 down to L4. Once this was done, the exposure was carried out to the tips of the transverse processes, and the facets in each area were stripped of their periosteum. After excellent exposure, laminotomies were made at the superior aspect of the L3 lamina and the superior aspect of the T12 lamina. A thoracic laminar hook was placed in a downgoing fashion over the T12 lamina, and a lumbar laminar hook was placed over the L3 lamina in a downgoing fashion. The ligamentum flavum separator was then placed beneath the lamina at L4 and at L1. The appropriate-sized lumbar laminar hooks were then used. All hook sites were prepared and felt to be excellent. At this point, the wound was packed with sponges and attention was directed towards the right posterior iliac crest. Electrocautery dissection was carried out over to the posterior iliac crest, and an iliac crest bone graft was then obtained in the usual fashion using a series of gouges, osteotomes and curets. After excellent bone grafts had been obtained without complication, the wound was copiously irrigated with irrigation solution. The fascia over the iliac crest donor site was then closed tightly with #1 Vicryl in a running fashion. Attention was then directed back to the main wound where the wound was copiously irrigated with irrigation solution. Once this had been obtained, the right portion of the spine was decorticated using a combination of osteotomes and rongeurs. The spinous processes were then removed using a combination of osteotomes and bone cutters. Once this had been done, bone graft was then placed in the posterolateral gutter from L4 through T12.

The right-sided hooks were then placed in the following fashion: There was a closed thoracic laminar hook in a downgoing fashion on the superior aspect of T12 and upgoing open lumbar laminar hook on the inferior aspect of L1, a downgoing open lumbar laminar hook on the superior aspect of L3, and a closed lumbar laminar hook in an upgoing fashion on the inferior aspect of L4. A 14-mm Cotrel-Dubousset rod was then bent into excellent lordosis. This was then threaded through the hooks with appropriate blockers. Some correction was obtained using the intraoperative in situ benders. All hooks were then secured and tightened. An identical process was then performed on the left side with decortication using osteotomes and rongeurs. The bone graft was placed in the posterolateral gutter, and the hooks were then placed in a similar fashion. Once again, the rod was prebent[4] and positioned into the hooks with correction with in situ benders. The hook sites were all tightened in compression across the claws. There appeared to be excellent restoration of lumbar lordosis and excellent position of the hooks. Intraoperative SSEPs[5] remained excellent. At this point, the DDTs were then placed and tightened. All nuts were then placed and tightened. Remaining bone graft was then placed throughout the wound after copious irrigation. The deep fascia was then approximated using #1 Vicryl in a running fashion. The iliac crest donor site and the paraspinal muscles were then injected with a total of 30 cc of 0.25% Marcaine with 1:200[6] epinephrine. The wound was copiously irrigated with irrigation solution and a 1/4-inch Hemovac drain placed over the fascia. The subcutaneous tissue was approximated using 0 Vicryl in a running fashion. The skin was closed using 3-0 Vicryl in a subcuticular fashion. A dressing of Benzoin, Steri-Strips, Xeroform, dressing sponges, and foam tape with Reston foam was then applied. The patient was then positioned supine on her intensive care unit bed. The patient was then awakened from general anesthesia and extubated without complication. She was able to move her feet in the operating room. She was then taken to the surgical intensive care unit for recovery. There were no noted intraoperative complications. Total estimated blood loss was 2000 cc. The patient received 3 units of autologous packed red blood cells and 325 cc of Cell Saver. She received 1000 cc of Hespan and had 700 cc of urine out by Foley catheter.

Footnotes:

1. 1.Thoracolumbar = Relating to the thoracic and lumbar portions of the vertebral column.
2. 2.A good surgical word book is VERY helpful in filling in equipment blanks and verifying equipment information is accurate.
3. 3.*Morcellized* means to crush so as to be able to remove piece by piece. This can also be spelled morselized.
4. 4.This word reads better with a hyphen, although it is not required. Pre-bent, as in bent before it is inserted.
5. 5.SSEPs = somatosensory evoked potentials.
6. 6.This is dictated as "one to two hundred epinephrine."

SPELLING.

Determine if the following words are spelled correctly. If the spelling is correct, leave the word as it has already been entered. If the spelling is incorrect, provide the correct spelling.

1. thoracolumbar _____   2. end plates _____

3. cancellus _____   4. facets _____

5. autologus _____

Multiple Choice.
Choose the best answer.

1. The patient was positioned in the lateral (○ decubitis, ○ decubitus) position.

2. Patient has a history of (○ lordosis, ○ lordosus).

3. The wound was cleaned with (○ copius, ○ copious) irrigation.

4. The facets in each area were stripped of their (○ periosteum, ○ periostium) .

5. A thoracic (○ laminar, ○ laminer) hook was placed.

NEUROLOGY REPORT 8 – DISCHARGE SUMMARY

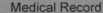

HISTORY OF PRESENT ILLNESS: The patient is a 32-year-old white male who was in his usual state of excellent health until March 2003[1] when he suffered bilateral maxillary sinus pain with yellow-green mucus production. He presented to the emergency room and was placed on Augmentin and Tylenol No. 3 with some relief. On followup appointment, the patient complained of nausea and vomiting and was treated with Tigan. The patient was not experiencing fever or chills. On March 28,[2] the patient suffered sudden onset of diplopia while working, followed by a headache which was bitemporal and bioccipital and was relieved by covering one eye. The patient denied a change in visual acuity, confusion, paresthesias, motor weakness, syncope, seizures, gait disturbances, history of syphilis, history of herpes simplex virus, or a history of TB.

PAST MEDICAL HISTORY: Habits: 15-pack-year smoking history, and 6 to 12 beers per week. Family history: Negative. Childhood illnesses: Usual. Travel: History of travel to France. Past medical illnesses: Astigmatism as an adult. Past surgical history: T&A at age 3. Injuries: No history of trauma.[3]

ALLERGIES: QUESTION REACTION TO ERYTHROMYCIN AS A CHILD, WHICH PRODUCED A RASH.

MEDICATIONS: Augmentin, Tylox, Tylenol No. 3, Tigan.

PHYSICAL EXAMINATION: Temperature 98.0, pulse 68, respiratory rate 12, blood pressure 120/80. In general, the patient was a well-developed, well-nourished white male in no acute distress, alert and oriented times 3. Head, eyes, ears, nose, throat: NC/AT,[4] bilateral esotropia with PERRLA, fundi benign, full visual fields bilaterally by confrontation. Nares: Unobstructed. TMs: Clear. Oropharynx: Clear. Sinuses: Nontender. Neck: Supple without lymphadenopathy or thyromegaly. Lungs: Clear to auscultation bilaterally. Cardiac: Regular rate and rhythm with a normal S1, S2, and no murmurs, gallops, or rubs. Abdomen: Soft, nondistended, nontender, no hepatosplenomegaly, no masses, positive bowel sounds. GU: Deferred. Rectal: Deferred. Extremities: No cyanosis, clubbing, or edema. Neuro: Cranial nerves 2-12 intact, except for bilateral 6 nerve palsy. Vision: 20/20 bilaterally. Sensory: Grossly intact. Strength: 5/5 in all groups. DTRs: 2+ and symmetric bilaterally. Toes are downgoing. Cerebellar function is intact by testing. Skin: Without lesions.

HOSPITAL COURSE: The patient was admitted for evaluation on the general medicine service for further evaluation of headaches and bilateral 6 nerve palsy. The patient underwent an MRI of the head which showed diffuse meningeal irritation/inflammation. An LP was performed and showed 28 red blood cells, 3 white blood cells, protein 91, glucose 51. Cryptococcal antigen was negative. Cultures for AFB, fungus, and bacteria were negative on the spinal fluid at discharge. To rule out chronic meningitis, 3 large volume LPs were performed, and cultures for TB, fungal, and anaerobes were negative at discharge. A repeat MRI on hospital day 10 showed no progression of meningeal inflammation. The patient's examination was unchanged throughout hospitalization. He felt well, except for mild headaches and continued diplopia, requiring a patch over 1 eye. The patient was seen by the neurology service. They agreed with the above workup. Also of note was a TSH which was normal, an RPR which was negative, FTA-ABS which was negative, ACE level within normal limits, India ink of the CSF negative, KOH prep of the CSF negative. Visually-evoked responses were performed bilaterally and were probably within normal limits. Bilateral BAERs were also symmetrical, and there was a suggestion of a bilateral peripheral 8 nerve disorder that was symmetrical. Cytology of the CSF was negative for malignant cells. The infectious disease service was also consulted. They requested a PPD with anergy panel, which was negative with positive controls. They also required Lyme, mycoplasmas, CMV, and EBV serologies. Cerebrospinal fluid IgG[5] was 6.7, which is elevated. Albumin was 47.7, which is elevated. IgG SYN was 8.2, which is slightly elevated. IgG IND was 0.7, which was normal. CSF BAN was 2, which is elevated. Myelin protein was less than 1, which is normal. The CSF FTA was negative. The CSF RPR was negative. The CSF cryptococcal antigen was negative. The CSF RPR, repeated, was negative. The CSF cryptococcal antigen, repeated, was negative.

DISCHARGE DIAGNOSIS

1. Bilateral 6 nerve palsy with meningeal inflammation of unknown etiology.

SPECIAL PROCEDURES

1. MRI of the head.
2. Lumbar puncture.
3. PPD and anergy panel.
4. MRI of the head.

DISCHARGE MEDICATIONS: Tylenol 650 mg p.o. q. 4 h. p.r.n. headaches.

DISPOSITION AND FOLLOWUP: Diet: Regular. Activity: As tolerated. The patient will follow up in the neurology clinic with Dr. Shepherd at 8:15 a.m. on April 3. The patient is to return to the Seattle Grace Emergency Room for confusion, worsening of the headache, visual symptoms, neck stiffness, fever, chills, nausea, vomiting, weakness, sensory changes, or any other new symptoms. The emergency room physician is to call the neurologist on call immediately should the patient present to the emergency room. A stat CT of the head and LP will likely be needed should new symptoms develop. The neurology service will draw viral titers on or about April 2. Audiometry is to be performed in the ENT clinic. Tests pending on discharge also include the serologies/mycoplasmas, Lyme, and EBV. Also pending is a CSF multiple sclerosis panel.

Footnotes:

1. 1.Generally, you do not use a comma after the year when a month and year are dictated together. If a day was also dictated, you would use commas (March 17, 2003,).
2. 2.Also regarding dates, do not edit days of the month as ordinals, even if dictated that way (March 28th would be a "no no").
3. 3.Grouping all this information under PMH is a style issue. It could easily be separated out under additional headings.
4. 4.NC/AT = normocephalic, atraumatic.
5. 5.The abbreviation *Ig* or *IG* stands for immunoglobulin. Lab studies include several Ig classifications. These are designated by alpha letters: A, D, I, IgG, IgA, IgD, IgM, IgM-RF, and others.

SPELLING.
Determine if the following words are spelled correctly. If the spelling is correct, leave the word as it has already been entered. If the spelling is incorrect, provide the correct spelling.

1. hepatosplenomegaly _____

2. Lime _____

3. dyplopia _____

4. biocipital _____

5. meningeal _____

Matching.

Match the correct abbreviation to the expansion.

1. ____ TB

2. ____ LP

3. ____ AFB

4. ____ TSH

5. ____ RPR

6. ____ FTA-ABS

7. ____ CSF

8. ____ ACE

9. ____ KOH

10. ____ BAER

11. ____ PPD

12. ____ CMV

13. ____ EBV

A. rapid plasma reagin

B. fluorescent treponemal antibody absorption

C. lumbar puncture

D. brainstem auditory-evoked response

E. cytomegalovirus

F. tuberculosis

G. potassium hydroxide

H. thyroid stimulating hormone

I. acid-fast bacillus

J. Epstein-Barr virus

K. purified protein derivative

L. angiotensin-converting enzyme

M. cerebrospinal fluid

NEUROLOGY REPORT 9 – OPERATIVE NOTE

PREOPERATIVE DIAGNOSIS: Recurrent left L4-5 herniated nucleus pulposus.

POSTOPERATIVE DIAGNOSIS:

1. Recurrent left L4-5 herniated nucleus pulposus.
2. Lateral recess stenosis.

OPERATION PERFORMED:

1. L4-5 hemilaminotomy with L4-5 discectomy.
2. Left L5 foraminotomy.
3. Left L4-5 partial facetectomy.

INDICATIONS: The patient is a 48-year-old male with a history of recurrent left L4-5 herniated nucleus pulposus. The patient's care has been refractory to nonoperative therapy, to include steroids, nonsteroidals, and narcotic analgesics. The patient has not improved since symptoms began and desires immediate surgical care due to progressive pain.

DESCRIPTION OF PROCEDURE: The patient was taken to the operating suite where he was given a general endotracheal anesthetic without complication. The patient was then positioned prone on a Toronto frame. All bony prominences were well padded. His skin was then prepped and draped in a sterile fashion. A longitudinal incision was then made in the midline away from his previous incision. Electrocautery was carried out through the subcutaneous tissue and additional paravertebral musculature. Cobb elevators were then used to strip the paravertebral musculature subperiosteally. Adequate hemostasis was obtained using electrocautery.

Intraoperative radiograph was taken to confirm positioning at the L4-5 level. At this time, the L4-5 interspace[1] was cleared using a series of Cobb elevators and curets. At this point, an L4-5 hemilaminotomy was performed to expose the retained ligamentum flavum and dura. The lateral recesses were found to be quite tight, confirming the diagnosis of lateral recess stenosis. At this point the bony window was widened. Partial facetectomy needed to be performed. As this was performed, a large bulging disc was identified. The scar tissue was separated from the disc with gentle blunt dissection. The annulus was then incised using a cruciate incision with an 11 blade. The disc space was entered, and herniated nucleus pulposus was excised. This portion of the bulging fragment was taken. There appeared to be some retained disc fragments slightly more centrally which were sequestered beneath the posterior longitudinal ligament. Blunt dissection with Penfield 4, dental, and Woodson elevators was then used to loosen these fragments, which were then removed with a pituitary rongeur. The largest single fragment measured approximately 12 mm x 8 mm across. The disc space was cleared of all loose pieces of nucleus with pituitary rongeurs. The L4-5 foramen was also cleared of loose pieces of disc fragment. It should be noted that the L5 nerve root appeared to be quite scarred, and the L5 foramen appeared to be quite tight. A partial foraminotomy was then performed over the area of the L5 nerve root. In addition, the medial border of the pedicle was removed partially to further decompress the L5 nerve root. A Woodson elevator was placed then into the L5 foramen, and the L5 nerve root appeared to be adequately decompressed. There were no retained fragments either superior or inferior to the nerve root, as well as no fragments anterior or posterior to the nerve root. The wound was copiously irrigated with irrigation solution. Thrombin-soaked Gelfoam was then placed into the spinal canal, while a fat graft was taken in the usual fashion. The Gelfoam was removed, and adequate hemostasis appeared to be obtained. Then 1 cc of 80 mg Depo-Medrol was placed in the spinal canal and the fat graft placed over the dura. The paravertebral musculature and fascia were then closed using 1-0 Vicryl in a running fashion. The paravertebral musculature was then injected with a total of 20 cc of 0.25% Marcaine with epinephrine. The subcutaneous tissue was once again irrigated and the subcutaneous tissue reapproximated with 0 Vicryl. The skin was then closed using 3-0 Vicryl. A dressing of Benzoin, Steri-Strips, Xeroform, dressing sponges, and microform tape was then applied. Total blood loss estimated at 250 cc. The patient was then positioned supine on the recovery room bed and awakened from general anesthesia. He was moving both feet well in the operating room. He was then taken to the recovery room in stable condition.

Footnotes:

1. 1.Notice this is "interspace" and not "innerspace." It is the space "between."

Multiple Choice.
Choose the correct spelling of the term.

1. Narrowing of a canal or passageway.
   - ○ stinosis
   - ○ stenosis
   - ○ stinoses
   - ○ stenosus

2. Marked by fibrous tissue.
   - ○ scarred
   - ○ scared
   - ○ scharred
   - ○ schared

3. Medication used to relieve pain.
   - ○ anilgesic
   - ○ anelgisic
   - ○ anelgisec
   - ○ analgesic

4. Ring-like structure.
   - ○ anuluss
   - ○ annulus
   - ○ anulis
   - ○ annulis

5. Structure protruding through an opening.
   - ○ herniated
   - ○ herneated
   - ○ hernnieated
   - ○ hernieted

Matching.
Match the correct term to the definition.

1. ____ Recurring again and again.

2. ____ Not responding to treatment.

3. ____ A small projection or protuberance.

4. ____ An instrument shaped like a scoop used to remove tissue from a body cavity.

5. ____ The outermost of the three meninges.

A. prominence

B. recurrent

C. dura

D. refractory

E. curet

UNIT 6
Obstetrics/Gynecology

OBSTETRICS AND GYNECOLOGY – INTRODUCTION

Obstetrics is the branch of medicine dealing with management of pregnancy, labor, delivery, and the period following labor and delivery (the postpartum period).

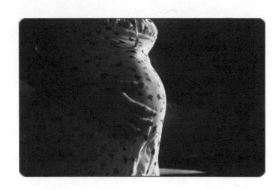

Obstetric reports describe the various stages of pregnancy, labor and delivery, and post-delivery of a baby, as well as conditions and procedures related to terminated pregnancies:

- prenatal care
- neonatal vaginal deliveries
- cesarean sections
- missed or spontaneous abortions
- therapeutic or elective abortions
- postpartum tubal ligations

This specialty also utilizes ultrasounds for following fetal development and is concerned with the detection and treatment of problems related to pregnancy—such as:

- gestational diabetes and hypertension
- surgery on the fetus
- toxemia
- premature rupture of membranes
- bleeding during pregnancy
- complications of birth

Admissions for some of the gynecological issues mentioned below often require the transcription editing of the "big four"—consultations, H&P's, operation reports, and discharge summaries. Records for a routine delivery would include an H&P and discharge summary, while complicated or difficult deliveries might also include an operative summary or consultation visits for mom and/or baby.

Gynecology is the branch of medicine that treats diseases of and problems with the female reproductive system.

These conditions might include:

- dysmenorrhea
- menometrorrhagia
- uterine prolapse
- cervical or uterine cancers
- ectopic or tubal pregnancies
- infertility
- fertility

Surgeries for gynecological problems include:

- laparoscopies
- hysterectomies
- oophorectomies
- salpingectomies
- tubal ligations
- hysterosalpingograms
- in-vitro fertilization

While there are two different technical terms for these specialties, a physician who treats the medical problems of women is frequently certified in both obstetrics and gynecology (OB/GYN).

OB/GYN LANGUAGE WORKSHOP

Before we begin this OB/GYN FOMS unit, we will take some time to review common OB/GYN terminology. The following is meant to be a review of word-building terms and abbreviations that you have already been exposed to in the Medical Word Building module and Abbreviations unit of the Mastering Medical Language module.

Common Obstetrics/Gynecology Root Words and Combining Forms

Root Word & Combining Form	Meaning	Example
amni/o	amnion	amniocentesis/amniotic
cervic/o	cervix, neck	endocervicitis
chori/o (chorion/o)	chorion	choriogenesis/chorionic
colp/o	vagina	colporrhaphy/colposcopy
culd/o	cul-de-sac	culdocentesis
episi/o	vulva	episiotomy
galact/o	milk	galactorrhea
gynec/o	woman, female	gynecogenic
hyster/o	uterus, womb	hysterectomy/hysteroscopy
lact/o	milk	lactogenesis/lactation
mamm/o	breast	mammary/mammoplasty
mast/o	breast	mastitis/mastectomy
men/o	menses, menstruation	amenorrhea/dysmenorrhea oligomenorrhea/menorrhagia
metr/o (metri/o)	uterus	metrorrhagia menometrorrhagia
my/o	muscle	myometrium
myom/o	muscle tumor	myomectomy
nat/i	birth	perinatal
obstetr/o	midwife	obstetric
oo/o	egg	oogenesis
oophor/o	ovary	bilateral oophorectomy
ov/o	egg	ovum
ovari/o	ovary	ovarian
ovul/o	egg	anovulatory
perine/o	perineum	perineorrhaphy
phor/o	to bear	oophoritis
salping/o	fallopian tubes	salpingectomy
uter/o	uterus	uterine prolapse
vagin/o	vagina	vaginal orifice/vaginitis
vulv/o	vulva	vulvovaginitis

Common Obstetrics/Gynecology Prefixes

Prefix	Meaning	Example
ante-	before, forward	antenatal/anteversion
dys-	painful	dyspareunia
endo-	within	endometritis
in-	in	involution
intra-	within	intrauterine device
multi-	many	multipara/multigravida
nulli-	no, not, none	nulligravida/nullipara
primi-	first	primiparous
retro-	backward	retroflexion

Common Obstetrics/Gynecology Suffixes

Suffix	Meaning	Example
-arche	beginning	menarche
-cyesis	pregnancy	pseudocyesis
-gravida	pregnancy	primigravida
-parous	to bear, bring forth	primiparous
-rrhea	discharge	leukorrhea
-salpinx	uterine tube	pyosalpinx
-tocia	labor, birth	dystocia/oxytocia
-version	act of turning	cephalic version

Common Obstetrics/Gynecology Abbreviations

Abbreviation	Expansion
A/AB	abortion
AC	abdominal circumference
AFP	alpha-fetoprotein
AI	artificial insemination
BPD	biparietal diameter
BSE	breast self-examination
BSO	bilateral salpingo-oophorectomy
CIN	cervical intraepithelial neoplasia
CIS	carcinoma in situ
CMG	cystometrogram
CPD	cephalopelvic disproportion
CS or C-section	cesarean section
CVS	chorionic villus sampling
D&C	dilatation or dilation and curettage
DES	Diethylstilbestrol

DUB	dysfunctional uterine bleeding
ECC	endocervical curettage
EDC	estimated date of confinement
EFW	estimated fetal weight
EMB	endometrial biopsy
EGA	estimated gestational age
ERT	estrogen replacement therapy
FHR	fetal heart rate
FHT	fetal heart tone
FL	femur length
FSH	follicle-stimulating hormone
FTND	full-term normal delivery
G	gravida
GC	Gonorrhea culture
GYN	gynecology
HC	head circumference
hCG	human chorionic gonadotropin
HPV	human papilloma virus
HSG	hysterosalpingography
HSV	herpes simplex virus
IUD	intrauterine device
IUGR	intrauterine growth rate/intrauterine growth retardation
IVF	in vitro fertilization
LAVH	laparoscopic-assisted vaginal hysterectomy
LEEP	loop electrocautery excision procedure
LGA	large for gestational age
LH	luteinizing hormone
LMP	last menstrual period
LSO	left salpingo-oophorectomy
MSAFP	maternal serum alpha fetoprotein
NSVD	normal spontaneous vaginal delivery
OCPs	oral contraceptive pills
P	para
PAP/Pap	Papanicolaou smear
PID	pelvic inflammatory disease
PMP	previous menstrual period
PMS	premenstrual syndrome
ROM	rupture of membranes
RSO	right salpingo-oophorectomy
SAB	spontaneous abortion

SGA	small for gestational age
SIDS	sudden infant death syndrome
SROM	spontaneous rupture of membranes
SSVD	sterile, spontaneous vaginal delivery
STD	sexually transmitted disease
TAB	therapeutic abortion
TAH	total abdominal hysterectomy
TAH-BSO, TAHBSO	total abdominal hysterectomy with bilateral salpingo-oophorectomy
TBLC	term birth, living child
TSS	toxic shock syndrome
TVH	total vaginal hysterectomy
VBAC	vaginal birth after cesarean section

REVIEW: OB/GYN LANGUAGE

TRUE/FALSE.
Mark the following true or false.

1. The abbreviation *FL* stands for femur length.

   ○ true

   ○ false

2. *Mastectomy* is defined as removal of the breast.

   ○ true

   ○ false

3. A patient described as "nulliparous" has given birth.

   ○ true

   ○ false

4. *Prenatal* means before birth.

   ○ true

   ○ false

5. *Colposcopy* is a procedure that involves viewing of the vagina with a scope.

   ○ true

   ○ false

6. The abbreviation *D&C* stands for dilatation and colposcopy.

   ○ true

   ○ false

Fill in the Blank.
Using the word(s) in the box, enter the appropriate term in the space provided.

cephalopelvic	
papilloma	
bilateral	
inflammatory	
metrorrhagia	
galactorrhea	

1. _____ is the spontaneous flow of milk from the nipple at any time other than during nursing.

2. _____ disproportion is a condition in which the baby's head will not fit through the mother's pelvis.

3. Human _____ virus is a sexually transmitted disease that causes genital warts and may even lead to eventual cervical cancer.

4. _____ salpingo-oophorectomy is the removal of tubes and ovaries on both sides.

5. _____ is irregular uterine bleeding between menstrual periods.

6. Pelvic _____ disease is a general term that refers to infection of the uterus (womb), fallopian tubes (tubes that carry eggs from the ovaries to the uterus), and other reproductive organs.

Multiple Choice.

Choose the best answer.

1. (◯ Menarche, ◯ Menopause) is the beginning of menstruation.

2. (◯ Perineorrhaphy, ◯ Perineotomy) is surgical repair of the perineum.

3. An (◯ alfa, ◯ alpha) -fetoprotein test is often done during pregnancy to help determine if the fetus has neural tube defects.

4. (◯ Pseudocyesis, ◯ Pseudoparous) means false pregnancy.

OB/GYN REPORTS

Obstetrics and gynecology are the source of some of the most common transcription editing reports. Pregnancy is obviously a common condition and obstetric reports often include ultrasounds and the detection and treatment of problems related to pregnancy—such as gestational diabetes and hypertension, surgery on the fetus, toxemia, premature rupture of membranes, bleeding during pregnancy, complications of birth, and other problems. Gynecology problems include dysmenorrhea, menometrorrhagia, cervical or uterine cancers, ectopic or tubal pregnancies, infertility, fertility. Surgeries and other procedures for these problems include laparoscopies, hysterectomies, oophorectomies, salpingectomies, tubal ligations, and hysterosalpingograms. Following are typical OB/GYN reports.

OB/GYN REPORT 1 – OPERATIVE NOTE

PREOPERATIVE DIAGNOSIS: Endometriosis of ovary, endometriosis of the pelvic peritoneum.

MATERIAL TO LABORATORY: Cyst and biopsy from right ovary.

OPERATION PERFORMED: Exploratory laparotomy, left ovarian cystotomy with cyst oversew, and right ovarian cystectomy with ovarian biopsy.

INDICATIONS: Pelvic mass.

FINDINGS: The left ovary was noted to have an approximately 8-cm endometrioma and was covered with diffuse material consistent with powder burns of endometriosis. The cyst was incised and drained, and the cystotomy incision was oversewn. Fulguration[1] of endometrial implants was performed. The right ovary was also noted to contain an endometrioma which was approximately 2-3 cm; this was excised. An area of the ovary that contained multiple large powder-burn-like lesions with stellate contractions was included with the cyst. The cul-de-sac was also noted to have multiple implants consistent with endometriosis and stellate scarring of the peritoneum. The appendix was visualized fully and noted to be without visible pathology.[2]

> A **chocolate cyst** is an ovarian cyst with hemorrhage inside the cavity and formation of a hematoma containing old brown blood.

DESCRIPTION OF OPERATION: After informed consent was obtained, the patient was taken to the operating room where she was placed under general endotracheal anesthesia. She was given an abdominal and vaginal prep, and a Foley catheter was placed. A Maylard incision was made through the abdomen. A Turner-Warwick retractor was used for visualization of the pelvic contents. The bowel was packed using moistened laparotomy sponges. The left ovary was bluntly dissected from the pelvic sidewall, to which it was adherent. The mass in the left ovary was noted to be approximately 8 cm in size. While bluntly dissecting the ovary, material consistent with a chocolate cyst was noted to discharge from the ovary. Copious irrigation was performed of this chocolate cyst. A cystotomy was performed for drainage of the cyst, and the edges of the cystotomy were oversewn. Endometrial implants were fulgurated. The left fallopian tube was noted to be without obvious pathology, as was the right fallopian tube. The right ovary was also noted to be adherent to the ovarian fossa and was bluntly dissected away. An ovarian biopsy and wedge resection with cyst removal was performed using Metzenbaum scissors and careful dissection of the ovarian cyst. Included in the biopsy were several very large areas of endometrial implants and powder-burn-like lesions. Hemostasis was achieved using electrocautery and 4-0 Vicryl sutures in a figure of 0[3] fashion. The pelvis was copiously irrigated, and endometrial implants were again fulgurated. The appendix was inspected and noted to be without obvious pathology. The peritoneum was then closed with a running suture of 3-0 PDS, and a subfascial drain was placed. Fascia was closed with a running suture of 0 Vicryl, and the subcutaneous layer was copiously irrigated. Hemostasis was achieved using electrocautery, and the skin was closed using staples. Estimated blood loss: 300 cc. Complications: None. Condition: Stable. Disposition: The patient will be taken to the post-anesthesia care unit.

Footnotes:

1. 1.*Fulguration* is the destruction of living tissue by electric sparks generated by a high frequency current (similar to electrocautery).
2. 2.This means the appendix looked normal.
3. 3.Also acceptably edited as figure-of-eight.

SPELLING.
Determine if the following words are spelled correctly. If the spelling is correct, leave the word as it has already been entered. If the spelling is incorrect, provide the correct spelling.

1. endometriosis _____
2. fullguration _____
3. Maylard _____
4. Turner-Warnick _____

5. Metzanbaum

_____

Matching.
Match the term to the equipment type or procedure.

1. ___ Metzenbaum   A. retractor

2. ___ Maylard   B. catheter

3. ___ Turner-Warwick   C. incision

4. ___ Foley   D. scissors

5. ___ subfascial   E. drain

128

OB/GYN REPORT 2 – DISCHARGE SUMMARY

CHIEF COMPLAINT: This patient is a 20-year-old white female, gravida 1, para 0[1] at 32-5/7 weeks, being transferred with preterm labor.

HISTORY OF PRESENT ILLNESS: She presented to labor and delivery on July 10, 2007, at approximately 1030 hours, with a complaint of suprapubic and low back discomfort and cramping since early morning. There was no blood or fluid loss at that time. On exam, she was 3 cm, 90%, vertex presentation, and she received 1000 cc of lactated Ringer's and 0.25 mg[2] of subcutaneous terbutaline. She received her second dose of subcutaneous terbutaline at 1100 hours. She continued to contract, and was given a 4 gm bolus of magnesium sulfate, followed by a 2 gm per hour magnesium sulfate drip.[3] She arrived here at approximately 1345 hours. Her blood type is A+. She is rubella immune. Serology was nonreactive. Her prenatal course was complicated by first trimester spotting. She was also treated for a urinary tract infection in late February. She had continued spotting to the 20-week period, and this was attributed to cervical friability. She was also noted to have a low-lying anterior placenta without evidence of a previa. There was also an admission for uterine contractions and some brownish discharge and questionable bleeding. This resolved with bedrest. The patient was discharged to home with instructions for pelvic rest. There was a complaint of vaginal bleeding, but none was found. However, the patient was noted to have spotting and some cramping which continued on July 9, 2007. On July 10, 2007, the patient presented with the aforementioned acute complaint. It was noted that she was contracting every 3-4 minutes at that time. An ultrasound was done at 17-2/7 weeks, which was consistent with dates. On admission she was noted to have an estimated fetal weight of 1999 grams.

PAST MEDICAL HISTORY: She has no allergies. Medications: Prenatal vitamins. Past medical history: Questionable pyelonephritis in June of 2001. Past surgical history: T&A as a child. Tobacco: None. Ethanol: None. Sexually transmitted diseases: None.

PHYSICAL EXAMINATION: Unremarkable. Cervix was 3 cm, 80%, -2 station.

LABORATORY DATA: Chlamydia negative, RPR nonreactive, GC negative, urine culture negative, cervix positive for group B beta hemolytic Strep. Hemoglobin was 14.2 and 14.8, respectively. The hematocrit was 38.8 and 35.4. Platelets were 363 and 316. Cord gases were 7.23 and 7.30. Electrolytes were normal. UA was yellow, clear, 1.017, ketones 80-160, pH of 7.5. PT, PTT were normal.

HOSPITAL COURSE: This 20-year-old white female was admitted with preterm labor and a rule out abruption status. She was given ampicillin 2 gm IV piggyback q.6 hours, along with 12.5 mg of betamethasone IM.[4] Her magnesium sulfate was increased to 3 gm an hour secondary to continued uterine contractions. At 2120 hours on July 10,[5] the patient was still continuing to have uterine contractions every 5 minutes which were very strong in nature, in spite of the double tocolytics. The magnesium sulfate had been increased to 3.5 gm an hour, along with subcutaneous terbutaline. The plan at that time was to discontinue the tocolytics at 5 cm, which the patient was at that time. She continued to dilate, artificial rupture of membranes was to be performed with close monitoring. The patient continued to progress, and her membranes were ruptured at 0110 on July 11. At 0237, the patient had a 2070 gm male spontaneously, over a midline episiotomy. The infant was taken to the neonatal intensive care unit for observation. Pediatrics was in attendance. The postpartum course was unremarkable. The patient was placed on self care. She was discharged to home on July 13, 2007, with a recommendation for a 6-week checkup.

DISCHARGE DIAGNOSES

1. A 32-5/7 weeks intrauterine pregnancy, 2070 gm male, 5 and 7 Apgars.
2. Preterm labor.
3. Failed tocolysis.
4. Group B beta hemolytic Streptococcus of the cervix.

PROCEDURES

1. Internal and external fetal and uterine monitoring.
2. Tocolysis with magnesium sulfate.
3. Spontaneous vaginal delivery.
4. Midline episiotomy and repair.
5. Ampicillin antibiotics for cervical infection.
6. Betamethasone, intramuscular.

ANESTHESIA: Local.

PATHOLOGY: None.

CONSULTS: None.

Footnotes:

1. 1.*Gravida* means number of pregnancies and *para* is number of births of viable offspring.
2. 2.Even if the dictator says ".25 mg," the leading zero is edited in order to not confuse 0.25 with 25 mg.
3. 3.This could be acceptably edited with hyphens as well. Although meaning is clear without them.
4. 4.*IM*, of course, is intramuscular.
5. 5.We do not typically edit ordinals with dates, even when dictated (July 10th).

SPELLING.

Determine if the following words are spelled correctly. If the spelling is correct, leave the word as it has already been entered. If the spelling is incorrect, provide the correct spelling.

1. turbutaline _____

2. Chlamidia _____

3. betamethazone _____

4. taucolytics _____

5. Streptococus _____

Matching.

Match the correct term to the definition.

1. ____ Number of pregnancies.

2. ____ Number of births of viable offspring.

3. ____ A beta-2 adrenergic agonist drug that relaxes smooth muscles and therefore interferes with uterine contractions.

4. ____ Small colorless crystal that decreases the frequency and force of contractions.

5. ____ The placenta is positioned over the cervical os.

A. terbutaline

B. placenta previa

C. gravida

D. magnesium sulfate

E. para

OB/GYN REPORT 3 – PROCEDURE NOTE

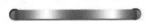

PREOPERATIVE DIAGNOSIS: Abnormal uterine bleeding.

POSTOPERATIVE DIAGNOSIS: Abnormal uterine bleeding.

OPERATION PERFORMED

1. Endocervical curettage.
2. Endometrial curettage with cervical dilation.

ESTIMATED BLOOD LOSS: Minimal.

FLUIDS: 700 cc electrolytes.

ANTIBIOTICS: Prophylactic ampicillin and Gentamicin.

FINDINGS: This patient is a 30-year-old white female G5, P 1-3-1-4[1] with an LMP of December 19, 2006, who has had heavy bleeding on and off since that time. Her hematocrit had dropped from 37.5 on January 3, to 30.7 on January 7, 2007. A Vabra biopsy and administration of Provera were both unsuccessful at stopping her bleeding. She was taken to the operating room and prepped and draped in a sterile manner following general anesthesia with mask ventilation. A weighted speculum was placed into the vagina, and a tenaculum was used to grasp the anterior portion of the cervix. The bladder had previously been straight cathed and emptied. A sharp curet was used to obtain an endocervical curettage. The uterus was then sounded to 9.5 cm. It should be noted that on bimanual exam, there were no adnexal masses and the uterus was sharply retroverted and firmly held into the cul-de-sac. The cervix was then dilated with Hank dilators to #20. Randall stone forceps were used, and no polyps were removed from the endometrial lining. The walls of the endometrium were then curetted, and a good uterine cry was noted in all quadrants. There were no complications with the procedure. The patient was then taken to the recovery room in stable condition.

Footnotes:

1. 1.The numbers following the *P* (for para) are numbers commonly referred to as TPAL. This gal's TPAL is 1-3-1-4 and it breaks down to T (term infants) 1, P (premature infants) 3, A (abortions) 1, and L (living children) 4. So she was pregnant 5 times (that is the G), and has 4 living children.

SPELLING.
Determine if the following words are spelled correctly. If the spelling is correct, leave the word as it has already been entered. If the spelling is incorrect, provide the correct spelling.

1. curatage _____

2. Vabra _____

3. Proveara _____

4. speculam _____

5. tenaculum _____

6. retroverted _____

7. Randal _____

8. uterine cry _____

TRUE/FALSE.
Mark the following true or false.

1. A female who is G1, P1 is currently pregnant.

   ○ true

   ○ false

2. A female who is G1, P 0-2-0-2 was pregnant one time.

   ○ true

   ○ false

3. A female who is G2, P 2-1-0-3 delivered term multiples.

   ○ true

   ○ false

4. A female who is G3, P 2 is currently pregnant.

   ○ true

   ○ false

5. A female can be G0, P1.

   ○ true

   ○ false

OB/GYN REPORT 4 – OPERATIVE NOTE

PREOPERATIVE DIAGNOSIS: Symptomatic pelvic relaxation.

POSTOPERATIVE DIAGNOSIS: Symptomatic pelvic relaxation.

DRAINS: Foley catheter.

MATERIAL TO LAB: Uterus, tubes, ovaries, and vaginal mucosa.

OPERATION PERFORMED: Total vaginal hysterectomy, bilateral salpingo-oophorectomy, anterior and posterior colporrhaphy, and McCall's culdoplasty.[1]

INDICATIONS: This patient is a 57-year-old white female gravida 4, para 4 with a long history of symptomatic pelvic relaxation. The patient also has stress urinary incontinence secondary to her cystocele. The patient has been using a pessary,[2] but has developed discomfort from pelvic relaxation and little success with the pessary.

FINDINGS: Normal uterus, tubes, and ovaries, normal vaginal mucosa, third degree cystocele, second degree rectocele.

DESCRIPTION OF OPERATION: After adequately being counseled, the patient was taken to the operating room and placed in the supine position. General endotracheal tube anesthesia was induced, and the patient was placed in the high lithotomy position. The vagina was prepped and draped in the usual sterile fashion and a weighted speculum placed in the posterior fornix with a Diva retractor placed anteriorly. The cervix was grasped with a single-tooth tenaculum, and a posterior colpotomy incision was made with Mayo scissors. A figure-of-eight stitch using #1 chromic was placed in the posterior vaginal cuff, incorporating the peritoneum to the posterior vaginal cuff. A Heaney-Ballantine clamp was placed on the left side incorporating the uterosacral ligament. The pedicle was then cut and suture ligated with #1 chromic. This was then performed on the left side. The cardinal ligament was taken down in a similar fashion using #1 chromic to tie off the pedicle. The uterine arteries were clamped off using Heaney-Ballantine clamp, suture ligated after cutting with #1 chromic. A semilunar incision was made from 9 o'clock to 3 o'clock using a scalpel. A finger was used to dissect the bladder off the lower uterine segment and cervix. The anterior colpotomy was performed using Mayo scissors, and the tubo-ovarian round ligament was clamped using Heaney-Ballantine clamps, cut, and suture ligated with #1 chromic, first with a free tie then with a suture ligature. The ovaries were brought down, including the fallopian tubes on both sides, and clamped proximally with the Heaney-Ballantine clamp. First a free tie was placed, then a suture ligature of #1 chromic. This was performed on both sides. Good hemostasis was noted, and the peritoneal lining was closed in a pursestring suture using 0 chromic. The McCall's culdoplasty stitch was placed incorporating the posterior vaginal cuff to the uterosacral ligament on both sides. This was performed with 2 sutures of #1 chromic. This closed off the cul-de-sac and also suspended the vagina to the uterosacral ligaments. Two Allis clamps were placed at either angle of the vaginal cuff, and Metzenbaum scissors were used to dissect the vaginal mucosa off the underlying pubovesical cervical fascia. The vaginal mucosa was incised in the midline up to 1 cm distant from the urethral meatus. Pratt clamps were used to grasp the edge of the vaginal mucosa, and the vaginal mucosa was dissected off the underlying pubovesical cervical fascia sharply with Metzenbaum scissors. A Kennedy-Kelly stitch was placed using 0 chromic by placing a stitch on either side of the urethra and bringing them together. This was done with interrupted stitches until the bladder, urethra, and bladder neck were suspended. The vaginal mucosa was closed using a running locking stitch of 2-0 chromic. Next, 2 Allis clamps were placed at either side of the vaginal introitus, and an episiotomy was performed using a scalpel. The vaginal mucosa was incised in a triangular fashion on the base of the vagina. This was performed up to the prior culdoplasty stitches. The vaginal mucosa was dissected off the underlying perirectal fascia. Then several interrupted stitches of 0 chromic were used to bring together the perirectal fascia, also incorporating the levator muscles. The vaginal mucosa was then trimmed and brought back together using a running locking stitch of 2-0 chromic. The remaining portion of the episiotomy was repaired using 2-0 chromic in a running nonlocking fashion for the subcuticular stitch. A vaginal pack was placed, and the Foley catheter was also placed. The patient was awakened and extubated in the operating room and taken to the recovery room in good condition. No complications were noted.

Footnotes:

1. 1. The use of 's with McCall is the possessive eponym form. Some clients, even when dictated, do not allow the use of the possessive form of an eponym and would require this be edited as McCall culdoplasty. Without instruction, either is acceptable.
2. 2. If you are unsure what a pessary is, now would be a good time to look it up and add it to your word list. If you don't have a word list, now would be a GREAT time to start one!

Multiple Choice.
Choose the best answer.

1. The patient had little benefit from the (○ pessiary, ○ pessary).

2. The vaginal (○ mucosa ○ mucous) was incised.

3. Clamps were placed at either side of the vaginal (○ introitus, ○ introitis).

4. The anterior (○ colpotomy, ○ colpotimy) was performed using scissors.

5. A finger was used to (○ disect, ○ dissect) the bladder off the lower uterine segment.

Matching.
Match the proper name to the common term that it belongs with.

1. ____ Kennedy-Kelly		A. scissors
2. ____ Metzenbaum		B. stitch
3. ____ Heaney-Ballantine		C. tenaculum
4. ____ single-tooth		D. retractor
5. ____ Diva		E. clamp
6. ____ Allis		
7. ____ Mayo		

OB/GYN REPORT 5 – DISCHARGE SUMMARY

CHIEF COMPLAINT: Uterovaginal prolapse.

HISTORY OF PRESENT ILLNESS: This patient is a 76-year-old white female, gravida 2, para 3, last menstrual period at age 47. The patient is not currently on hormone replacement therapy. The patient complains of pelvic and vaginal pressure symptoms and urinary frequency and urgency. The patient has incomplete bladder emptying by history. The patient denies a history of stress urinary incontinence. The patient has no history of digitalization to remove stool. The patient was seen by Dr. Johnson, and postvoid residual was found to be 155 cc. An IVP shows a left pelvic kidney. The patient's last Pap smear was in 1987, and was found to be normal. The patient has no past GYN history.

PAST MEDICAL HISTORY: Essential hypertension controlled with medications, and degenerative joint disease. The patient's past surgical history is significant for bilateral cataract surgery and an exploratory laparotomy. The patient has no known drug allergies. Tobacco use: One pack per day times ten to fifteen years.[1] The patient stopped several years ago. The patient denies a history of alcohol use. Present medications include Ditropan 10 mg p.o. t.i.d., Minipress 1 mg p.o. t.i.d., Maxzide 1/2 tablet p.o. q.d.

REVIEW OF SYSTEMS: Noncontributory.

PHYSICAL EXAMINATION: On admission, vital signs were stable, blood pressure 140/80, afebrile. In general, this patient is a well-developed, well-nourished white female in no apparent distress. HEENT exam was normal. Cardiovascular: Regular rate and rhythm, normal S1, S2, without murmurs or gallops. Lungs are clear. Abdomen: Benign. Pelvic exam: EGBUS[2] within normal limits. Vagina: Atrophic with a third degree cystocele and first to second degree rectocele. The cervix is without lesions. The uterus is small. Adnexa are nonpalpable. Rectovaginal exam is confirmatory. Extremities are without cyanosis, clubbing, or edema.

LABORATORY DATA: On admission, hematocrit was 42.3%. Postoperative hematocrit was 32%. All other labs were within normal limits. Chest x-ray and EKG were both normal.

HOSPITAL COURSE: The patient was admitted to the GYN service with the above physical examination and laboratory evaluation. The patient was taken to the operating room and underwent a total vaginal hysterectomy with anterior and posterior colporrhaphy and McCall culdoplasty. The patient progressed through a normal postoperative course, was advanced to a regular diet, and had a bowel movement prior to discharge. The patient was discharged after passing a bladder challenge test. The patient was noted to be urinating without difficulty prior to discharge. Discharge medications include Tylenol No. 3,[3] Maxzide, Minipress, and Colace. Scheduled followup is in four to six weeks in the postoperative clinic with Dr. Carter.

DISCHARGE DIAGNOSES

1. Uterovaginal prolapse, incomplete.
2. Rectocele.
3. Cystocele.
4. Essential hypertension.

PROCEDURES

1. Total vaginal hysterectomy.
2. Bilateral salpingo-oophorectomy.
3. Vaginal suspension, fixation.
4. Repair of rectocele, cystocele.
5. Electrocardiogram.
6. Chest x-ray.

ANESTHESIA: General endotracheal tube.

Footnotes:

1. <u>1.</u>This could be edited using the Arabic numerals.
2. <u>2.</u>EGBUS is a medical acronym for External Genitalia, Bartholin's glands, Urethra & Skene's glands.
3. <u>3.</u>This could be edited as Tylenol #3 (although No. 3 is the tradename).

SPELLING.

Determine if the following words are spelled correctly. If the spelling is correct, leave the word as it has already been entered. If the spelling is incorrect, provide the correct spelling.

1. uterovaginal _____

2. McAll _____

3. couldoplasty _____

4. hematecrit _____

5. atrophic _____

Matching.
Match the correct term to the definition.

1. ____ Antihypertensive drug.

2. ____ Hernia in which the urinary bladder protrudes through the wall of the vagina.

3. ____ Stool softener.

4. ____ Protrusion of the rectum into the vagina.

5. ____ A bluish discoloration of skin and mucous membranes.

A. Colace

B. rectocele

C. Minipress

D. cyanosis

E. cystocele

OB/GYN REPORT 6 – OPERATIVE NOTE

PREOPERATIVE DIAGNOSIS: Secondary infertility, secondary to bilateral tubal ligation.[1]

POSTOPERATIVE DIAGNOSIS: Secondary infertility, secondary to bilateral tubal ligation.

DRAINS: Foley catheter.

MATERIAL TO LAB: Small portion of right fallopian tube and left fallopian tube, small adhesions.

OPERATION PERFORMED: Tubal reanastomosis.

ESTIMATED BLOOD LOSS: 50 cc.

FLUIDS: 2000 cc crystalloid.

INDICATIONS: This patient is a 29-year-old female, gravida 1, para 1 with a history of bilateral tubal ligation in 2003. Diagnostic laparoscopy revealed 4-5 cm of distal tube and 1 cm of proximal tube on both sides. There were also adhesions noted on diagnostic laparoscopy. The patient is remarried and wishes to have further childbearing potential.

FINDINGS: Exploration of the abdomen revealed a normal liver edge, normal gallbladder, normal bowel, normal appendix, and normal size uterus. The left fallopian tube had adhesions between the ovary and the fallopian tube and the ovary and the left pelvic sidewall. The right ovary was essentially normal. Both fimbriated ends of the fallopian tubes appeared normal.

DESCRIPTION OF OPERATION: After adequately being counseled, the patient was taken to the operating room and placed in the supine position. The abdomen and vagina were prepped and draped in the usual sterile fashion and the HUMI manipulator placed in the cervix. A Foley catheter was also placed. A Pfannenstiel[2] skin incision was made with a scalpel and taken down to the fascia. The fascia was nicked with a scalpel and the fascial incision taken laterally on both sides with Mayo scissors. Straight Kochers were used to grasp the superior edge of the fascia, and the fascia was dissected off the rectus muscle both sharply and bluntly. This was then performed in a similar fashion inferiorly. The peritoneal lining was incised bluntly with the digits, and the peritoneal incision taken superiorly and inferiorly with Metzenbaum scissors. A Turner-Warwick retractor was placed in the incision, and two moistened laparotomy tapes were used to pack the rectus muscle, and curved blades were placed. The bowel was packed using 3 moistened laparotomy tapes. The adhesions on the left side were taken down with electrocautery, and the right tubal reanastomosis was begun by undermining the mesosalpinx beneath the fallopian tube on both sides using electrocautery. A small portion of the fallopian tube was removed from the proximal and distal segments of fallopian tube left over, and the mesosalpinx was reapproximated using interrupted stitches of 5-0 Vicryl. The mucosa of the fallopian tubes was reapproximated using interrupted stitches of 7-0 Vicryl in an interrupted fashion at 6 o'clock, 10 o'clock, 2 o'clock, and 4 o'clock. The serosa was reapproximated using interrupted stitches of 7-0 Vicryl. This was performed in a similar fashion on the left side. All laparotomy tapes and the retractor were removed from the incision and the peritoneal lining closed using a running nonlocking stitch of 0 chromic. The fascia was closed using 0 Vicryl. Staples were placed, closing the skin, and a pressure dressing was applied. The patient was awakened and extubated in the operating room and taken to the recovery room in good condition.

Footnotes:

1. 1.Secondary infertility refers to the case in which a person has conceived one or more children in the past but now is unable to conceive a child. In this person's situation, her inability to conceive a child is due to (secondary to) her previous tubal ligation.
2. 2.Pfannenstiel incision is a type of surgical incision that allows access to the abdomen. The surgeon cuts on a generally horizontal (slightly curved) line just above the pubic symphysis. This incision is commonly called the "bikini line incision" and is quite frequently used in a Cesarean section.

SPELLING.
Determine if the following words are spelled correctly. If the spelling is correct, leave the word as it has already been entered. If the spelling is incorrect, provide the correct spelling.

1. reanastimosis _____ 2. proximal _____

3. scalple _____ 4. mesosalpynx _____

5. serosa _____

Multiple Choice.
Choose the best answer.

1. There were (○ adhesions, ○ adheshuns) noted on laparoscopy.

2. Both (○ fimbriated, ○ fimbricated) ends of the fallopian tubes appeared normal.

3. The HUMI manipulator placed in the (○ cervex, ○ cervix).

4. The peritoneal lining was incised with (○ Metzenbaum, ○ Metzinbaum) scissors.

5. The bowel was packed using three moistened (○ laparatomy, ○ laparotomy) tapes.

OB/GYN REPORT 7 – OPERATIVE NOTE

PREOPERATIVE DIAGNOSIS: Transverse lie.

OPERATION PERFORMED: Primary low transverse cesarean section for transverse lie.

FINDINGS: Fetus in transverse lie with back up, with the left arm and shoulder as the presenting part and moderately difficult extraction in the breech position. Otherwise, normal anatomy and routine surgery.

COMPLICATIONS: None.

ESTIMATED BLOOD LOSS: 1000 cc.

INDICATIONS: This is a 29-year-old, now gravida 8, para 7, AB 1, Caucasian female at 34 weeks' gestation[1] by an LMP of December 21, 2006, and EDC of September 26, 2007, who presented to Dr. McArthur's office this morning at 8:30 a.m. stating that she had been contracting for the previous 7 hours. Terbutaline was administered subcutaneously which arrested the contractions. Then arrangements were made for the patient to come to Alaska Regional Hospital. Due to snowy weather and poor visibility, physicians were unable to fly out and get her. She was administered more Terbutaline, and a high-risk OB/GYN physician was in constant contact with Dr. McArthur. Finally there was a plane available in a nearby village, and the pilot agreed to pick her up and bring her to the hospital. This was done. On presentation to the hospital she was found to be completely dilated with a bulging bag. At that time vaginal exam revealed no presenting part and then an appendage was felt. Ultrasound confirmed a transverse lie. The patient was then prepared for surgery. She consented to cesarean section. Foley catheter was placed and intravenous fluids administered, and she was taken to the OR.

DESCRIPTION OF OPERATION: The patient was taken to the OR and placed in the dorsolithotomy position. General anesthesia was then administered. Her abdomen was prepped and draped in the usual sterile fashion. A Pfannenstiel skin incision was then made with a #10 scalpel and sharp dissection was used down to the fascial layer. Fascial plane was identified and then opened with scalpel and then extended with Mayo scissors laterally on both sides. Midline was identified. Peritoneum was identified with hemostats and entered with Metzenbaum scissors. The peritoneum was then extended cephalad and then caudad. Bladder flap was identified and then well developed. The lower uterine segment was well developed, and an incision was made in the lower uterine segment with some brisk bleeding at the incision site. Uterine incision was then extended manually, and initially it felt like placenta, but then a bulging bag protruded through the opening. Membranes were ruptured revealing clear fluid. The fetus' left hand and arm then came down through the opening. Exam intrauterinely revealed the fetus in a somewhat oblique position with the head in the left upper quadrant and the back up, with difficulty identifying the legs. The left leg was then identified and extracted through the uterine opening. Then with moderate difficulty the right leg was finally identified and freed from an already contracting uterus, brought through the opening, and then gently the body, right arm, and head in flexed position were eased through the uterine incision. The fetus was somewhat lethargic on the perineum and was handed off to a waiting pediatrician. It then perked up quickly in the pediatric warmer. The placenta was then manually extracted from the uterus. The placenta was explored with a clean lap. Then the uterine repair was begun. The uterine corners were identified, and then with 2 layers of 0 chromic sutures, the first interlocking and running and the second an imbricating layer, the uterine incision was closed with good hemostasis. We then found that we did have a bleeder in the left corner, quite close to the left uterine artery. This finally took 2 sutures to create hemostasis. The uterine artery was palpable adjacent to but lateral to the sutures that were placed. The gutters, cul-de-sac, and bladder flap were then irrigated and meticulously observed for any bleeders. None were found. The uterus was returned to the abdomen, and then the muscle layer was observed for any bleeders, and none were found. The fascial edges were then identified, and the fascial layer was closed with a running 0 Vicryl suture with good hemostasis. The subcutaneous tissues were then copiously irrigated, and then the skin was closed with surgical staples. A mild amount of clots were then expressed from the uterus, and the cervix was examined, and there were no clots. The patient had about 150 cc of urine out during the procedure after 4 liters of IV fluids and was presumed to be somewhat dehydrated prior to the surgery. The urine was not blood stained. The patient was somewhat slow to wake up from anesthesia, due to prolonged response to the succinylcholine, which is common in this Alaskan Native[2] population. However, approximately 20 minutes after finishing the surgery, the patient was awake enough to be transferred to the recovery room. At this time she was making clear yellow urine, was alert and oriented, and her vitals were stable. Foley catheter was in place, and she will be kept in the recovery room for an hour and then transferred to the OB unit for frequent vital signs and checking of her blood count on the first and third postoperative days. By the end of the surgery the baby was doing well and was in the newborn nursery. She was active and moving all extremities and had an initial newborn exam by the pediatricians consistent with 34 weeks' gestation.

Footnotes:

1. 1.If you can replace the possessive form ("s'") with "of" without changing the meaning, then the possessive form is correct. (34 weeks of gestation is correct and therefore the s' works.)
2. 2.The patient information in this report has been made up. The Chinese race is generally associated with a prolonged succinylcholine response.

SPELLING.

Determine if the following words are spelled correctly. If the spelling is correct, leave the word as it has already been entered. If the spelling is incorrect, provide the correct spelling.

1. sucinylcholine _____   2. fascial _____

3. cul-de-sac _____   4. bleader _____

5. Trebutaline _____

TRUE/FALSE.

Mark the following true or false.

1. The patient received no IV fluids.

   ○ true

   ○ false

2. Terbutaline was administered subcutaneously.

   ○ true

   ○ false

3. Membranes were ruptured revealing thick meconium.

   ○ true

   ○ false

4. A Pfannenstiel skin incision was made in the abdomen.

   ○ true

   ○ false

5. The placenta was then manually extracted from the uterus.

   ○ true

   ○ false

OB/GYN REPORT 8 – DISCHARGE SUMMARY

CHIEF COMPLAINT: Rule out pregnancy-induced hypertension.

HISTORY OF PRESENT ILLNESS: The patient is a 19-year-old G 1, P 0 black female with a history of very late prenatal care and an estimated date of confinement of 4 July[1] based on a 30-week ultrasound. She was seen in complicated OB clinic with an elevated blood pressure of 144/90 on the day of admission. The patient's initial blood pressures were 130s over 90s. She was noted to have a uric acid of 4.5 from a prior admission on 29 May. The patient denies headache, scotomata, right upper quadrant pain, nausea, vomiting, leakage of fluid, or vaginal bleeding.

PAST MEDICAL HISTORY: Negative, except as in HPI.

PAST SURGICAL HISTORY: Molar extractions at 14 years of age.

ALLERGIES: The patient has no known drug allergies.

REVIEW OF SYSTEMS: As per HPI.

PHYSICAL EXAMINATION: Vital signs: Temperature 98.3, pulse 116, blood pressure 144/90, height 54 inches, and weight 134 lb. Physical exam was within normal limits with the exception of abdominal exam that revealed a gravid abdomen that was nontender with active bowel sounds. Neuro exam revealed deep tendon reflexes of 3+, symmetric, without clonus.

LABORATORY DATA: Prenatal labs included a maternal blood type of B+ and a history of a positive HSV culture. Prenatal antibody screen was negative, HIV negative, rubella immune, RPR nonreactive. Laboratories on admission showed white count 12.8, hematocrit 37.3%, platelets 372,000. All other laboratories were within normal limits.

HOSPITAL COURSE: The patient was admitted to labor and delivery where she was initially monitored and found to be stable with decrease in her blood pressures from 140s over 100s to 120s over 60s with reactive fetal heart tones and no uterine activity. The patient was then transferred to 6 West. A 24-hour urine collection was begun, and the patient was begun on Aldomet and baby aspirin. The patient's blood pressures remained somewhat labile. She had an AFI of 4-5 cm with a BPP 8/8 and normal cord Dopplers. The 24-hour urine results returned with 665 mg of protein in 24 hours. The patient remained on the ward and had relatively stable blood pressures, but required an increased dose of Aldomet to 250 mg t.i.d. and persistent relative oligohydramnios. The patient had an attempted amniocentesis for LSPG which was unsuccessful. The patient's AFI remained in the 8-10 cm and antenatal testing was reassuring. On 21 May, the patient had a repeat 24 hour urine for protein with 1153 mg/24 hours noted at that time. The patient's blood pressures remained in the 130/80 range, and uric acid on 25 May was 4.5, and deep tendon reflexes were 2+/4 symmetrically. On 25 May, the patient had an ultrasound for growth scan and was noted to have an amniotic fluid index of 3.5. In the face of elevated blood pressures, proteinuria, elevated uric acid, and significantly decreased AFI, the patient was transferred to labor and delivery for possible induction. Cervical exam at the time of transfer was 4 cm, 80%, -2 station, anterior and soft for a Bishop score of 10. A bright light exam was also performed which revealed no lesions. The patient then had amniotomy and placement of internal monitors and was started on Pitocin induction. The patient progressed steadily and after a 4 hour and 48 minute first stage of labor and a 15 minute second stage of labor, went on to deliver a 2250 gm female infant with Apgars of 8/1 and 9/5.[2] The patient did require manual extraction of the placenta which was extracted intact, and there was a 3-vessel cord noted. On the first postpartum day, the patient developed a temperature to 101.4 and had minimally tender abdomen and nontender fundus. A pelvic exam revealed no masses or hematomas that were apparent and no erythema of the skin. Cultures for group B Strep, GC, Chlamydia, were obtained at that time, as were blood cultures, CBC, and UA. The patient was then started on Unasyn 1.5 gm IV q.6 hours. The patient was noted to have a white count of 23.8 and a urinalysis that revealed only 4 white blood cells and 25 red blood cells per high-powered field. All cultures taken were negative. After 2 days of antibiotics, they were stopped and the patient remained afebrile and was discharged home on postpartum day 6 in stable condition. The patient was given prescriptions for Colace, iron, Motrin, prenatal vitamins, and given instructions for regular diet, pelvic rest, and no heavy lifting for 6 weeks. The patient is to follow up with Dr. Mitchell in 6 weeks for postpartum appointment.

DISCHARGE DIAGNOSES

1. Intrauterine pregnancy at 34-4/7 weeks, delivered a 2240 gm female infant with Apgars of 8/1 and 9/5 minutes.
2. Preeclampsia, suspected.
3. Oligohydramnios.
4. Febrile morbidity, resolved.

PROCEDURES

1. Spontaneous vaginal delivery.
2. Manual extraction of the placenta.
3. Amniotomy.
4. External fetal and uterine monitoring.
5. Internal fetal and uterine monitoring.
6. Midline episiotomy and repair.
7. Obstetrical ultrasounds.
8. Antenatal testing.
9. Intravenous antibiotics.

ANESTHESIA: Local.

PATHOLOGY: None.

CONSULTS: None.

Footnotes:

1. 1.This is the military style presentation of a date. You do not use commas, but you do use Arabic numerals (4 July or even 4 July 2007).
2. 2.This would mean an Apgar score of 8 at 1 minute and 9 at 5 minutes.

SPELLING.

Determine if the following words are spelled correctly. If the spelling is correct, leave the word as it has already been entered. If the spelling is incorrect, provide the correct spelling.

1. scotomata _____

2. clonous _____

3. Aldomette _____

4. oligohydramnios _____

5. preclampsia _____

Fill in the Blank.

The following abbreviations and/or terms are used in the previous reports. Fill in the appropriate blank with either the abbreviation or its expansion.

1. EDC_____

2. HPI_____

3. AFI_____

4. deep tendon reflexes_____

5. P_____

6. SVD_____

7. gonorrhea culture_____

8. BPP_____

OB/GYN REPORT 9 – OPERATIVE NOTE

PREOPERATIVE DIAGNOSIS: Chronic pelvic pain, CIN III.[1]

POSTOPERATIVE DIAGNOSIS: Same as above.[2]

MATERIAL TO LAB: Cervical conization specimen.

OPERATION PERFORMED

1. Cervical conization.
2. Diagnostic laparoscopy.

INDICATIONS: 37-year-old white female gravida 3, para 3 with recent Pap smear in March 2005 showing high grade squamous intraepithelial lesion and colposcopically directed biopsies consistent with CIN III, with positive endocervical curettings for dysplasia. She is also describing left-sided chronic abdominal pelvic pain for greater than six months' duration.

FINDINGS: Grossly normal appearing cervix with examination under anesthesia benign. Laparoscopic examination showed a normal pelvis without evidence of adhesions, endometriosis, mass lesions, or other significant pelvic pathology. No fimbrial agglutination was noted. Fallopian tubes and ovaries bilaterally appeared normal. Cul-de-sac was free of disease.

DESCRIPTION OF OPERATION: After obtaining informed consent, the patient was taken to the operating room, and after adequate general anesthesia was induced, was placed in the low lithotomy position, prepped and draped in the usual sterile fashion. Weighted speculum was placed in the posterior vaginal fornix and a Sims retractor used to expose the cervix which was then grasped on its anterior and posterior lips using single-tooth tenacula. Hemostatic sutures of #1 chromic were used in a figure-of-eight pattern in the lateral fornices and left and right sinus to establish hemostasis. A circumferential incision of the cervical mucosa was performed, outlining the transformation zone. This was carried down to the endocervical canal using a scalpel to produce a cone-shaped cervical biopsy specimen which was submitted as a fresh specimen tagged at the 12 o'clock position. A suction Bovie device was used to obtain hemostasis which was then judged adequate at the end of the procedure. Hulka tenaculum was then placed into the uterine cavity and the retractors removed from the vagina. An infraumbilical skin incision approximately 1 cm in length was performed, through which a 10 mm trocar and sleeve were inserted into the abdominal cavity. The diagnostic laparoscope was inserted and its position inside the abdominal cavity verified by direct visualization. Approximately 3 liters of carbon dioxide gas was then insufflated, and a brief survey of the pelvic contents was performed. Suprapubic skin incision approximately 5 mm in length was performed, through which a 5 mm trocar and sleeve were inserted. The trocar was removed and a pelvic manipulator inserted. Formal survey of the pelvic contents was performed with the above-noted findings. At the end of the procedure, the operating instruments were removed from the patient's abdomen and as much carbon dioxide gas was allowed to escape as possible. The skin incisions were closed using 4-0 Vicryl suture subcutaneously in an interrupted fashion. Hulka tenaculum was removed from the patient's vagina. She was taken out of low lithotomy position. General anesthesia was reversed. She was extubated in the operating room, transported to the recovery room having tolerated the procedure well. Estimated blood loss: 100 cc. No complications. Sponge, needle, and instrument counts were correct.

Footnotes:

1. 1.Often abbreviations are expanded in the diagnosis heading. *CIN* stands for cervical intraepithelial neoplasia. This is also referred to as cervical dysplasia and caused by a sexually transmitted virus called the human papillomavirus. CIN III is the most severe precancerous change in the cervix.
2. 2.Again, many clients will require this be expanded, but some will allow the simple transcription of "same" or "same as above."

Multiple Choice.
Choose the best answer.

1. An (○ intraumbilical, ○ infraumbilical) skin incision was made.

2. Examination under anesthesia was (○ B9, ○ benign).

3. Speculum was placed in the posterior vaginal (○ fornix, ○ fornex).

4. A cone-shaped (○ cervical, ○ cervicle) biopsy specimen was submitted.

5. She was taken out of low (○ lithotimy, ○ lithotomy) position.

Matching.
Match the correct term to the definition.

1. ____ Scaly.

2. ____ A surgical clamp designed to hold or grasp tissue.

3. ____ The clumping together of cells.

4. ____ The presence of endometrium elsewhere than in the lining of the uterus.

5. ____ An instrument used for dilating.

A. speculum

B. tenaculum

C. agglutination

D. squamous

E. endometriosis

UNIT 7

Ophthalmology

OPHTHALMOLOGY – INTRODUCTION

Ophthalmology is the medical specialty that diagnoses and treats problems related to the anatomy, physiology, and pathology of the eyes and related structures.

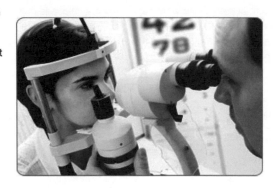

With the exception of vision correction by glasses or contact lenses, probably the most common ailment ophthalmologists diagnose and treat is cataracts. Cataract extraction with phacoemulsification and lens implantation is the most commonly performed eye surgery. A more recent development in the treatment of vision problems has been the LASIK procedure, which corrects vision anomalies by the use of lasers. In fact, the abbreviation *LASIK* is expanded as "laser-assisted in situ keratomileusis."

Other eye problems or conditions are also treated by eye specialists:

- strabismus
- glaucoma
- diplopia
- exotropia
- retinopathy

"Eye plastics" is the term used to describe the specialty of those who perform surgeries on the structures that surround the eye. Such procedures include:

- blepharoplasties
- excision of xanthelasmas and other eyelid growths
- fat pad resections
- operations on the muscles that control eye movement

Many treatments and procedures related to the eye do not require admission to the hospital. However, some do. In addition, consultations with ophthalmologists for patients who are hospitalized are not uncommon.

OPHTHALMOLOGY LANGUAGE WORKSHOP

Ophthalmology has what seems to be a language of its own. Particularly different are the ophthalmology surgical equipment terms. You will find it quite helpful to have your surgical word book or even ophthalmology word book handy as you work through this FOMS unit. If you do not have an ophthalmology word book, do not despair—there are a variety of useful and helpful online resources devoted to surgical equipment terms and ophthalmology terms.

Common Ophthalmology Root Words and Combining Forms

Root Word & Combining Form	Meaning	Example
angi/o	vessel	angiokeratoma
anter/o	anterior, before	anterograde degeneration
blephar/o	eyelid	blepharitis
canth/o	canthus	epicanthal
capsul/o	capsule	capsulorrhexis
conjunctiv/o	conjunctiva	conjunctivitis
dextr/o	right	dextrocular
dist/o	far/distant from origin	distally, distortion
hom/o	common, same	homonymous
irid/o	colored circle/iris	iridectomy
kerat/o	cornea	keratoplasty
kor/o / cor/o	pupil	anisocoria
lacrim/o	tear, crying	lacrimal
my/o	muscle	myopic
odyn/o	pain, distress	odynometer
ophthalm/o	eye	ophthalmology
phac/o / phak/o	lens	phacoemulsification
phot/o	light	photophobia
scler/o	sclera	scleritis
stigmat/o	point or mark	astigmatism
tempor/o	temple	temporalis

Common Ophthalmology Prefixes

Prefix	Meaning	Example
dys-	difficult, abnormal	dysgenesis
exo-	outside	exophthalmic
hyper-	greater than normal	hypermature
hypo-	below normal	hypopyon
iso-	equal	isometric
macro-	large	macrophthalmous
micro-	small	microvasculopathy

Common Ophthalmology Suffixes

Suffix	Meaning	Example
-algia	pain	ophthalmalgia
-cele	hernia	keratocele
-ectasia	dilation	telangiectasia
-edema	swelling	corneal edema
-ism	condition	astigmatism
-itis	inflammation	dacryocystitis
-megaly	enlargement	trichomegaly
-opia/-opsia	vision	diplopia
-pathy	disease	retinopathy
-plasty	surgical repair	blepharoplasty
-rrhexis	rupture	capsulorrhexis
-spasm	twitching	blepharospasm

Common Ophthalmology Abbreviations

Abbreviation	Expansion
BSS	balanced salt solution
DCR	dacryocystorhinostomy
ECCE	extracapsular cataract extraction (ECCE)
IOL	intraocular lens
I&A	irrigation and aspiration (irrigation-aspiration)
KPE	Kelman phacoemulsification
MVR	microvitreoretinal
OD	right eye (oculus dexter)
OS	left eye (oculus sinister)
OU	both eyes (oculus unitas)
PKP	penetrating keratoplasty

REVIEW: OPHTHALMOLOGY LANGUAGE

FIll In the Blank.
Using the word(s) in the box, enter the appropriate term in the space provided.

1. Oculus _____, or the left eye, was considered in ancient times to be the "evil eye."

2. The _____ duct is also known as the tear duct.

3. _____ means inflammation of the eyelid.

4. BSS stands for balanced _____ solution.

5. _____ is a term meaning intolerance, fear of, or aversion to light.

lacrimal
sinister
salt
photophobia
blepharitis

Multiple Choice.
Choose the best answer.

1. (○ Phacoemulsification, ○ Vitreoemulsification) is a procedure involving the lens of the eye.

2. (○ Ophthalmology, ○ Neurology) is the branch of medicine that deals with the anatomy, functions, pathology, and treatment of the eye.

3. A spasm or twitching of the eyelid is called a (○ conjunctivospasm, ○ blepharospasm).

4. Inflammation of the conjunctiva is called (○ conjunctivitis, ○ polycystitis).

5. (○ Iridectophy, ○ Iridectomy) is removal of the iris.

6. (○ Retinopathy, ○ Retinoplasty) means disease of the retina.

TRUE/FALSE.
Mark the following true or false.

1. *Hypopyon* means swelling of the eyelid.
   - ○ true
   - ○ false

2. *Dextrocular* means right ocular dominance.
   - ○ true
   - ○ false

3. *Capsulorrhexis* literally means rupture of a capsule.
   - ○ true
   - ○ false

4. Cor/o is the root word and combining form for cornea.
   - ○ true
   - ○ false

5. OD refers to both eyes.
   - ○ true
   - ○ false

OPHTHALMOLOGY REPORTS

Initially, ophthalmology is perhaps one of the most difficult specialties to edit. As with anything else, the more you do, the easier it becomes, and there is much repetition of the terms in ophthalmology reports.

One advantage to transcribing and editing ophthalmology reports is that there tends to be a limited number, perhaps only one or two, of ophthalmology doctors in any given hospital. Therefore, you can easily become familiar with the doctor's style and voice, as well as his/her standard formats, and the reports will be similar. (This, of course, may not ring true if you are transcribing and editing for a large teaching hospital.)

OPHTHALMOLOGY REPORT 1 – OPERATIVE NOTE

PREOPERATIVE DIAGNOSIS: Fracture of floor, left orbit.

ANESTHESIA: General.

POSTOPERATIVE DIAGNOSIS: Fracture of floor, left orbit.

OPERATION PERFORMED: Repair of the fracture of the floor of the left orbit.

INDICATIONS: The patient is a 32-year-old male who sustained an injury to his left orbit approximately 10 days prior to admission. He is noted to have diplopia and restriction of gaze secondary to entrapment of his inferior rectus in a fracture of the floor of the left orbit. He is here for release of the inferior rectus muscle and repair of the fracture.

DESCRIPTION OF PROCEDURE: The patient was taken to the operating room and placed in the supine position. General anesthesia was induced. The right eye was taped shut, and a shield was placed over the right eye. Prior to prepping, local anesthetic consisting of 2% Xylocaine with 1:200,000 epinephrine and 0.75% Marcaine[1] with 1 amp of Wydase was injected under the palpebral conjunctiva of the lower lid; approximately 1 cc was used. Next, the left periorbital region was prepped and draped in the normal sterile fashion. A corneal shield was placed over the globe. A malleable retractor was used to superiorly place the globe. The lower lid was retracted. The lower lid retractors and conjunctiva were incised with cutting cautery. Hemostasis was achieved with cautery. The inferior orbital rim was then exposed. A #15 blade was used to incise the periorbit along the inferior orbital rim. A Freer elevator was used to elevate the periosteum[2] from the floor of the orbit. There was noted to be a linear fracture just medial to the infraorbital groove, extending approximately 8 mm. There was noted to be soft tissue entrapped within the fracture site. The Freer elevator was used to depress the fracture nasally, and bayonet forceps were used to free the soft tissue from the fracture site. This was accomplished without difficulty. The fracture was then completely exposed and found to extend for a total of approximately 10 mm in a linear fashion. There was noted to be a slight depression over the bony fragment nasally. However, the temporal aspect of the floor was intact, as was the extreme nasal aspect of the floor. The conjunctiva was then closed with 6-0 plain gut in a running suture fashion. The corneal shield was removed. Maxitrol ointment was placed between the lids. A 4-0 silk Frost suture was placed in the lower lid and affixed to the forehead with Steri-Strips. The eye was patched. The patient tolerated the procedure well. There were no complications, and he was taken to the recovery room in good condition.

Footnotes:

1. 1. This would likely be dictated as "one to two-hundred thousand epinephrine and three-quarters percent Marcaine."
2. 2. Periosteum = The thick fibrous membrane covering the entire surface of a bone except its articular cartilage. Not to be confused with perineum or peritoneum.

SPELLING.
Determine if the following words are spelled correctly. If the spelling is correct, leave the word as it has already been entered. If the spelling is incorrect, provide the correct spelling.

1. diplopia _____

2. Marcane _____

3. Wydase _____

4. palpibral _____

5. conjunctiva _____

6. malliable _____

7. bayonette _____

8. Maxitrol _____

Matching.
Match the correct terms.

1. ____ bayonet
2. ____ Freer
3. ____ Frost
4. ____ corneal
5. ____ malleable

A. suture
B. elevator
C. shield
D. forceps
E. retractor

OPHTHALMOLOGY REPORT 2 – OPERATIVE NOTE

PREOPERATIVE DIAGNOSIS: Dislocated lens, OS,[1] with cortical cataract.

POSTOPERATIVE DIAGNOSIS: Dislocated lens, OS, with cortical cataract.

OPERATION PERFORMED
1. Kelman phacoemulsification of lens, OS.
2. Anterior vitrectomy, OS.
3. Insertion of posterior chamber intraocular lens in the sulcus with haptics at 12 o'clock and 6 o'clock.[2]

PROSTHETIC DEVICE: AMO pc11MB posterior chamber intraocular lens 6.0 mm[3] optic size, power 20.0 diopters, serial number 8675309.[4]

INDICATIONS: The patient is a 57-year-old white female with a history of trauma to the left eye as a child resulting in a slightly dislocated lens, as well as a small cortical cataract. The patient has been noticing decreasing visual acuity in the left eye with increasing glare over the past 1-2 years. Lens was removed in an attempt to improve visual acuity and decrease glare.

DESCRIPTION OF PROCEDURE: The patient was brought into the operating room and placed in the supine position. After general anesthesia was administered to the patient, Lacri-Lube was instilled under the right upper eyelid, and it was taped in place. A Fox shield was placed over the right periorbital region. The patient was then prepped and draped in the normal sterile fashion around the left periorbital region. A lid speculum was placed in the conjunctival fornices. A 4-0 silk bridle suture was then placed under the superior rectus tendon. A limbal peritomy was performed between 11 o'clock and 2 o'clock with sharp Westcott dissection. Hemostasis was maintained with cautery. A 5.5 mm partial thickness scleral incision was made between 12:30 and 11:30, approximately 2 mm posterior to the surgical limbus, with a 64 Beaver blade.[5] A tunnel incision was created the full width of this incision into clear cornea with a 66 Beaver blade. A paracentesis was made at 2:30 with a Supersharp blade into clear cornea. Using a 3-mm 5510 keratome, a V-flap incision was created at the end of the scleral tunnel into the anterior chamber. The anterior chamber was then inflated with Healon on a blunt-tip cannula. A capsulorrhexis was then performed without difficulty utilizing a bent 25-gauge cystotome needle. Hydrodissection and hydrodelineation were carried out with BSS on a 30 gauge blunt-tip cannula. The lens nucleus was phacoemulsified with the Storz premier phacoemulsification handpiece with a 30 degree phaco tip, 40% surging control maximum power. This was done without difficulty. Average phaco power was 5% with a phaco time of 38 seconds. Cortical cleanup was attempted with the irrigation/aspiration handpiece. It was noted partway through the cortical cleanup that some vitreous had come around the nasal portion of the lens where it had been dislocated, so the cortical cleanup was stopped. An anterior vitrectomy was then performed through the scleral tunnel incision with the vitrectomy handpiece. Cut rate was 400 cuts per minute with an aspiration of 115 mmHg. After this was performed, cortical cleanup again was performed. There was some difficulty getting the superior and superonasal cortical material. The capsular bag was then inflated with Healon on the blunt-tip cannula. Utilizing a J-shaped cannula on a 3 cc syringe of BSS, the superior and superonasal lens material was stripped from the capsule. The loose cortical material was then aspirated with the automated irrigation and aspiration handpiece. The vitrectomy handpiece was then inserted into the anterior chamber near the nasal aspect of the capsular bag, and a vitrectomy was performed to make sure that no other additional vitreous strands were coming around the lens. Healon was then used to push back any vitreous near the nasal portion of the capsule and also to inflate the potential space between the anterior capsule leaflet and the posterior aspect of the iris, notably the sulcus. The wound was then opened to 6 mm with the 5.1 keratome and a Supersharp blade. The pc11MB was then inserted into the anterior chamber with the inferior haptic in the sulcus with the Shepard lens forceps. The superior haptic was then gently inserted into the superior sulcus with the Kelman-McPherson forceps. The haptics were left at 6 o'clock and 12 o'clock, the IOL centered. Healon was then removed from the anterior chamber with the automated irrigation and aspiration handpiece. No vitreous was seen coming around the nasal aspect of the capsular bag. The wound was checked with a Weck-Cel[6] to make sure that all vitreous was removed from the wound and the wound was clean. The wound was then closed with a running 10-0 nylon suture in a baseball stitch fashion. The anterior chamber was then inflated with Miochol. The wound was checked and found to be watertight. It was noted that the iris constricted in a circular fashion over the edge of the optic. The silk bridle suture was removed, and the conjunctiva was closed with coaptation cautery. Dexamethasone 5 mg/mL 0.5 mL was given subconjunctivally in the inferior fornix and Fortaz 50 mg in 1/2 cc was given in the same fashion. Both were on 30-gauge needles. The patient was undraped after removing the lid speculum, and the left periorbital region was cleansed of remaining Betadine.

A collagen shield soaked in Ancef and Solu-Medrol was then inserted on top of the corneal epithelium, and Maxitrol ophthalmic ointment was instilled into the left upper eyelid. An eyepad and Fox shield were then placed over the closed left eyelid. The patient was awakened from general anesthesia. The patient tolerated the procedure well. There were no complications. The patient was transferred to the recovery room in stable condition.

Footnotes:

1. 1.OS is the abbreviation for left eye. This is considered a "dangerous abbreviation" by ISMP. Some clients may require this be expanded out to "left eye," but many will not.
2. 2.Remember when indicating location, "o'clock" is used instead of the ":00." However, when the clock-face orientation is expressed as a partial hour, omit the word o'clock, even if dictated.
3. 3.A trailing zero (a zero after a whole number) is used frequently with precision measurements.
4. 4.This serial number has been changed to protect patient identity—did you recognize Jenny's number?
5. 5.There is a "Beaver" blade typically used with the eye (although not exclusively) and a "Deaver" blade used vaginally. Sometimes it is hard to tell what is being dictated by sound alone, but context should help you make the call between Beaver and Deaver.
6. 6.This is a trademark name and should be spelled "Weck-Cel," although some resource books may have it listed as Weck-cel.

SPELLING.
Determine if the following words are spelled correctly. If the spelling is correct, leave the word as It has already been entered. If the spelling is incorrect, provide the correct spelling.

1. McPhearson _____

2. vitrectomy _____

3. Lacri-Lube _____

4. Veeflap _____

5. decsamethasone _____

6. Fortaz _____

Multiple Choice.
Choose the correct spelling of the term.

1. The making of a continuous circular tear in the anterior part of the lens capsule.

   ○ cappsulorrhexis

   ○ cappsulorrhexis

   ○ capsullorhexis

   ○ capsulorrhexis

2. The mucous membrane that lines the inner surface of the eyelids.

   ○ conjunctiva

   ○ conjuncteva

   ○ conjuntiva

   ○ conjentiva

3. Clouding of the natural lens of the eye.

   ○ catiract

   ○ cateract

   ○ catarect

   ○ cataract

4. The protein substance of the white fibers of skin, tendon, bone, cartilage and all other connective tissue.

   ○ colligen

   ○ collagen

   ○ collagan

   ○ collegan

5. Relating to or based on the sense of touch.

   ○ haptac

   ○ haptec

   ○ haptic

   ○ haptaec

OPHTHALMOLOGY REPORT 3 – DISCHARGE SUMMARY

CHIEF COMPLAINT: Epiphora,[1] OD.

HISTORY OF PRESENT ILLNESS: The patient is a 30-year-old Hawaiian female who complains of constant tearing from her right eye since November 2001. She is status post ethmoidectomy and sphenoidectomy on the right in June 1999 in Korea. She is also noted to have a blocked nasal lacrimal duct by examination at Sacred Heart Hospital and was sent here for further evaluation.

PAST MEDICAL HISTORY: She denies the use of tobacco or alcohol. Family history is positive for diabetes in her father. Past medical history: Chronic sinusitis; allergic rhinitis; reactive airway disease, exercise induced; recurrent hives, idiopathic; and hypertension. Past surgical history: Right ethmoidectomy, sphenoidectomy June 1999. She is also status post maxillary sinus drainage in January 1999. She is status post bilateral maxillary windows, status post appendectomy, TAH/BSO secondary to fibroids in 1996. Her medications include Premarin 0.625 mg q.d., Hismanal 10 mg q.d., Enalapril 10 mg q.a.m. and 5 mg q.p.m., normal saline nasal spray, Vancenase nasal spray, Septra 1 p.o. b.i.d., Afrin 1 spray t.i.d. SHE IS ALLERGIC TO CEPHALOSPORIN.[2]

PHYSICAL EXAMINATION: Physical exam other than ocular was within normal limits. Visual acuity with correction 20/20-, OU, tonometry of applanation at 14, 15, 11, and 14 mmHg respectively. External exam is normal, OU. Lids, lashes are normal OU. Puncta appear to be open. Lid margins are well opposed to the globe. She does have an increased tear lake temporally in the right eye. Conjunctivae: She has a pinguecula, OD, clear OS. Cornea: Clear OU, anterior chamber deep and quiet OU, lens clear OU. Dilated fundus exam: Cup-to-disc 0.2, OU, with a normal rim, OU. Macula is normal, OU. Nasal lacrimal duct probe and irrigation noted in the right eye. She is noted to have a hard stop with probing of the inferior canaliculus. Irrigation of the superior puncta: There is backflow through the inferior puncta; with irrigation inferiorly, there is noted to be backflow through the superior puncta, OS. Nasal lacrimal canaliculus was probed easily. With irrigation, she is noted to have flow in her nasopharynx. Schirmer's with fluoros are 15 mm and 20 mm respectively.

REVIEW OF SYSTEMS: Positive for chronic nasal congestion with a yellow discharge since November 2001. Otherwise noncontributory.

HOSPITAL COURSE: She is admitted for right dacryocystorhinostomy. Her preoperative evaluation including CBC and chem-7[3] was normal. Chest x-ray reveals no acute disease. EKG shows no change from June 1999. She is noted to have normal sinus rhythm, possible left atrial enlargement with a nonspecific T-wave abnormality and a prolonged QT. She was taken to the operating room on December 22, 2001. Procedure performed was right DCR. She tolerated the procedure well. There were no complications. Her postoperative course was without complication. During her hospitalization she was also evaluated by the ENT service and they placed her on antibiotics for her perioperative period. She was also evaluated by the allergy service during her hospitalization. They increased the Vancenase and recommended followup with the allergist at home following her discharge. On December 28, she was discharged using Maxitrol drops and ointment twice a day in her right eye and along the incision. She has done well and has noted resolution of her symptoms of epiphora. She notes slight discomfort near the scar. Her exam prior to discharge: Visual acuity 20/20-, OU. Examination of the incision: There is no erythema or induration. There is a slightly raised firm area under the scar which is consistent with scar formation. The silicone tubes placed during surgery were in good position between the puncta. The pinguecula is noted nasally, and the conjunctiva appears to be slightly enlarged. Her exam is otherwise unchanged from her preoperative evaluation.

DISCHARGE DIAGNOSES

1. Epiphora.
2. Chronic sinusitis.
3. Hypertension.
4. Reactive airway disease secondary to exercise.
5. Idiopathic hives.
6. Allergic rhinitis.

PROCEDURES: Right dacryocystorhinostomy.

DISCHARGE MEDICATIONS: Tears as needed. She is to continue her medications as noted in her past medical history.

Footnotes:

1. 1.If you aren't sure what this is, look it up. It is the chief complaint of this patient and if you don't know what it is, you won't be able to follow the report.
2. 2.Some clients will prefer allergy information always be separated out and presented under an ALLERGY heading. Without specific instruction, there are a variety of ways this information could be presented correctly.
3. 3.Chem-7 is an older term for the BMP (basic metabolic panel).

SPELLING.

Determine if the following words are spelled correctly. If the spelling is correct, leave the word as it has already been entered. If the spelling is incorrect, provide the correct spelling.

1. epifora _____

2. premaren _____

3. Hismannle _____

4. Vancenase _____

5. sephalosporin _____

6. tonometry _____

7. aplanation _____

8. puncta _____

9. pingucula _____

10. maccula _____

11. Schirmer's _____

12. dacrosistorrhinostomy _____

Fill in the Blank.

The following abbreviations and/or terms are used in the previous reports. Fill in the appropriate blank with either the abbreviation or its expansion.

1. no acute distress_____

2. OS_____

3. mmHg_____

4. complete blood count_____

5. OD_____

6. TAH/BSO_____

7. ears, nose, and throat_____

OPHTHALMOLOGY REPORT 4 – OPERATIVE NOTE

PREOPERATIVE DIAGNOSIS: Left epiretinal membrane.

OPERATION PERFORMED: Left pars plana vitrectomy and membrane peeling.

INDICATIONS: The patient is a 58-year-old man with progressive decreased visual acuity in the left eye associated with distorted vision. The cause of vision loss is epiretinal membrane. The natural history of his condition and the risks and benefits of surgical treatment were reviewed with him, including possible risk of total loss of vision in the eye or loss of the eye, as well as complications from anesthesia. He expressed his understanding of these issues and asked that the following operation be performed.

DESCRIPTION OF PROCEDURE: In the supine position under general anesthesia, the left eye was prepped and draped. A lid speculum was placed. A 3-port pars plana vitrectomy was performed through limited conjunctival peritomies. First a 4-mm infusion cannula was secured in the inferotemporal quadrant with a preplaced 6-0 Vicryl suture. The cannula tip was identified through the pupil before beginning infusion of BSS+, and then 2 superior sclerostomies were made. Each of the sclerostomies was 3.5 mm from the limbus. A Landers contact lens system was used. The contact lens ring was secured at the corneal limbus with 3 partial thickness 6-0 Vicryl sutures. Goniosol provided interface between contact lens and cornea. Pars plana vitrectomy was then done. The vitreous anatomy was that of a synergetic liquid vitreous cavity in front of the macula. No definite posterior vitreous detachment was seen; rather, cortical vitreous was still present on the surface of the temporal macula. After removing the central vitreous gel, Grieshaber mini-diamond-dusted end-biting forceps were used to grasp the epiretinal membrane in the temporal macula. The membrane was then slowly and gently elevated from the retina. It separated from the center of the macula. The membrane had peripheral attachments along the superior and inferior arcades. As the membrane was lifted, it tore, leaving peripheral macular epiretinal membranes. These were regrasped with the forceps and completely separated from the macula. A membrane remnant was left at the inferior temporal arcade, but this area did not have any distortion of the retinal anatomy and therefore was felt to be clinically insignificant, and no further peeling was performed. During the membrane peeling, 2 small petechial hemorrhages occurred in the superior nasal macula and a small self-limited epiretinal hemorrhage occurred in the temporal macula. This was so small it only appeared as a rose-colored blush. The membranes were removed from the eye with forceps or with the vitrectomy instrument. The contact lens ring was removed. The sclerostomies were closed with 7-0 Maxon suture. The infusion cannula was removed and that sclerostomy also sutured. Small knuckles of vitreous gel were trimmed from each sclerostomy site before closure. Indirect ophthalmoscopy confirmed that the retina was completely attached, and there were no retinal tears behind the sclerostomies. Next, 4 cc of 0.75% Marcaine[1] solution were irrigated in the inferotemporal and superotemporal meridians into posterior sub-Tenon space using 19-gauge cannula. Conjunctiva was closed with 6-0 plain collagen suture. Subconjunctival Fortaz 50 mg and Kenalog 20 mg were injected. The eye was dressed with Atropine[2] eyedrops and Maxitrol ointment. An eye patch was placed, and the patient was awakened and taken to recovery room in good condition. At the beginning of surgery, the patient received 500 mg IV Vancomycin and 125 mg IV Solu-Medrol. Throughout the operation, the retina was protected as much as possible from light sources.

Footnotes:

1. 1.This is likely dictated as three-quarters percent Marcaine, but should always be edited as 0.75%.
2. 2.Both atropine and vancomycin are generic drugs and should be transcribed in lower case letters. However, these are actual reports from the workplace and it may be that an employer is not going to be too concerned with the capitalization.

Fill in the Blank.
Using the word(s) in the box, enter the appropriate term in the space provided.

epiretinal membrane
ophthalmoscope
peritomy
sclerostomy
vitrectomy

1. The surgical formation of an external opening in the sclera is called a _____ .

2. Surgical extraction of the contents of the vitreous chamber of the eye is called a

   _____ .

3. Surgical incision of the conjunctiva and subconjunctival tissue about the whole circumference of the

   cornea is called a _____ .

4. A membrane or scar on the vitreal surface of the retina often resulting in marked loss of vision is

   called _____ .

5. A/an _____ is a medical instrument for examining the retina of the eye.

True/False.
Mark the following true or false.

1. The patient has decreased vision in the right eye.

    ○ true

    ○ false

2. DeBakey mini-diamond-dusted forceps were used to grasp the epiretinal membrane.

    ○ true

    ○ false

3. The patient was given 4 cc of Marcaine solution at the end of the procedure.

    ○ true

    ○ false

4. Kenalog was given in tablet form.

    ○ true

    ○ false

5. The patient was taken to the recovery room in good condition.

    ○ true

    ○ false

OPHTHALMOLOGY REPORT 5 – DISCHARGE SUMMARY

CHIEF COMPLAINT: Decreasing visual acuity, OD, secondary to a retinal detachment.

HISTORY OF PRESENT ILLNESS: The patient is a 65-year-old white male who is status post PKP[1] for a bullous keratopathy of his right eye in February. On followup exam in March he complained of decreasing visual acuity. Dilated fundus exam was positive for rhegmatogenous retinal detachment with a retinal hole at 10 o'clock. He was treated with cryotherapy and pneumatic retinopexy. On followup evaluation, the fundus exam showed a residual inferior bullous retinal detachment. He is admitted for repair of the retinal detachment with a scleral buckle and cryotherapy or diathermy as needed.

PAST MEDICAL HISTORY: Positive for 2 vessel coronary artery bypass graft, positive for hypertension. He has a history of colon polyps with multiple benign biopsies. He has no diabetes and no history of a myocardial infarction.

PAST SURGICAL HISTORY

1. Left total knee arthroplasty.
2. Status post PKP, OD in February.
3. Status post intracapsular cataract extractions with secondary intraocular chamber IOLs, OU.
4. Status post appendectomy.
5. Status post bilateral inguinal hernia repair.
6. Status post right shoulder and right foot surgery.

SOCIAL HISTORY: He admits to occasional alcohol use and 1 pack per day times 50 years of smoking.[2]

ALLERGIES: HE IS ALLERGIC TO PENICILLIN.

MEDICATIONS: His medications include Colace 100 mg b.i.d., Cimetidine 400 mg b.i.d., Enalapril 10 mg q.d., hydrochlorothiazide 25 mg 1/2 tablet p.o. q.d.

REVIEW OF SYSTEMS: Noncontributory.

PHYSICAL EXAMINATION: Other than ocular, within normal limits except to have noted a 3/6 systolic ejection murmur on his cardiovascular exam. Visual acuity without corrections: Count fingers in his right eye; with correction his left eye is 20/25. Tonometry with a Tono-pen at 1350 is 20 mmHg. Slit lamp exam OD: Conjunctiva is 2+, subconjunctival hemorrhage. The corneal epithelium is noted to be intact. The graft is clear. Anterior chambers: Deep and quiet, dilated for this exam. There is an inferior bullous detachment located inferotemporally. A hole is not identified preoperatively. The patient is admitted for repair of the retinal detachment.

LABORATORY DATA: EKG shows normal sinus rhythm with first degree AV block and a nonspecific interventricular block. T-wave abnormality. There is no change from February. He was evaluated preoperatively by Cardiology,[3] and there is found to be no contraindication to surgery. Chest x-ray reveals no acute disease. CBC and BMP are within normal limits. With his history of total knee arthroplasty, he will be given SBE prophylaxis using 500 mg of IV vancomycin intraoperatively and Keflex p.o. postoperatively.

HOSPITAL COURSE: The patient was taken to the operating room on March 17. Procedures performed included right scleral buckle, cryopexy, and drainage of subretinal fluid. The patient tolerated the procedure well, and there were no complications. His hospital course was without complications. His exam prior to discharge revealed visual acuity without correction 20, light perception with projection OD. Tonometry with a Tono-pen at 1600 was 16 mm of mercury. Slit lamp exam OD. Lid, lashes: Decreasing edema. Conjunctiva: 2+ injection. Cornea: Epithelium is intact. Anterior chamber: There is noted to be vitreous at 2 o'clock and 8 o'clock in the anterior chamber. The ACIOL is in good position. The anterior chamber is otherwise deep with 1+ cell and flare. Dilated fundus exam: He is noted to have a residual frontal detachment with choroidal effusions noted superiorly.

DISCHARGE DIAGNOSES

1. Rhegmatogenous retinal detachment, OD.
2. Coronary artery disease.
3. Hypertension.

PROCEDURES

1. Scleral buckle.
2. Cryopexy.
3. Drainage of subretinal fluid, OD.

DISCHARGE MEDICATIONS: The patient is to include the oral medications as noted in his past medical history. His ocular medications include Maxitrol drops q.i.d. OD, scopolamine 0.25% b.i.d. OD, Pred Forte 1% b.i.d. OD. He is to take Tylenol with codeine 1-2 p.o. q.4-6 hours p.r.n. pain. He is to follow up on March 29, 2002, with Ophthalmology.

Footnotes:

1. 1.PKP = penetrating keratoplasty.
2. 2.This is the equivalent of a 50-pack-year smoking history. Although the way it was edited and 50-pack-year is the same thing, you wouldn't convert to this way of presenting the information unless your account required it be presented this way. You should always present the information the way it is dictated.
3. 3.This is capped because they are referring to it as an entity. This, however, is a style issue. Without specific instruction on capping clinic or department names, it would be perfectly acceptable for it to be edited with initial lower cap.

SPELLING.
Determine if the following words are spelled correctly. If the spelling is correct, leave the word as it has already been entered. If the spelling is incorrect, provide the correct spelling.

1. karatopathy _____
2. regmatogenous _____
3. retinopexy _____
4. diathermy _____
5. Simetidine _____
6. Scopolamine _____
7. Preid Fort _____

Fill in the Blank.
The following abbreviations and/or terms are used in the previous reports. Fill in the appropriate blank with either the abbreviation or its expansion.

1. myocardial infarction_____
2. PKP_____
3. AV_____
4. intraocular lens_____
5. OD_____
6. DCR_____
7. left eye_____
8. OU_____
9. anterior chamber intraocular lens_____
10. millimeters of mercury_____

OPHTHALMOLOGY REPORT 6 – OPERATIVE NOTE

PREOPERATIVE DIAGNOSIS: Bilateral upper lid ptosis.

POSTOPERATIVE DIAGNOSIS: Bilateral upper lid ptosis.

OPERATION PERFORMED: Bilateral upper lid levator aponeurosis tuck.

PROSTHETIC DEVICES: None.

INDICATIONS: The patient is a 49-year-old white male who complains of droopy upper eyelids that have interfered with his vision for most of his life.

DESCRIPTION OF PROCEDURE: The patient was brought to the operating room and placed in the supine position. The patient received 1 drop of Tetracaine anesthetic in his cornea, and his upper and lower eyelids were cleaned with 70% isopropyl alcohol on both sides. Utilizing brilliant green dye, the pupil position as straight ahead gaze was marked on both upper lids and onto both eyebrows. The natural eyelid crease in both eyes was approximately 8 mm and equal so both upper eyelid creases were marked with brilliant green dye starting at the lateral to the medial lash margins. The patient received local anesthesia. Approximately 0.3 cc was[1] used per side infiltrated subcutaneously along the eyelid crease markings. The anesthesia mixture consisted of 50% of 2% Xylocaine with 1:100,000 epinephrine and 0.75% Marcaine with 1 amp of Wydase per 10 cc and 8.4 mEq of bicarb per 10 cc. The patient was prepped and draped in the standard sterile fashion and corneal shields placed over both corneas. The patient's right upper eyelid was incised with a #15 blade along the brilliant green dye eyelid crease marking. The subcutaneous tissue was tented with 0.5 forceps and sharply dissected with Westcott scissors down to the orbital septum. At all times the fat bulge from the preaponeurotic fat was identified. The orbital septum was incised and bluntly dissected with Westcott scissors and cut along the eyelid markings to free up the preaponeurotic fat. This fat was retracted with a Desmarres retractor and the levator aponeurosis identified. Any remaining thin membranous connective tissue connecting fat to levator aponeurosis was bluntly dissected away with Westcott scissors. A 6-0 nylon suture on a cutting CE-2 needle was placed horizontally starting approximately 2 mm nasal to the pupillary marking into the levator aponeurosis at approximately the level of the superior edge of the tarsus. This suture was also run through the levator aponeurosis approximately 10 mm superior to the original stitch. This was then pulled tight and tied with a slipknot, effectively folding the levator aponeurosis. The patient's skin was laid in its natural position and the corneal shield was removed. The patient was evaluated in all positions of gaze, and his current eyelid height was approximately superior limbus with good eyelid contour. This incision site was covered with saline-soaked gauze and a similar procedure performed on the left upper lid. The skin was incised with a #15 surgical blade, and while maintaining visualization of the preaponeurotic fat bulge, the orbicularis was sharply dissected down to preaponeurotic fat. This was bluntly dissected and the orbicularis cut with Westcott scissors along the upper eyelid incision site. The preaponeurotic fat was retracted back with Desmarres retractor, and any remaining membranous tissue between fat and levator aponeurosis was bluntly dissected with Westcott scissors. The inferior edge of the incision site, which consisted of the edge of the orbicularis overlying the levator and tarsus, was bluntly dissected away from the levator aponeurosis to free up the mobility. In a similar procedure, a 6-0 nylon suture on a cutting CE-2 needle was placed horizontally a few millimeters inferior to the superior edge of the tarsus through the levator aponeurosis. The suture was placed approximately 2 mm nasal to the pupillary marking. A similar stitch was placed superiorly into the levator aponeurosis and tied with a slipknot, effectively tucking the levator aponeurosis. Corneal shields were removed, and the patient's lid heights were evaluated in all positions of cardinal gaze. The height evaluated was then adjusted by removing the slipknot and taking deeper, shallower bites as needed through the levator aponeurosis. Once the final lid height was determined to be at superior limbus and good contour was obtained, the 6-0 nylon suture was tied and cut. The slipknot on the right upper eyelid was also tied and cut at this time. Skin edges were approximated on both sides with running suture of 6-0 fast absorbing gut on a conventional cutting PC-1 needle. The patient was dressed with bacitracin ophthalmic ointment and no patches were placed.

The patient was discharged in the postoperative recovery room after tolerating this procedure well. Immediately in the postop recovery room ice packs were placed on both upper lids. The patient was instructed to keep ice on as much as possible at least 1/2 hour per hour for the remaining waking hours tonight. Following recovery, the patient was discharged to home with instructions to follow up with Dr. Baker at 11:15 a.m. on 11 March 2003 in the ophthalmology clinic. The patient was given further instructions to return to the emergency room if there was any significant pain, swelling, or discharge. The patient's discharge medications include bacitracin ophthalmic ointment to be placed along the incision sites q.i.d. and Tylenol #3 take 1-2 tablets p.o. q.4-6 hours as needed for pain.

Footnotes:

1. 1.Units of measurement are treated as a singular collective group. You wouldn't say 2 cc **were**, rather 2 cc **was**.

SPELLING.

Determine if the following words are spelled correctly. If the spelling is correct, leave the word as it has already been entered. If the spelling is incorrect, provide the correct spelling.

1. pitosis _____

2. preaponeurotic _____

3. pupilary _____

4. orbicularis _____

5. limbis _____

Matching.
Match the correct terms.

1. ____ Desmarres

2. ____ Westcott

3. ____ Tetracaine

4. ____ corneal

5. ____ saline-soaked

A. anesthetic

B. shields

C. scissors

D. gauze

E. retractor

OPHTHALMOLOGY REPORT 7 – DISCHARGE SUMMARY

CHIEF COMPLAINT: Glaucoma.

HISTORY OF PRESENT ILLNESS: The patient is a 67-year-old male with a history of glaucoma. He is status post trabeculectomy OS in September 1996. He is noted to have continued increased ocular pressure in his right eye despite medications which include Timoptic, Pilogel, and Neptazane.

SOCIAL HISTORY: The patient denies the use of alcohol and tobacco.

FAMILY HISTORY: Negative for glaucoma.

PAST MEDICAL HISTORY: Positive for PPD test secondary to a vaccine, positive for glaucoma.

PAST SURGICAL HISTORY: Trabeculectomy OS September 1996.

ALLERGIES: No known drug allergies.

MEDICATIONS: Timoptic 0.5% b.i.d. OD, Pilogel q.h.s. OD, Diamox[1] 500 mg p.o. b.i.d.

REVIEW OF SYSTEMS: Noncontributory.

PHYSICAL EXAMINATION: Other than ocular is within normal limits. Ocular exam: Visual acuity with correction 20/20 OU. Tonometry: By applanation at 1612, 20, and 12 mm of mercury respectively. Lid, lashes: Normal OU. Conjunctiva: Clear OD. He is noted to have a diffuse bleb with a cystic bleb noted at 11 o'clock OS. There is a remaining suture at 11 o'clock which has been covered with epithelium. Cornea is clear OU. There are no Krukenberg's spindles. Iris is normal OU. No transillumination OU. He has a PI at 11 o'clock OS. Gonioscopy: 360 degrees of 3+ open angle to ciliary body OU. Sclerostomy is open at 11 o'clock OS. Dilated fundus exam: Cup-to-disc 0.4 OD, 0.9 OS. Macula is normal in both eyes.

HOSPITAL COURSE: The patient was taken to the operating room on October 18, 1997. Procedure performed: Trabeculectomy with 5 fluorouracil OD. The patient tolerated the procedure well, and there were no complications. The patient's postoperative course during hospitalization was complicated with continued positive Seidel's sign which necessitated wound revision, on October 20, and again on October 23, 1997. Following the second bleb revision, he had a persistent epithelial defect; however, the Seidel's remained negative. He was treated with antibiotic soaked collagen shields, as well as topical Pred Forte, Voltaren, and antibiotic drops alternating between Ciloxan and TobraDex. Once the epithelial defect healed, he received subconjunctival 5 fluorouracil injections for a total of 52.5 mg of 5FU. Each injection was 7.5 mg of 5FU. The patient tolerated this well and maintained an intraocular pressure of approximately 11 mm of mercury, and his epithelium remained intact. His exam prior to discharge was visual acuity in his right eye of 20/40, pinhole to 20/20-. Tonometry by applanation was 10 and 13 mm of mercury respectively. The pupil is noted to be round in his right eye. Slit lamp exam of his right eye is noted to have a shallow bleb at approximately 2 o'clock with a PI at 2 o'clock. The anterior chamber is deep and quiet. There is irregular corneal epithelium noted midperipherally at approximately 8 o'clock. The epithelium is otherwise intact.

DISCHARGE DIAGNOSIS: Glaucoma.

PROCEDURES

1. Trabeculectomy OD.
2. Bleb revision.
3. Repeat bleb revision.
4. Multiple injections of 5 fluorouracil for a total of 52.5 mg.

DISCHARGE MEDICATIONS: Pred Forte q.2 hours OD.

DISPOSITION: The patient is discharged to follow up with Dr. Perry Cox in Ophthalmology one week following his discharge.

Footnotes:

1. 1.Report shows Neptazane in HPI and Diamox under Medications. It might make sense to flag this for clarification from the client since they are not the same medication.

SPELLING.

Determine if the following words are spelled correctly. If the spelling is correct, leave the word as it has already been entered. If the spelling is incorrect, provide the correct spelling.

1. Pillogel _____

2. Neptazane _____

3. Krukenburg's _____

4. gonioscopy _____

5. florouracil _____

6. Seidel's _____

7. Voltaren _____

Multiple Choice.
Choose the best answer.

1. Glaucoma is increased pressure in the eyeball due to (◯ obstruction, ◯ increases) of the outflow of aqueous humor.

2. The patient had a persistent (◯ epithelial, ◯ collagen) defect.

3. Exam revealed no (◯ Kreutzmann, ◯ Krukenberg's) spindles.

4. Slit lamp exam of his right eye is noted to have a shallow (◯ blurb, ◯ bleb) .

5. Conjunctivae are clear (◯ OD, ◯ AD) .

OPHTHALMOLOGY REPORT 8 – OPERATIVE NOTE

PREOPERATIVE DIAGNOSIS: Lower lid dermatochalasis, OU.

POSTOPERATIVE DIAGNOSIS: Fat prolapse lower eyelids, OU.

OPERATION PERFORMED: Bilateral transconjunctiva lower lid blepharoplasty.

PROSTHETIC DEVICES: None.

INDICATIONS: The patient is a 33-year-old white male complaining of fat prolapse in both lower lids for years.

DESCRIPTION OF PROCEDURE: The patient was brought into the operating room and placed in the supine position. The patient received Tetracaine anesthetic drops to both corneas, and corneal shields were placed. The patient's upper and lower eyelids were cleaned with 70% isopropyl alcohol on both sides. The patient received local anesthesia consisting of a 50% mixture of 2% Xylocaine with 1:100,000 epinephrine and 0.75% Marcaine with 1 amp of Wydase and 8.4 mEq of bicarb per 10 cc. The patient received an infraorbital nerve block on both sides with approximately 2 cc of local anesthesia per side. Following this, the patient received a subconjunctival injection into both lower eyelids through the lid retractor muscles with approximately 1.5 to 2 cc per side. The patient also received subcutaneous infiltration into both lower eyelids of approximately 2 cc per side. The patient was prepped and draped in the standard sterile fashion. Utilizing electrocautery, the conjunctiva of his right lower lid was incised inferior to the tarsal plate. This incision was continued with electrocautery through the lower lid retractors. This incision site was sharply dissected while maintaining position over the fat bulge. Sharp dissection continued down to fat. Any membranes around the fat lobules were bluntly dissected away to free up the fat. Tarsal fat was clamped with hemostats, cut with Westcott scissors, cauterized with thermocautery unit, and finally cauterized with electrocautery after removal of the hemostats. Good hemostasis was maintained throughout the operation. This procedure was continued with the remaining fat bulges until sufficient amount of fat was removed. Fat was identified at all times, as well as the inferior oblique muscle. Following removal of what was determined to be an adequate amount of fat, the patient's eyelid was placed in its natural position and covered with a saline-soaked gauze. Using a similar procedure, the left lower eyelid was incised through the conjunctiva inferior to the tarsal plate, using the electrocautery unit, through the lid retractor muscles. This incision site was bluntly and sharply dissected down to fat while maintaining position over the fat bulge. Again, the inferior oblique muscle was identified and care taken not to incise the muscle. The fat was removed using a similar procedure as with the right eyelid, consisting of clamping and cutting followed by thermocautery and electrocautery. Once a sufficient amount of fat was removed and found to be approximately equivalent to the amount of fat removed from the right lower lid, the skin in the left lid was placed in its natural position. Following assurance of good hemostasis and visual evaluation of the amount of fat removed and the skin position, the patient was dressed with bacitracin ophthalmic ointment to both lower cul-de-sacs. The patient was transferred to the postop recovery room in stable condition. The patient tolerated the procedure well. The patient was discharged to home following recovery. Discharge instructions include bacitracin ophthalmic ointment to both lower cul-de-sacs q.i.d. and ice to both lower lids as much as possible for the rest of the day while awake. Discharge medicines include bacitracin ophthalmic ointment and Tylenol No. 3 one to two tablets p.o. q.4-6 hours as needed for pain. Additional instructions include to return to the emergency room if there is any significant pain, swelling, or discharge.

SPELLING.
Determine if the following words are spelled correctly. If the spelling is correct, leave the word as it has already been entered. If the spelling is incorrect, provide the correct spelling.

1. dermatichalasis _____

2. oblicque _____

3. thermocautery _____

4. blephiroplasty _____

5. infraorbital _____

Multiple Choice.
Choose the best answer.

1. (○ Ice, ○ Heat)is to be used on both lower lids for the rest of the day.

2. The patient received(○ topical, ○ local)anesthesia consisting of Xylocaine with epinephrine and Marcaine.

3. Utilizing (○ scissors, ○ electrocautery)the conjunctivae of the right lower lid was incised inferiorly.

4. The patient received (○ tetracaine, ○ lidocaine)anesthetic drops to both corneas.

5. Discharge medications included bacitracin ointment and (○ Tylenol, ○ Lortab)as needed for pain.

OPHTHALMOLOGY REPORT 9 – PROCEDURE NOTE

INDICATIONS: Decreased visual acuity.

DESCRIPTION OF PROCEDURE: The patient was brought to the surgical suite in the supine position. After IV sedation was given, a retrobulbar injection of a 50/50 mix of 0.75% Marcaine and 2% Xylocaine with 1:200,000 epinephrine and 150 units of Wydase was given. Gentle palpation on the globe after this injection failed to reveal any evidence of retrobulbar hemorrhage. After adequate akinesia had been verified, Honan's cuff was placed over the eye and left in place for approximately 10 minutes. The patient was then scrubbed and draped in the usual sterile fashion. Lid speculum was placed and a bridle suture placed in the superior rectus of the right eye. A superior conjunctival peritomy was then placed. A 64 surgical blade was used to remove residual tenons and episcleral vessels, followed by wet-field cautery, assuring good hemostasis across the surgical field. Calipers were set and verified at 5 mm. This was measured off at a position 2 mm back from the surgical limbus. A partial thickness scleral groove using 64 surgical blade was then placed at that position. A 66 surgical blade developed a scleral tunnel from this initial incision to clear cornea. A Supersharp blade was used at the 2 o'clock position to enter the anterior chamber. A 55-10 blade keratome was then used to enter the anterior chamber at the 12 o'clock position through the scleral tunnel. This allowed introduction of the 25 gauge cystotome on a Healon syringe and reformation of the anterior chamber with Healon. After this step a continuous tear circular capsulorrhexis capsulotomy was then placed. Hydrodissection was then conducted with visualization of good posterior fluid wave. Phacoemulsification of the lens nucleus was then conducted with automated irrigation/aspiration of residual cortex material. This was without violation of the posterior capsule. Healon was then reintroduced into the anterior chamber and into the capsular bag. This allowed safe placement of the intraocular lens, specifically a Pharmacia model 810 F power +22 diopter intraocular lens, rotating this lens and leaving the haptics in a horizontal position. Residual Healon was removed using the automated irrigation/aspiration unit. Miostat was then introduced into the anterior chamber through the paracentesis site. The paracentesis site was noted to have a positive Seidel's, necessitating placement of an interrupted suture at this position. Additionally, horizontal 10-0 nylon suture was placed in the scleral tunnel. After these maneuvers the wounds were noted to be watertight. Bacitracin, gentamicin, and Maxitrol ointment were placed in the conjunctival fornices. Soft pressure patch was placed over the eye, and a Fox shield was placed. The patient tolerated the procedure well and was transported to the recovery room in stable condition.

SPELLING

Determine if the following words are spelled correctly. If the spelling is correct, leave the word as it has already been entered. If the spelling is incorrect, provide the correct spelling.

1. retrobulber _____

2. akinesia _____

3. scleril _____

4. capsulorhexis _____

5. Miostat _____

True/False.
Mark the following true or false.

1. The patient was seen for decreased visual acuity.

   ○ true

   ○ false

2. A full thickness sclera groove was placed 2 mm back from the surgical limbus.

   ○ true

   ○ false

3. A +32 diopter intraocular lens was placed.

   ○ true

   ○ false

4. The Honan's cuff was left in place for approximately 10 minutes.

   ○ true

   ○ false

5. The keratome entered the anterior chamber at the 3 o'clock position.

   ○ true

   ○ false

UNIT 8

Orthopedics

ORTHOPEDICS – INTRODUCTION

Orthopedics is the medical specialty concerned with the preservation and/or restoration of the function of the skeletal system, its articulations (joints), and associated structures such as ligaments and muscles. The orthopedic specialist evaluates and treats primarily the bones of the limbs—the arms and legs. The bones of the spine and the cranium are sometimes evaluated and treated by **neurologists**. Depending on the institution, however, spinal surgery may be performed by the neurosurgeon, the orthopedist, or the two working together.

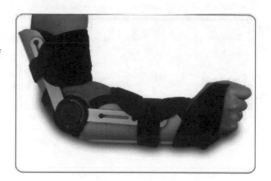

Orthopedists deal with diseases and injuries of the bones and joints, such as:

- degenerative joint disease
- developmental and/or congenital anomalies of the musculoskeletal system
- sports or stress injuries
- traumatic accidents
- fractures
- bone malignancies
- osteomalacia and osteoporosis
- arthritis
- bone infections such as osteomyelitis

The somewhat recent development of a new subspecialty, *sports medicine*, combines both orthopedics and *physiatry* (physical medicine and rehabilitation).

Common orthopedic procedures include:

- fracture repairs (open reduction, internal fixation, and closed reduction) and casting
- placement and revision of prosthetics (such as a total or partial knee, shoulder, or hip replacement)
- arthroscopies
- amputations
- trigger finger releases
- excisional biopsies from bone or related structures
- carpal or tarsal tunnel releases
- spinal surgeries (fusions, laminectomies, hemilaminectomies, facetectomies, diskectomies, etc.)
- repairs of structures in the knees and shoulders

Some of the orthopedic procedures mentioned are day surgeries; others require a hospital stay of several days.

Physiatry (or physiatrics) is closely related to the field of orthopedics and is the branch of medicine that deals with the ongoing treatment for physical problems, such as severely broken bones, torn ligaments, knee and hip replacements, amputations, rehab for spinal injuries, postsurgical rehabilitation, and similar conditions. The physician who specializes in physical medicine and rehab is called a physiatrist.

Physical therapy and rehabilitation also constitute an important part of medical management for damage to internal structures, such as reconditioning for a patient who is status post a heart attack, a stroke, or a lung replacement—conditions unrelated to orthopedics.

Physical medicine includes the subspecialties of physical and occupational therapy. Sports medicine is often a subspecialty of this field, especially when associated with orthopedics. Physical medicine can be part of a short hospital course, as well as outpatient treatment for prolonged periods of time—weeks, months, or years—depending on the nature of the rehabilitation required.

As you might expect, the terminology involved in physical medicine includes many orthopedic terms. Some maneuvers, positions, devices, and procedures are unique to physical therapy.

Podiatry is also closely related to orthopedics. **Podiatry** is concerned with the care and study of the feet—the anatomy and pathology, as well as the medical and surgical treatment of problems related to the feet. The specialist in podiatry is a podiatrist.

ORTHOPEDICS LANGUAGE WORKSHOP

Orthopedic terminology is quite specialized, and thorough exposure to orthopedic word-building terms will help you get the most out of this FOMS unit. As you work through the reports in this unit, it is important to stop and research terms you are unfamiliar with. Also, if you have not already begun to do so, now is a GREAT time to start a word list. A word list is a resource you will use not only throughout this training program, but also when you become a productive MTE.

Common Orthopedics Root Words and Combining Forms

Root Word & Combining Form	Meaning	Example
acr/o	extremities	acromegaly
ankyl/o	crooked or fused	ankylodactyly
arthr/o	joint	arthroplasty
articul/o	joint	articulation
brachi/o	arm	brachiocephalic
burs/o	bursa	bursectomy
calc/i	calcium	calcification
carp/o	carpus/wrist	carpometacarpal
cervic/o	neck	cervicothoracic
chondr/o	cartilage	chondromalacia
cleid/o	clavicle	sternocleidomastoid
cost/o	rib	costochondritis
dactyl/o	fingers or toes	dactyledema
disc/o	disc/disk	discogenic
femor/o	femur	femoral
fibul/o	fibula	fibulotibial
ili/o	ilium (hip bone)	sacroiliac
ischi/o	ischium	ischiodynia
lumb/o	lower back	lumbosacral
my/o	muscle	myotomy
odyn/o	pain	arthrodynia
orth/o	straight	orthopedic
oste/o	bone	osteopathic
patell/o	patella (kneecap)	patellofemoral
phalang/o	phalanx or phalanges	interphalangeal
proxim/o	nearest point of origin	proximal
spondyl/o	vertebra	spondylolisthesis
stern/o	sternum	retrosternal
tars/o	tarsal (ankle bone)	metatarsal

Common Orthopedics Prefixes

Prefix	Meaning	Example
ab-	away from	abduct
ad-	toward	adduct
dia-	through, between	dialysis
hemi-/semi-	half, partly	hemilaminectomy
infra-	beneath	infraorbital
inter-	between	intercondylar
peri-	around, near	periventricular
retro-	behind, backward	retroareolar
syn-/sym-	together, union	symphysis

Common Orthopedics Suffixes

Suffix	Meaning	Example
-algia	pain	fibromyalgia
-edema	swelling	lymphedema
-itis	inflammation	arthritis
-kinesia/-kinesis	movement, motion	hypokinesis
-lysis	loosening, freeing	adhesiolysis
-malacia	softening	chondromalacia
-penia	deficiency	osteopenia
-plasty	surgical repair	arthroplasty
-tome	a cutting instrument	osteotome
-tomy	incision (cutting into)	craniotomy

Common Orthopedics Abbreviations

Abbreviation	Expansion
AC	acromioclavicular
ACL	anterior cruciate ligament
C1-7	cervical vertebrae 1-7
C-spine	cervical spine
CMC	carpometacarpal (joint)
CPM	continuous passive motion
CTS	carpal tunnel syndrome
DIP	distal interphalangeal (joint)
IP	interphalangeal
IT	iliotibial
L1-5	lumbar vertebrae 1-5
L-spine	lumbar spine
LS	lumbosacral (spine)
MCP	metacarpophalangeal (joint)
MTP	metatarsophalangeal (joint)
PCL	posterior cruciate ligament
PIP	proximal interphalangeal (joint)
SI	sacroiliac (joint)
T1-12	thoracic vertebrae 1-12
T-spine	thoracic spine
TMJ	temporomandibular joint

REVIEW: ORTHOPEDICS LANGUAGE

Multiple Choice.
Choose the best answer.

1. An instrument used to cut bone is an (○ osteophyte, ○ osteotome).

2. The term *osteochondritis* refers to inflammation of bone and (○ muscles, ○ cartilage).

3. Bursitis is (○ removal, ○ inflammation) of the bursa.

4. A tear of the ACL, or anterior (○ clavicular, ○ cruciate) ligament, is a frequently seen injury in professional football players.

5. The term (○ osteopathy, ○ osteopenia) literally means bone deficiency.

TRUE/FALSE.
Mark the following true or false.

1. *CTS* stands for carpal tunnel syndrome
   - ○ true
   - ○ false

2. Swelling of the fingers is called dactyledema.
   - ○ true
   - ○ false

3. *Femoroiliac* pertains to both the femur and the ilium.
   - ○ true
   - ○ false

4. The term *craniotomy* means removal of the cranium.
   - ○ true
   - ○ false

5. *Patellofemoral* relates to the knee cap and femur.
   - ○ true
   - ○ false

Fill in the Blank.
Using the word(s) in the box, enter the appropriate term in the space provided.

1. _____ is a term meaning incision into muscle.

2. The term _____ means inflammation of ribs and cartilage.

3. The _____ (MCP) joint is also known as the knuckle.

4. _____ tunnel syndrome is a condition in which one of the major nerves that controls the functioning of the hand and fingers becomes compressed inside a "tunnel" in the wrist.

5. _____ is surgical repair of a joint.

costochondritis
myotomy
carpal
arthroplasty
metacarpophalangeal

ORTHOPEDICS REPORTS

Although orthopedic surgical procedures are often long and detailed, they are also common. The terminology is quite similar regardless of where the procedure is being performed, with the exception of anatomy terms. This is why in the Anatomy, Pathophysiology and Disease Processes modules of the training program you were required to learn the major bones of the body.

A note of interest: The MTE who first becomes exposed to orthopedic reports may think he/she has stumbled into a carpentry shop. Much of the terminology is the same:

- mortises and beveled edges
- chamfers
- drills and drill bits
- pins
- saws
- hammers
- cutters
- jigs
- screws
- burs
- planers
- reamers
- pulleys
- gauges

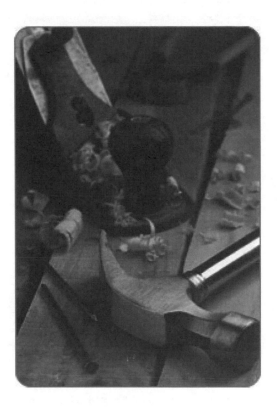

ORTHOPEDICS REPORT 1 – OPERATIVE NOTE

PREOPERATIVE DIAGNOSIS: Left thigh abscess secondary to chronic left femoral osteomyelitis, status post irrigation and debridement x2.[1]

POSTOPERATIVE DIAGNOSIS: Left thigh abscess secondary to chronic left femoral osteomyelitis, status post irrigation and debridement x2.

DRAINS: 1/4 inch[2] Hemovac, left thigh wound.

OPERATION PERFORMED: Irrigation and debridement and delayed primary closure, left thigh wound.

FLUIDS: 2500 cc of crystalloid.

ESTIMATED BLOOD LOSS: 50 cc.

INDICATIONS: The patient is a 38-year-old white male who noted a 2-month history of progressive left thigh pain without any trauma. He was seen and evaluated by the orthopedic service and was admitted with a presumptive diagnosis of left femoral abscess secondary to flare of quiescent left femoral osteomyelitis. He was taken to the operating room and underwent irrigation and debridement of his left thigh abscess x2. He now returns to the operating room with the intent of delayed primary closure of his left thigh wound. He has remained afebrile, has negative cultures and a normal white count heading into the operating room today.

DESCRIPTION OF PROCEDURE: The patient was taken to the operating room and placed in the supine position. After satisfactory spinal anesthesia was obtained, the patient was prepped and draped in the usual sterile manner. The wound was opened and noted to have some turbid purulent drainage of the sinus tract, approximately 3 cm below the left thigh wound. Anaerobic, aerobic, fungal and TB cultures were obtained. The left thigh wound itself was noted to be clean and free of any purulent discharge. The underlying tissue was healthy and vascular. The wound was debrided and irrigated copiously with 6 liters of sterile normal saline. The wound edges came together easily without any undue tension. The wound was then closed using interrupted 2-0 Vicryl sutures in the subcutaneous tissue. Then an interrupted vertical mattress 3-0 nylon suture was used to approximate the skin edges. The sinus tract approximately 3-4 cm inferior to the left thigh wound was then extended with a longitudinal incision, approximately 1-2 cm on each side of the sinus tract. This was then copiously irrigated and packed with fine mesh gauze soaked in Betadine. A 1/4 inch Hemovac drain was placed into the left thigh wound prior to its closure and connected to Hemovac suction drainage. The wounds were then covered with a compressive dressing. The patient was then taken from the operating room to the recovery room without any apparent complications, in stable condition.

Footnotes:

1. 1.Also acceptably edited as x 2 and times 2. When the word *times* is dictated and means the number of times a thing was done, the letter *x* can be used. Only use *x* with numerals—you wouldn't say x two. And x is lowercase. Sometimes you will see this with a space between the x and numeral for easier readability, but this is a style preference issue.
2. 2.It is rarely acceptable to edit " for inch. Without specific instruction, always go with spelling out *inch* or *inches*.

SPELLING.
Determine if the following words are spelled correctly. If the spelling is correct, leave the word as it has already been entered. If the spelling is incorrect, provide the correct spelling.

1. fungal _____

2. quiesent _____

3. commpresive _____

4. anarobic _____

5. Hemovac _____

Multiple Choice.
Choose the best answer.

1. Anaerobic, aerobic, (◯ fungal, ◯ fundal) and TB cultures were obtained.

2. The abscess was secondary to chronic (◯ osteomyelitis, ◯ osteomyolitis).

3. The wound was irrigated with (◯ copius, ◯ copious) amounts of normal saline.

4. The thigh wound was clean and free of any (◯ purulent, ◯ purralent) discharge.

5. Interrupted 2-0 Vicryl sutures were used in the (◯ subcutaneus, ◯ subcutaneous) tissue.

ORTHOPEDICS REPORT 2 – OPERATIVE NOTE

PREOPERATIVE DIAGNOSIS: Right distal humerus fracture.

POSTOPERATIVE DIAGNOSIS: Right distal humerus fracture.

OPERATION PERFORMED: Open reduction and internal fixation, right distal humerus fracture.

INDICATIONS: The patient is a 22-year-old white male who sustained a right distal humerus fracture in a motorcycle accident approximately 12 days ago. He has intraarticular comminution and displacement, and is scheduled for open reduction.

DESCRIPTION OF PROCEDURE: Patient was brought to the operating room, and general endotracheal anesthesia was performed. After adequate anesthesia, patient was placed prone on the operating table with all bony prominences well padded. His right upper extremity was then prepped and draped in the usual sterile manner. Limb was exsanguinated using an Ace wrap and tourniquet brought to 275 mmHg. A midline longitudinal incision was made over the elbow and carried sharply down through the skin and subcutaneous tissue. The triceps[1] was identified. The edge of the triceps was then identified, being careful to identify the ulnar nerve and protect it. The olecranon was then isolated and an osteotomy was performed using an oscillating reciprocating saw through the olecranon. This was predrilled with a 4.5 cortical screw. The triceps was then stripped up off the distal humerus, and the fracture was exposed. There was a large lateral fragment, a central fragment, and a large medial fragment. These were reduced and held in place using a 4.5 cortical screw. This reduced the joint quite well. The ulnar and radial columns were then reconstituted. The radial column was reduced and held in place using a 6.0 one-third tubular plate. The ulnar column was then reduced and held in place using a 3.5 recon plate, approximately 7 holes in length. This gave adequate reduction of the joint and good stable construction. The elbow was brought through a range of motion, and traction was found to be stable. The wound was then irrigated profusely. Radiographs revealed good alignment of the fracture fragments. The olecranon was then fixed back in place using the 4.5 cortical screw in a tension band wire technique. The wound was then irrigated. The wounds were then closed using 2-0 Vicryl in the fascia, 2-0 Vicryl subcutaneous, and staples on the skin. A 1/8-inch Hemovac drain was placed along the medial aspect of the wound, beneath the fascia. Xeroform, fluffs, Kerlix, Ace wrap, and dressing were applied. The patient was placed in a posterior splint. Tourniquet times: The first tourniquet time was 123 minutes; the second was 32 minutes. He had brisk return of capillary flow and radial pulse upon letting down the tourniquet. The patient was brought to the recovery room in stable condition.

Footnotes:

1. 1.Triceps is always triceps (singular or plural); it is never tricep.

TRUE/FALSE.
Mark the following true or false.

1. No staples were used in wound closure for this patient.

   ○ true

   ○ false

2. The surgery was performed under general endotracheal anesthesia.

   ○ true

   ○ false

3. The humerus fracture was repaired with closed reduction.

   ○ true

   ○ false

4. Exposure of the fracture revealed 4 fragments.

   ○ true

   ○ false

5. Total tourniquet time was 155 minutes.

   ○ true

   ○ false

Matching.
Match the type of tool to its name.

1. ____ Xeroform

2. ____ Ace

3. ____ Hemovac

4. ____ cortical

5. ____ oscillating reciprocating

A. screw

B. wrap

C. saw

D. drain

E. gauze

ORTHOPEDICS REPORT 3 – DISCHARGE SUMMARY

CHIEF COMPLAINT: Failed left patella of total knee arthroplasty.

HISTORY OF PRESENT ILLNESS: The patient is a 73-year-old white female with complaint of left knee pain for the past 2 weeks, as well as crepitus. The patient is 9 years status post total knee arthroplasty which was noncemented. The patient was noted on routine followup radiographs to have failure of a metal-backed patella. The patient has a history of a prior patella revision in May of 1999.

PAST MEDICAL HISTORY: Irritable bowel syndrome, degenerative joint disease.

PAST SURGICAL HISTORY: See HPI, cholecystectomy in June of 1995.

OCCUPATION: She is retired.

SOCIAL HISTORY: Smoking: None. Ethanol: None.

MEDICATIONS: Erythromycin and Premarin.

CHILDHOOD DISEASES: Jaundice.

DRUG ALLERGIES: FLAGYL, PENICILLIN, AND SULFA.

REVIEW OF SYSTEMS: Noncontributory.

PHYSICAL EXAMINATION: Height 5 feet 1 inch, weight 145 pounds. General: The patient is a well-developed, well-nourished white female who ambulates with 2 crutches. Head, ears, eyes, nose, and throat: Appropriate for age, negative dentures, positive myopia. Lungs: Clear to auscultation times four. Cardiovascular: Heart rate regular and rhythmical, without murmur, S3 or S4. The abdomen has a right upper quadrant scar, bowel sounds times four. Left knee: There is a well-healed midline scar, active range of motion 0 to 90 degrees, a mild amount of effusion, crepitus[1] with patellar grind. The MCL and LCL are intact with varus and valgus stressing, negative tibial sag, negative Lachman's.[2]

LABORATORY DATA: Routine preoperative labs: CBC, PT/PTT, UA, and a general health profile were all within normal limits. Discharge H&H was 13.7 and 40.8. Radiographs reveal patellar dissociation with fragmentation of the patella; the other components appear well fixed. Chest x-ray: No active disease. EKG: Sinus tachycardia, otherwise within normal limits.

HOSPITAL COURSE: The patient was admitted for revision of the left patella. She underwent this on 6 November. The previously placed left total knee arthroplasty was found to be intact. The left patella with a polyethylene insert was noted to have abnormal wear. There was inadequate remaining bone for revision, and therefore a primary patellectomy was performed. The patient was noted to have a quite thinned patellar tendon and quadriceps tendon upon repair of the region. The patient started in physical therapy in which she was prevented from doing any active extension or leg lifts of that lower extremity. She was placed in a postoperative DonJoy Legend ACL knee brace[3] locked at 0-45 degrees. The patient was cleared by PT and OT upon discharge.

FINAL DIAGNOSES

1. Failed left patellar component of total knee arthroplasty.
2. Degenerative joint disease.
3. Irritable bowel syndrome.

OPERATION: Left knee patellectomy.

COMPLICATIONS: None.

CONSULTATIONS

1. Physical therapy.
2. Occupational therapy.

DISCHARGE MEDICATIONS: No change from admission medications with the exception of Tylenol No 3. one to two p.o. q.4-6 hours p.r.n. pain, dispensed #20.

DISPOSITION/RECOMMENDATIONS: The patient was discharged to home with vital signs stable, afebrile, the wound clean, dry and intact, and staples in place. The patient will follow up on a routine basis with Physical Therapy as per protocol. The patient will follow up in the clinic on 26 November at 0900 hours for staple removal. The patient is to avoid any active extension or leg lifts of the left lower extremity times eight weeks. At eight weeks we plan on increasing her range of motion from 0-45 to 0-90 degrees.

Footnotes:

1. 1.The term *crepitus* is the same as *crepitation*. You may sometimes hear docs say "crepitance," which will probably eventually make it to the medical dictionary. (Of note, in a verbatim account, edit crepitance as dictated when dictated. In an account that allows editing, you would probably change it to crepitus or crepitation.)
2. 2.Lachman's, of course, is the possessive form of Lachman test. Some accounts will not allow possessive eponyms and in this case it would be edited as Lachman or Lachman test.
3. 3.Any really good surgical word book will have this term in it for quick and easy spelling verification.

Fill in the Blank.
Using the word(s) in the box, enter the appropriate term in the space provided.

1. ACL – anterior _____ ligament
2. OT – _____ therapy
3. H&H – hemoglobin and _____
4. MCL – _____ collateral ligament
5. DJD – _____ joint disease
6. IBS – irritable _____ syndrome

| bowel |
| cruciate |
| degenerative |
| hematocrit |
| medial |
| occupational |

True/False.
Mark the following true or false.

1. The patient is 19 years status post total knee arthroplasty.
   - ○ true
   - ○ false

2. The patient has no drug allergies.
   - ○ true
   - ○ false

3. A primary patellectomy was performed.
   - ○ true
   - ○ false

4. Occupational therapy did not clear the patient upon discharge.
   - ○ true
   - ○ false

5. The patient is to avoid active extension for 8 weeks.
   - ○ true
   - ○ false

ORTHOPEDICS REPORT 4 – OPERATIVE NOTE

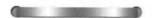

Medical Record

PREOPERATIVE DIAGNOSIS: Degenerative joint disease, right knee.

OPERATION PERFORMED: Right total knee arthroplasty, press-fit[1] with cemented patella.

INDICATIONS: This is a 58-year-old female with severe limitation of activities of daily living with pain, despite conservative therapy for her right knee with degenerative changes in 3 compartments.

DESCRIPTION OF PROCEDURE: The patient was taken to the operating room. After successful administration of a general anesthetic, she was prepped and draped in the usual sterile manner. She was draped in a routine manner after a tourniquet had been placed high on her leg. The limb was exsanguinated. A midline incision was made through the skin and subcutaneous tissues. The extensor tendon was identified, and an incision was made through the extensor tendon. The patella was dislocated laterally, and the osteophytes were removed off the intercondylar notch. The femur was then gouged. A 9-mm drill[2] was then introduced, irrigation followed down the canal, and an intramedullary reamer was introduced with 7-degree, 3-inch stem. After this was accomplished, the distal femoral cutting guide was utilized to remove the femur. It was then planed smooth. A medium jig was then placed and appropriately positioned. The anterior cut was then made without difficulty. Anterior chamfer, posterior, and posterior chamfer cuts were then performed. She was in a mild amount of varus at this time.[3] The deep medial collateral ligament was then subperiosteally released. The anterior cruciate ligament was then incised. A posterior retractor was placed, and an intramedullary rod was placed down the tibia. This was also followed with copious irrigation. The intramedullary cutting guide was then placed, and the tibia was resected at the appropriate level. Trials were then utilized. The patellar groove was then placed without difficulty. After the trials were positioned, it was noted that she had excellent fit. Therefore it was elected to go with a press fit. The tibial base plate, a small +, was then utilized and screwed into position utilizing 4 screws. After this was accomplished, the femoral component was placed. The patella was prepared in a routine manner, being offset with a 25-mm high dome patella, which was cemented into position. All osteophytes all around the patella were removed. The osteophytes were also removed around the femur and tibia. There was excellent fit. Trial with 8-mm tray revealed there to be good stability. There was good ligament balance. Therefore an 8-mm tray was packed into position. An 1/8-inch drain was then placed into the knee. The wound was then closed in layers with 1-0 Vicryl closing the extensor mechanism, 0 Vicryl closing the deep subcutaneous tissues, and staples closing the skin. Dressing consisted of Xeroform, dressing sponges, Kerlix, and an Ace wrap. The patient tolerated the procedure well and was taken to the recovery room in stable condition. The patient received 1 g of Ancef preoperatively.

Footnotes:

1. 1.While this can also be referenced as "Press-Fit," in this instance it makes contextual sense to use the lowercase "press-fit." The dictator does not (apparently) say specifically a Press-Fit component.
2. 2.This could easily be edited as 9 mm drill. The meaning is clear with or without the hyphen. This is not a risk management issue (meaning something that could negatively impact the patient).
3. 3.Varus = An abnormal position in which part of a limb is twisted inward toward the midline; opposite of valgus.

SPELLING.
Determine if the following words are spelled correctly. If the spelling is correct, leave the word as it has already been entered. If the spelling is incorrect, provide the correct spelling.

1. varus _____

2. intercondilar _____

3. cruciate _____

4. pateller _____

5. kerlex _____

TRUE/FALSE.

Mark the following true or false.

1. The high dome patella was cemented in place.

    ○ true

    ○ false

2. The patient is 85 years old.

    ○ true

    ○ false

3. The wound was covered with 4 x 4's.

    ○ true

    ○ false

4. Osteophytes were removed around the femur and tibia.

    ○ true

    ○ false

5. A small (+) jig was used to make the chamfer cuts.

    ○ true

    ○ false

ORTHOPEDICS REPORT 5 – OPERATIVE NOTE

OPERATIVE DIAGNOSIS: Osteomyelitis, left femur.

POSTOPERATIVE DIAGNOSIS: Osteomyelitis, left femur.

OPERATION PERFORMED: Incision and debridement of left femur.

BLOOD LOSS: 500 cc.

FLUIDS: 2500 cc lactated Ringer's, 500 cc Hespan.

INDICATIONS: The patient is a 33-year-old white male with approximately 1-1/2 years of left thigh pain. This was originally thought to be secondary to muscle necrosis and stress fracture from an injury while weightlifting. He subsequently had increasing pain and cellulitis in his posterior thigh and what appears to be a large area of abscess and sequestrum formation in the left femoral diaphysis with necrosis of the vastus intermedius, as well as tracking posteriorly and laterally along the intermuscular septum to the posterior part of the thigh. Preoperatively his WBC was 7.5.

DESCRIPTION OF PROCEDURE: The patient was taken to the operating room, placed in the supine position, and general endotracheal anesthetic was successfully induced. He was positioned in the lateral decubitus position. Care was taken to pad his axilla, as well as underneath his right bottom leg. He was prepped and draped in sterile fashion. A posterolateral incision was made along the intermuscular septum. This was carried down through the fascia, and the vastus lateralis was identified anteriorly and the intermuscular septum posteriorly. The plane of dissection proceeded anterior to the intermuscular septum. The vastus lateralis was noted to be quite adhesed to the intermuscular septum, as well as the intermuscular septum being thickened and fibrotic. There was a hole in the septum which tracked posteriorly back to the area of cellulitis, and there was a large amount of purulent material, as well as gelatinous fibrous-type tissue posteriorly in the area of the biceps. This area also had a lot of loculations and with digital palpation this area was disrupted. Next the incision was carried down to the femur and the vastus lateralis elevated anteriorly. A large amount of periosteal reaction was identified, as well as a cloaca, which was located anteriorly. The vastus intermedius compartment also was noted to be filled with a lot of gelatinous and fibrous tissue. It appeared that the vastus intermedius was necrotic. This appeared to be a longstanding change. There was no active pus coming out of the cloaca in the femur. There was some fibrous tissue in this area. The vastus intermedius was debrided with removal of much of this tissue. Multiple cultures for aerobic, anaerobic, fungal, TB, and Gram stain were sent, as well as tissue for pathology from the vastus intermedius and the posterior thigh. Preliminary frozen section was consistent with chronic inflammatory tissue. Next, using the Anspach drill, a longitudinally oriented oval was made through the cortex to include the cloaca. This was removed to be sent down to Pathology for culture and tissue examination. A curet[1] was used to curet cortical bone, as well as medullary cavity through this area. Again specific cultures for aerobic, anaerobic, Gram stain, fungal, and TB, both swabs and tissue, were sent from and labeled "left femur." Again no active pus or pus under pressure was identified in the femur. Cortical bone appeared to be quite thick and of fairly normal quality, other than a great deal of periosteal reaction in this area. Next the pulse lavage was used to irrigate all the described compartments and areas, and a total of 6 liters was[2] used. The wound was then packed open using a Betadine-soaked Kerlix, and a 1/4-inch Hemovac drain was placed. The skin was loosely reapproximated using 4 interrupted 1-0 Prolene sutures. Dressing was then applied. The patient tolerated the procedure well and was extubated in the operating room and taken to the recovery room in stable condition.

Footnotes:

1. 1.Also acceptably edited as curette.
2. 2.Again, units of measurement are treated as singular. This would not be "6 liters were..."

SPELLING.
Determine if the following words are spelled correctly. If the spelling is correct, leave the word as it has already been entered. If the spelling is incorrect, provide the correct spelling.

1. debridement _____
2. celulitis _____

3. gelatinus _____   4. loculation _____

5. cloaca _____   6. lavage _____

Multiple Choice.
Choose the best answer.

1. Periostial reaction was identified anteriorly, as well as a (○ cloaca, ○ medullary) .

2. The pulse (○ lavage, ○ swab) was used to irrigate the compartments.

3. A (○ drill, ○ curet) was used to curet the cortical bone.

4. The (○ plane, ○ plain) of dissection proceeded anterior to the intermuscular septum.

5. Patient was positioned in the lateral (○ supine, ○ decubitus) position.

ORTHOPEDICS REPORT 6 – OPERATIVE NOTE

OPERATION PERFORMED: Below-knee amputation, left leg.

INDICATIONS: The patient is a 62-year-old Caucasian female who has had a prolonged hospital course for severe left lower extremity atherosclerotic peripheral vascular disease. The patient underwent a left lower extremity bypass procedure approximately 2 months ago to reestablish flow to her left leg and foot. Subsequently, she developed a thrombosis of her graft and underwent a urokinase infusion, which reestablished some flow to the graft and left leg. Since her initial bypass operation, she has continued to have intractable left leg and foot pain, as well as 2 large nonhealing ulcers on the foot and ankle area. After review of the angiograms with staff, it was decided that there were no further options for bypass or revascularization of the left lower extremity, and a below-knee amputation was therefore the only reasonable method of treatment of the patient's pain and nonhealing ulcerations. The patient was in agreement, and informed consent was obtained.

DESCRIPTION OF PROCEDURE: The patient was taken to the operating room and placed in a supine position with the left leg elevated. Her left lower extremity was then prepped and draped in the usual sterile fashion, with a tourniquet placed on the left thigh. While under general anesthesia and with the left lower extremity elevated, but no tourniquet used, a circumferential incision was created beginning anteriorly approximately 8-10 cm below the left tibial tuberosity. A 15-cm posterior muscle flap was developed. A Gigli saw was used to form a steeply angled, posterior to anterior transection of the tibia. An oscillating saw was then used to transect the fibula approximately 1-2 cm proximal to the end of the tibial segment. The remaining part of the lower leg and foot were amputated using sharp dissection. Hemostasis was quickly and temporarily controlled with hemostats, and eventually converted to permanent hemostasis with 2-0 and 3-0 silk ties. The tibial nerve and 2 other major nerve branches were identified. A high ligation and transection of each of these nerves was performed. After obtaining meticulous hemostasis, the wound was then irrigated with copious amounts of sterile saline with antibiotic solution. The posterior flap was then brought forward and trimmed to an appropriate length. This posterior-based flap was then closed over the stump using interrupted 0 silk ties. Prior to closure a Blake drain was laid into the stump area and brought out distal and medial to the knee. Xeroform gauze was then placed over the suture line, and a fluff dressing was placed. The prosthesis tech then applied a cast extending over the stump and to about midthigh. The patient was awakened from her general anesthetic and taken to the recovery room, having tolerated the operation well. The method of anesthesia was general endotracheal anesthesia. Complications were none. EBL was 300 cc. Fluids were 1900 cc of lactated Ringer's. Specimen was left leg and foot, BKA.

Spelling.
Determine if the following words are spelled correctly. If the spelling is correct, leave the word as it has already been entered. If the spelling is incorrect, provide the correct spelling.

1. anasthesia _____

2. Gigli _____

3. urokinase _____

4. ligashun _____

5. prostesis _____

Multiple Choice.
Choose the best answer.

1. The operation was a below-knee amputation, (○ right, ○ left) leg.

2. (○ Hemostasis, ○ Ligation) was quickly and temporarily controlled with hemostats.

3. The (○ Gigli, ○ oscillating) saw was used to transect the fibula.

4. The (○ operating room, ○ prosthesis) technician applied a cast extending over the stump.

5. The patient was placed in the (○ supine, ○ left-lateral) position.

ORTHOPEDICS REPORT 7 – DISCHARGE SUMMARY

CHIEF COMPLAINT: Bilateral knee pain.

HISTORY OF PRESENT ILLNESS: The patient is a 73-year-old African-American male with complaints of bilateral knee pain, right greater than left. The patient is status post arthroscopy on January 11, 2002, with a brief improvement in pain in the right knee. The patient uses crutches on occasion and takes nonsteroidal antiinflammatory drugs. The patient uses railings with stairs. The patient wears Ace wraps. He is status post a medial meniscectomy of the left knee in 1998. The patient lives on a ranch and is a vigorous man who requires full use of his lower extremities to keep his property running.

PAST MEDICAL HISTORY: Sick sinus syndrome, paced from 1994 to 2001, removed in 2001 and replaced in 2002 after a syncopal episode, asymptomatic since.

PAST SURGICAL HISTORY: See HPI, in 1989 a right hernia repair, in 1986 ulcers on the vocal cords x2.

ALLERGIES: The patient has no known drug allergies.

MEDICATIONS: Tylenol p.r.n.

SOCIAL HISTORY: A 10-pack-year history of smoking, quit in 1986. Ethanol: Drinks wine with dinner, 3-4 times per week.

REVIEW OF SYSTEMS: Noncontributory.

PHYSICAL EXAMINATION: Height 6 feet 1 inch, weight 186 pounds. General: A well-developed, well-nourished black male in no acute distress. Alert and oriented x3. HEENT: Extraocular muscles are intact. Pupils are equal and reactive to light and accommodation. No dentures. Neck: Full range of motion, supple, negative masses. Heart: Regular rate and rhythm. Lungs: Clear to auscultation throughout. The abdomen is soft and nontender, negative masses, negative bruits. Back: Negative costovertebral angle tenderness. Rectal: The prostate is smooth, small, soft. Guaiac negative, brown stool. The skin is warm and dry. Pulses are 2+/4+ in the dorsalis pedis and posterior tibial. Neurologic: He is intact to light touch, otherwise nonfocal throughout. Gait: Narrow-based, slow steady gait. Right lower extremity: Range of motion right knee is 10-120 degrees, negative Lachman, negative drawer, negative pivot, 2+ medial pseudolaxity, soft tissue mass superior pole, patella, and suprapatellar pouch, positive patellofemoral grind. Left knee range of motion is 5-120 degrees, negative Lachman, negative tibial sag, 2+ medial pseudolaxity, positive patellofemoral grind.

LABORATORY DATA: Routine preoperative labs reveal CBC, PT, PTT, UA, and a general health panel were within normal limits. On discharge, H&H was 7.7 and 22.3. Radiographs: Varus collapse and tricompartmental disease bilaterally with approximately 3 degrees varus anatomical axis, calcified Baker cyst noted, left knee. Knee score: 55/35 and 56/35 on the left. Chest x-ray: No focal disease, cardiomegaly noted with a pacemaker in place. Electrocardiogram: Normal sinus rhythm with a leftward axis. PFTs were within normal limits. ABGs: Saturation of 91.9.

HOSPITAL COURSE: The patient was admitted on April 3, for bilateral total knee arthroplasties. The patient was taken to the operating suite on April 4, where bilateral total knee arthroplasties were performed. The patient was admitted to the SICU for the first night. Postoperatively the patient was given Coumadin for DVT prophylaxis as well as TED hose and SCDs. The patient was given perioperative and postoperative antibiotics. The patient progressed fairly well in physical therapy, obtaining near 90 degrees range of motion. He required an infusion of 1 unit of autologous blood in the unit. The patient received his blood back via reinfusible drains. The patient was cleared by Cardiology, Dental, and Pulmonary[1] before the operation. The patient was seen by the home healthcare, PT, and OT during the hospital stay. The drains were removed on the second postoperative day. The wounds were found to be clean, dry, and well approximated. The staples were removed before discharge. The patient had a duplex ultrasound which revealed no clots. The remainder of the hospital course was uneventful.

FINAL DIAGNOSES

1. Bilateral knee degenerative joint disease.
2. Sick sinus syndrome.

OPERATIONS

1. Bilateral Ortholoc II total knee arthroplasties.
2. Transfusion 1 unit of autologous blood.

COMPLICATIONS: None.

CONSULTATIONS

1. Physical therapy.
2. Occupational therapy.
3. Home healthcare.
4. Cardiology.

DISCHARGE MEDICATIONS

1. Tylenol No. 3, dispensed 21, p.o. q.4-6 hours p.r.n. pain.
2. Prescriptions for an elevated toilet seat and CPM[2] were given.

DISPOSITION/RECOMMENDATIONS: The patient was discharged to home with vital signs stable, afebrile, wounds clean, dry and intact. The patient was cleared by PT and OT. The patient will receive physical therapy 3 times a week in his home as well as having a CPM at home, for which his family has been instructed on its appropriate use. The patient will follow up in the orthopedic clinic in 4 weeks for repeat radiographs and evaluation. The patient is to weightbear as tolerated with a walker. The patient is to have a repeat ultrasound at 3 weeks postoperatively.

Footnotes:

1. 1.These are capped because they are being referred to as entities. They would not be capped had they been presented as "by the cardiology, dental, and pulmonary departments." Again, this is style issue. Without specific instruction on how to handle department names, it would not necessarily be incorrect to uncap them as they are presented here.
2. 2.CPM = continuous passive motion.

Multiple Choice.
Choose the correct spelling for the term defined.

1. Symmetric instability.
   - ○ sudolaxity
   - ○ psudolaxity
   - ○ pseudolaxity
   - ○ pseudolaxaty

2. Preventative treatment.
   - ○ profalaxis
   - ○ prophalaxis
   - ○ prophalaxys
   - ○ prophylaxis

3. Blood that the donor has previously donated and then receives back.
   - ○ autologous
   - ○ autologus
   - ○ autolagus
   - ○ autologious

4. Above the patella.
   - ○ superpatelar
   - ○ superpatellar
   - ○ suprapatelar
   - ○ suprapatellar

5. Excision of a meniscus.
   - ○ meniscusectomy
   - ○ meniscectomy
   - ○ menescectomy
   - ○ meniscetomy

Fill in the Blank.
Using the word(s) in the box, fill in the blanks.

1. SCD – sequential _____ device
2. TED – thrombo_____ disease
3. CPM – _____ passive motion
4. DVT – deep vein _____
5. PFT – pulmonary _____ test

compression
continuous
embolic
function
thrombosis

ORTHOPEDICS REPORT 8 – OPERATIVE NOTE

PREOPERATIVE DIAGNOSIS: Left knee anterior cruciate ligament deficiency.

POSTOPERATIVE DIAGNOSIS

1. Left knee anterior cruciate ligament deficiency.
2. Grade 3[1] chondromalacial changes, lateral and medial femoral condyles.
3. Lateral meniscus tear in anterior horn and tear in posterior horn of medial meniscus.

OPERATION PERFORMED: Left knee anterior cruciate ligament reconstruction with partial lateral and medial meniscectomies.

FLUIDS: 1850 cc crystalloid.

ESTIMATED BLOOD LOSS: 150 cc.

TOURNIQUET TIME: 34 minutes.

INDICATIONS: The patient is a 42-year-old African-American male who sustained a remote injury to his left knee. Patient complains of left knee instability, giving way. Patient was seen in the orthopedic clinic and given an ACL derotational brace and sent to Physical Therapy for rehabilitation. Patient continued to have instability despite conservative management and desires left ACL reconstruction after having all options, risks and benefits explained to him.

DESCRIPTION OF PROCEDURE: Patient was taken to the operating room and placed in the supine position. After satisfactory general endotracheal anesthesia was obtained and 1 gram Ancef was given IV, the patient underwent an examination under anesthesia which revealed a 3B Lachman,[2] positive pivot shift, and a 2+ anterior drawer. The patient's left leg was then placed into a leg holder and a tourniquet placed on the upper aspect of the left thigh. The knee was then prepped and draped in the usual sterile manner. After initially exsanguinating the left leg with an Ace wrap, the tourniquet was then inflated to 300 mmHg. The central 3rd of the patellar tendon was harvested in an autograft equating to approximately 10 mm in width, with bone plugs on each end measuring 25 mm from the tibia and 20 mm from the patella. The bone plugs were predrilled with 1 drill hole in the patellar bone plug and 3 staggered holes in the tibial plug. The patellar plug was then fashioned on the back table to fit a 10-mm tunnel, and the tibial plug was fashioned to fit an 11-mm tunnel. One 5-0 Ethibond was placed through the drill hole in the patellar plug, and three 5-0 Ethibond sutures were placed through the tibial plug, and the autograft was then wrapped in a moist sponge. Attention was then directed toward arthroscopy of the left knee. Arthroscope was introduced, and the knee was examined sequentially. The suprapatellar pouch and the medial and lateral gutters were noted to be hyperemic, but otherwise within normal limits, without evidence of loose bodies. The medial compartment was then examined which revealed a posterior horn tear that was deemed irreparable and stable. The intercondylar notch was then examined, which revealed a midsubstance tear of the anterior cruciate ligament with a positive empty wall sign and cyclops lesion. The posterior cruciate ligament was noted to be intact. Attention was then directed towards the lateral compartment which revealed grade 3 chondromalacial changes in the lateral femoral condyle and a tear in the anterior horn of the lateral meniscus which was deemed irreparable as well. The anterior horn tear in the lateral meniscus and the posterior horn tear in the medial meniscus were debrided using suction punch and meniscal debridement. Attention was then directed towards the notch where the stump of the old torn ACL was excised. A notchplasty was then performed using a Dyonics bur. A tibial site was then selected using the PCL as a guide and the Acufex guide to align the K-wire into the selected tibial site. A Steinmann pin was then introduced into the tibial site which was approximately 7 mm anterior to the over-the-top position. The knee was then brought out into full extension which revealed the K-wire to be free of impingement. An 8-mm drill was then used to drill out tibial and femoral tunnels, and progressive sounds, ranging from 7 to 10 mm, were used to expand the tunnel. After insertion of the 8-mm sound, it was noted that the sound had pierced through the back of our femoral tunnel. We then decided to proceed with an arthroscopically assisted ACL reconstruction. A 5- to 6-cm longitudinal incision was made over the lateral aspect of the distal thigh. Sharp dissection was carried down to the level of the fascia which was sharply incised. A periosteal elevator was then used to elevate the vastus lateralis off the underlying lateral distal tibial cortex. A Beath pin was then placed up through the tibial tunnel and into the femoral tunnel and out the femoral cortex into the overlying soft tissue and skin. Using the Beath pin, the bone-tendon-bone autograft was then pulled up into the joint and femoral tunnel.

After being satisfied with the position of the graft to the femoral tunnel, the entry 0.2 drill bit was used to drill the distal femoral cortex. The 48-mm, 4.5-bicortical screw was then placed across the femur with a washer. The graft was tied over the screw before tightening and gauging the distal medial femoral cortex. The leg was then brought out to near full extension, and the tibial plug was then fixed using a 9 x 20 mm interference screw. After satisfactory purchase of the tibial plug, the patient was brought into full extension and assessed for stability. This revealed a negative Lachman at the termination of the procedure. The wound was then copiously irrigated with sterile normal saline, and a 1/8-inch Hemovac was then placed into the joint. The anterior half of the patellar tendon was then approximated using 3 interrupted 2-0 Maxon sutures, followed by a closure of the overlying peritenon with a running 2-0 Vicryl suture. The patellar defect was bone grafted before closing the peritenon using the bone obtained from fashioning the bone plugs from the autogenous graft. Staples were then used to close the skin, and 2 mg of Duramorph and 18 cc of 0.25% of Marcaine were injected into the joint through the inflow cannula. The cannula was then removed. The wound was then dressed using fluffs, followed by the application of an Icy Hot compressive cooling dressing. The patient was then placed into an EZ Wrap postop ACL brace and taken from the operating room to the recovery room in stable condition, extubated and without apparent complications. Tourniquet used to harvest the patellar tendon graft was deflated after procedure, and total tourniquet time was 34 minutes.

Footnotes:

1. 1.Grades are typically written in Arabic number format, although some clients may prefer these be presented using Roman numerals.
2. 2.The 3B here is a classification of the degree of Lachman.

Spelling.
Determine if the following words are spelled correctly. If the spelling is correct, leave the word as it has already been entered. If the spelling is incorrect, retype the word with the correct spelling.

1. _____   2. _____

3. _____   4. _____

5. _____

Matching.
Match the correct terms.

1. ____ Acufex   A. pin
2. ____ Dyonics   B. brace
3. ____ Beath   C. cannula
4. ____ Vicryl   D. guide
5. ____ inflow   E. bur
6. ____ EZ Wrap   F. suture

ORTHOPEDICS REPORT 9 – OPERATIVE NOTE

OPERATION PERFORMED: Left shoulder examination under anesthesia, glenohumeral and subacromial arthroscopy with subacromial decompression.

INDICATIONS: This is a 52-year-old white female with a long history of left shoulder impingement syndrome. She has had 2 subacromial steroid injections and intensive physical therapy. However, she has been refractory to these treatments and still has daily pain that impacts on her activities of daily living.

DESCRIPTION OF PROCEDURE: The patient was taken to the operating room, placed in the supine position for induction of general anesthetic. She was then repositioned to the right lateral decubitus position using the beanbag. An arm traction setup was then applied to her left arm, positioning her in approximately 20 degrees of flexion, 60 degrees of abduction. The rest of the limb was then sterilely prepped and draped. At that time, the surgical landmarks were palpated and delineated using the marking pen on the skin, showing both the posterolateral corner of the acromion, anterolateral corner, and the coracoid. The soft spot approximately 2 cm below the posterolateral corner of the acromion was then palpated. An 18-gauge spinal needle was inserted into the joint, and 30 cc of fluid was instilled into the joint. Free backflow was noted. The 11 blade was then used to make the stab wound incision in the region of the needle, and the sharp followed by dull trocars with scope were then introduced into the soft tissues and into the joint respectively. The glenohumeral joint was then inspected in a systematic fashion. No defects were noted. There was some tendinitis in the region of the biceps tendon. Scope was then removed from the glenohumeral joint, directed more superiorly into the subacromial bursa. It was noted there was marked bursal thickening, synovitis, and significant chronic inflammation of the bursa. The Dyonics debrider was then inserted into the bursa for subacromial soft tissue dissection. Following that, with the bone-cutting black Dyonics shaver, the acromion was shaved off level with its posterior aspect. Additional portals established for this procedure included an anterior portal and a lateral portal. Alternating the scope and the shavers in these portals, we were able to fully debride the acromion and do a subtotal bursectomy. The arthroscopic scissors were then inserted into the lateral portal, bringing them in line with the coracoacromial ligament. They were used to finish the resection of the coracoacromial ligament. After this and following inspection of the subacromial bursa with resection deemed adequate, all cannulas were removed. At the time, 15 cc of 0.5% Marcaine and 12 cc of 1% Xylocaine with epinephrine were infiltrated into the joint. The wound was then dressed with Xeroform, fluffs, ABDs, and foam tape. A shoulder immobilizer was applied prior to extubation. The patient was then extubated in the recovery room, having received a total of 14 cc of fluids, having 100 cc of blood loss. She was transported to the recovery room in stable condition.

Multiple Choice.
Choose the best answer.

1. The subacromial bursa showed marked (○ bursle, ○ bursal) thickening and synovitis.

2. The patient was then (○ exsanguinated, ○ extubated) in the recovery room.

3. The patient has daily pain that impacts on her (○ activities, ○ areas) of daily living.

4. The limb was then (○ sterilely, ○ sterily) prepped and draped.

5. The joint was infiltrated with Xylocaine with (○ epinephrine, ○ bacitracin) .

Multiple Choice.
Choose the best answer.

1. Lying down position
   - ○ decubitas
   - ○ decubitus
   - ○ decubitis

2. Behind and to one side, specifically to the outer side.
   - ○ posterolateral
   - ○ postorolateral
   - ○ postorrolateral

3. Situated beneath the acromial process of the scapula.
   - ○ subachromial
   - ○ subacromiol
   - ○ subacromial

4. In front and away from the middle line.
   - ○ anterolaterel
   - ○ anterolateral
   - ○ anteriolateral

5. Relating to the glenoid cavity and the humerus.
   - ○ glenohumeral
   - ○ glenohumerel
   - ○ glenohumoral

UNIT 9
Otorhinolaryngology

OTORHINOLARYNGOLOGY – INTRODUCTION

Otorhinolaryngology is a specialty of medicine that deals with disorders/operations of the ears, nose, and throat (ENT). As you remember, **oto** means ear, **rhino** means nose, and **laryngo** means throat. We will refer to this specialty as ENT and otorhinolaryngology interchangeably throughout this unit.

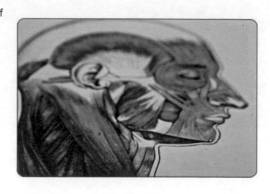

In ENT transcription editing you will encounter problems such as:

- tonsillitis
- laryngitis
- parotiditis
- pharyngitis
- snoring and sleep apnea
- ear infection (otitis media, otitis externa, and otitis interna)
- hearing loss
- dizziness
- conditions of the thyroid and parotid glands
- chronic sinusitis and rhinitis
- strep throat
- deviated septum
- nasopharyngeal carcinoma and other cancers
- common cold

Common ENT evaluative techniques include (but are certainly not limited to):

- physical examination
- hearing test
- sleep study
- culture
- various scope diagnostic studies
  - laryngoscopy
  - nasopharyngeal scope
- radiograph

And finally, typical procedures you may type in ENT include:

- myringotomy and tubes
- thyroidectomy
- rhinoplasty
- tympanoplasty
- ethmoidectomy
- tonsillectomy
- adenoidectomy
- functional sinus surgery
- turbinectomy
- nasoantral windows

Although not traditionally lumped in with ENT, Oral Surgery reports will be included as a mini-unit inside this ENT unit.

OTORHINOLARYNGOLOGY LANGUAGE WORKSHOP

Again, this list is in no way an exhaustive list of ENT word-building word parts and abbreviations. It is meant merely to be a review of words commonly associated with the ENT specialty—words you are likely to be exposed to in this FOMS unit, in the practicum modules of this training program, and as a successful working medical transcription editor.

Common Otorhinolaryngology Root Words and Combining Forms

Root Word & Combining Form	Meaning	Example
aden/o	gland	adenopathy
adenoid/o	adenoids	adenoidectomy
aer/o	air	aerosinusitis
aur/o	ear	auricle
bronch/o	windpipe	bronchoscopy
bucc/o	cheek	buccodistal
cephal/o	head	cephalostat
cervic/o	neck	cervicofacial
chondr/o	cartilage	chondroblast
dent/i, dent/o	teeth	dental
dips/o	thirst	polydipsia
gloss/o	tongue	glossopexy
gnath/o	jaw	gnathodynia
labi/o	lip	labiolingual
laryng/o	larynx	laryngopharynx
lingu/o	tongue	linguoaxial
medi/o	middle	mediolateral
muc/o	mucus	mucopurulent
nas/o	nose	nasopharyngeal
odont/o	teeth	odontoma
or/o	mouth	oronasal
ot/o	ear	otolaryngology
pharyng/o	pharynx	pharyngitis
phon/o	sound/voice	phonosurgery
rhin/o	nose	rhinology

Common Otorhinolaryngology Prefixes

Prefix	Meaning	Example
ab-	away from	abduct
ad-	toward	adduct
epi-	above/on	epicondylectomy
eu-	good/normal	euthyroid
hyper-	excessive, greater than normal	hyperesthesia
hypo-/sub-	below, beneath normal	hyponatremia
macro-	large	macrocephaly
meso-	middle or moderate	mesostructure
micro-	small	microblade
peri-	around/near	perivascular

Common Otorhinolaryngology Suffixes

Suffix	Meaning	Example
-centesis	procedure to aspirate fluid	paracentesis
-ectasia/ectasis	dilatation	telangiectasia
-edema	swelling	lymphedema
-emesis	vomiting	hematemesis
-gram	record	audiogram
-itis	inflammation	tonsillitis
-ium	membrane	sodium
-megaly	enlargement	acromegaly
-meter	instrument to measure	audiometer
-opia	vision	amblyopia
-phagia/-gic/-gy	eating/swallowing	dysphagia
-phasia	speech	dysphasia
-rrhage/-rrhagia	excessive flow or discharge	hemorrhage
-rrhea	flow or discharge	rhinorrhea
-scopy	examination with an instrument	otoscopy

Common Otorhinolaryngology Abbreviations

Abbreviation	Expansion
CSOM	chronic suppurative otitis media/chronic serous otitis media
ENT	ear, nose, and throat
EUA	exam under anesthesia
FB	foreign body
FESS	functional endoscopic sinus surgery
MUA	manipulation under anesthesia
OE	otitis externa
OM	otitis media
PACU	post-anesthesia care unit
PE	pressure equalization (tube)
PNS	postnasal space
SMD	sub-mucosal diathermy
SMR	submucous resection
T&A	tonsils and adenoids
TM	tympanic membrane
TO	tracheoesophageal
UPPP	uvulopalatopharyngoplasty

REVIEW: OTORHINOLARYNGOLOGY LANGUAGE

Fill in the Blank.
Using the word(s) in the box, fill in the blanks.

1. *PACU* stands for post-_____care unit.

2. In *CSOM*, or chronic _____otitis media, the patient suffers from a perforated tympanic membrane with persistent drainage from the middle ear.

3. Inflammation of the larynx is _____.

4. The term for examination of the ear with an instrument is _____.

5. *ENT* stands for ear, _____, and throat.

suppurative
anesthesia
otoscopy
laryngitis
nose

Multiple Choice.
Choose the best answer.

1. Term which literally means "bad speech" or inability to speak properly is (◯ dysphasia, ◯ polydipsia).

2. The term for vomiting blood is (◯ hematemesis, ◯ hematochezia).

3. The laryngoscope is an instrument used to examine the (◯ ears, ◯ larynx).

4. In the term *PE tube*, *PE* stands for pressure (◯ equalization, ◯ elimination).

5. A spasm in the windpipe is called a (◯ bronchospasm, ◯ vasospasm).

TRUE/FALSE.
Mark the following true or false.

1. *Tonsillitis* means inflammation of the adenoids.

   ◯ true

   ◯ false

2. Surgical procedure performed on the nose is called *rhinoplasty*.

   ◯ true

   ◯ false

3. The term *cephalad* means toward the head.

   ◯ true

   ◯ false

4. Term for inflammation of the pharynx is *pharyngitis*.

   ◯ true

   ◯ false

5. *Subglossal* means under the eyelid.

   ◯ true

   ◯ false

OTORHINOLARYNGOLOGY REPORTS

Although it is not always the case, as you will see in the reports in this unit, ENT reports do have a tendency to be quite short. The most frequently performed procedures are myringotomy with tubes and tonsillectomy and adenoidectomy. These are very common reports, with little variation as to technique and instruments. The terminology found in the history of present illness, physical examination, and hospital course for all types of ENT problems is quite similar. Following are samples of ENT reports. These may include procedure reports, as well as discharge summaries.

OTORHINOLARYNGOLOGY REPORT 1 – OPERATIVE NOTE

PREOPERATIVE DIAGNOSIS: Snoring, hypertrophic inferior turbinates.

ANESTHESIA: General.

POSTOPERATIVE DIAGNOSIS: Snoring, hypertrophic inferior turbinates.

MATERIAL FORWARDED TO LABORATORY: Right and left tonsils.

PROCEDURES PERFORMED

1. Uvulopalatopharyngoplasty.
2. Submucous resection of inferior turbinates.

INDICATIONS: The patient is a 23-year-old female who has a history of loud snoring at night. She has no symptoms or evidence of obstructive sleep apnea but wishes her snoring treated surgically. In addition, she has an ongoing history of nasal obstruction that has been unresponsive to medical therapy. On physical exam the patient has a very redundant soft palate and uvula. She also has very hypertrophic inferior turbinates. She is thus being taken to the operating room for definitive treatment of snoring and nasal obstruction.

DESCRIPTION OF PROCEDURE: After informed consent was obtained from the patient she was taken to the operating room and placed in the supine position. General endotracheal anesthesia was administered. The face was prepped and draped in the usual fashion.

The uvulopalatopharyngoplasty was addressed first. A McIvor mouth gag was placed in the patient's mouth, and the patient was suspended from the stand. A tonsillectomy was performed first to open up the oropharynx. On the left side, the tonsil was retracted medially, and Bovie cautery was used to dissect in the plane between the tonsil and underlying musculature. In this fashion, the tonsil was removed from its fossa and sent to Pathology. Essentially, no bleeding resulted from the tonsillectomy at this point. This procedure was repeated on the right side, and again, essentially no bleeding was encountered. Using palpation, the soft palate was pressed against the posterior wall of the oropharynx. In this fashion, the location of the cut for the soft palate was estimated such that after removal of the redundant tissue, the soft palate would still reach the posterior oropharyngeal wall for closure to prevent velopharyngeal insufficiency.[1] The edge of the soft palate was then grasped using a DeBakey forceps, and a beveled cut was made in the soft palate, using the Bovie cautery. This bevel was made such that the nasal mucosa could be pulled down and sewn to the oral side of the mucosa. This resulted in trimming approximately 1 cm off the soft palate, then 3-0 Vicryl sutures were used to sew the nasal mucosa to the oral side of the mucosa along the edge of the soft palate. In addition, the anterior and posterior tonsillar pillars were sewn together approximately three quarters of the way down towards the inferior pole. This resulted in excellent hemostasis, and the nasal mucosa was approximated to the oral mucosa along the edge of the soft palate. In addition, this opened up the oropharynx, both laterally and in the region of the soft palate. The wound was copiously irrigated with normal saline, and no further bleeding was noted. The mouth gag was let down for several seconds, and again, no further bleeding was noted. The patient was taken out of suspension and the mouth gag was removed.

The submucous resection of the inferior turbinates was then undertaken. The inferior turbinates were first infiltrated with 1% lidocaine with 1:100,000 epinephrine, and cocaine pledgets[2] were placed along the inferior turbinates for additional vasoconstriction. These pledgets were then withdrawn. An incision was made in the anterior edge of the inferior turbinates and along the inferior edge as well. A Freer elevator was used to elevate the mucoperiosteum from the turbinate bone. The turbinate bone was then infractured using a Sayre elevator. Turbinate scissors were then used to trim the turbinate bone along with the attached lateral mucoperiosteum. The remaining medial edge of the mucoperiosteum was then wrapped around the raw turbinate bone laterally and superiorly. This procedure was performed on both sides. Only minimal bleeding resulted from this procedure. Bacitracin impregnated Telfa dressing was then placed as a pack into either side of the nose, and these packs were sewn together anteriorly over the columella with a loose stitch to prevent aspiration of the packs. A nasal drip pad was then applied.

The patient was awakened and extubated in the operating room, and was taken to the recovery room in good condition. She tolerated the procedure well. Estimated blood loss: 30 cc. Fluids: Approximately 2200 cc crystalloid. Complications: None.

FINDINGS: Redundant soft palate, hypertrophic inferior turbinates.

Footnotes:

1. 1.Velopharyngeal insufficiency is incomplete closure of the velopharyngeal sphincter between the oropharynx and the nasopharynx.
2. 2.Cocaine pledgets are commonly used for topical vasoconstriction, to decrease the diameter of the blood vessels in the nose.

SPELLING.

Determine if the following words are spelled correctly. If the spelling is correct, leave the word as it has already been entered. If the spelling is incorrect, provide the correct spelling.

1. turbinates _____

2. uvulopalatopharyngoplasty _____

3. McIver _____

4. Bovie _____

5. vilopharyngeal _____

6. DeBaky _____

7. Vicryl _____

8. palate _____

9. epinephrine _____

10 vasoconstriction _____

11. pledguts _____

12. mucoperiosteum _____

13. Sayer _____

14. bacitracin _____

15. Telpha _____

16. columnella _____

17. crystalloid _____

Matching.

Match the correct terms.

1. ____ Sayre

2. ____ DeBakey

3. ____ McIvor

4. ____ Telfa

5. ____ Bovie

A. dressing

B. mouth gag

C. elevator

D. cautery

E. forceps

OTORHINOLARYNGOLOGY REPORT 2 – OPERATIVE NOTE

PREOPERATIVE DIAGNOSIS

1. Obstructive sleep apnea.
2. Chronic obstructive pulmonary disease.

POSTOPERATIVE DIAGNOSIS

1. Obstructive sleep apnea
2. Chronic obstructive pulmonary disease.

PROCEDURE PERFORMED: Tracheostomy.

ANESTHESIA: Local infiltration with IV sedation.

INDICATIONS: The patient is a 79-year-old white male with history of oxygen-dependent COPD with obstructive sleep apnea. The patient has undergone transtracheal oxygen catheterization x4 in the past. He now requires tracheostomy for increased oxygenation.

FINDINGS OF OPERATION: Marked pretracheal and tracheal scarring.

DESCRIPTION OF PROCEDURE: The patient was taken to the operating room, placed in a supine position, and anesthesia was induced with infiltration of 1% lidocaine with 1:100,000 epinephrine, and IV sedation. The patient was prepped with Betadine paint and scrub, and draped in the usual sterile fashion. The patient's cervical anatomy was reviewed, and a 4-cm transverse incision was made approximately 2 fingerbreadths[1] superior to the sternal notch. A pre-existing track from the transtracheal oxygen catheter[2] was included in the skin incision in an elliptical fashion. The skin incision was continued through the subcutaneous tissues using the scalpel with electrocautery utilized to maintain hemostasis. The TTO track[3] was then bluntly and sharply dissected to its origin at the first tracheal ring. Utilizing this landmark, the strap musculature was split in a midline plane, clearly revealing the pretracheal tissues. Marked scarring was noted throughout the pretracheal area. The thyroid isthmus was not visualized. A transverse incision was made through the second[4] tracheal interspace and continued laterally through the tracheal ring on each side, creating an inferior based flap. This flap was sutured to the subcutaneous layer of the inferior aspect of the skin incision. A #8 Shiley tufted non-fenestrated tracheostomy tube was then placed without difficulty, allowing excellent ventilation. The tracheostomy tube was then sutured to the skin in 4 places using 2-0 silk suture. The procedure was tolerated well by the patient. EBL: Less than 20 mL. Fluids: 750 mL of crystalloid. Complications: None. Disposition: To the surgical intensive care unit in stable condition.

Footnotes:

1. 1.Even when dictated as "fingersbreadth," the correct plural of fingerbreadth is fingerbreadths.
2. 2.Transtracheal oxygen therapy is a method for delivering oxygen directly to the lungs through a small, flexible tube (catheter) inserted into the windpipe.
3. 3.TTO track = transtracheal oxygen track.
4. 4.Also acceptably edited as 2nd. When available, account preference should be adhered to regarding ordinals.

SPELLING.
Determine if the following words are spelled correctly. If the spelling is correct, leave the word as it has already been entered. If the spelling is incorrect, provide the correct spelling.

1. fingersbreadth _____

2. scalple _____

3. Shiley _____

4. fennestrated _____

5. eliptical _____

TRUE/FALSE.
Mark the following true or false.

1. The procedure was done under general endotracheal anesthesia.

   ○ true

   ○ false

2. The pre-existing track from the TTO catheter was included in the skin incision.

   ○ true

   ○ false

3. Estimated blood loss was 750 mL.

   ○ true

   ○ false

4. The patient was taken to the surgical intensive care unit in stable condition.

   ○ true

   ○ false

5. Vicryl suture was used in this procedure.

   ○ true

   ○ false

OTORHINOLARYNGOLOGY REPORT 3 – OPERATIVE NOTE

PREOPERATIVE DIAGNOSIS[1]

1. Eustachian tube dysfunction.
2. Chronic right anterior ethmoid sinusitis.
3. Deviated nasal septum with accompanying nasal obstruction.
4. Compensatory turbinate hypertrophy.

ANESTHESIA: General endotracheal anesthesia.

POSTOPERATIVE DIAGNOSIS

1. Eustachian tube dysfunction.
2. Chronic right anterior ethmoid sinusitis.
3. Deviated nasal septum with accompanying nasal obstruction.
4. Compensatory turbinate hypertrophy.

MATERIAL FORWARDED TO LABORATORY: Right ethmoid sinus contents. Septal cartilage and bone.

PROCEDURE PERFORMED

1. Septoplasty.
2. Anterior ethmoidectomy on the right.
3. Right maxillary sinus antrotomy.
4. Cautery and outfracture of inferior nasal turbinates bilaterally.

INDICATIONS: The patient is a 14-year-old female with chief complaint of chronic eustachian tube dysfunction. This has not been relieved with trials of nasal sprays to include Vancenase AQ. The patient also complains of postnasal drip with chronic congestion.

FINDINGS OF OPERATION: The nasal septum is deviated to the right. The bony septum is deviated to the right, and there is an inferior cartilaginous spur on the right side. There is some thickened mucosa on the anterior ethmoid sinus on the right. The right maxillary sinus natural ostium was extremely small and covered with thickened mucosa. The inferior turbinates bilaterally were hypertrophic.

DESCRIPTION OF PROCEDURE: After having obtained consent, the patient was taken to the operative suite, where general endotracheal anesthesia was administered. After obtaining a satisfactory level of anesthesia, the table was turned, and a total of 4 cc of 4% cocaine was administered to each nostril on cottonoid pledgets. This remained in place for about 5 minutes. Subsequent to this, 1% lidocaine with 1:100,000 epinephrine was used to inject the following areas: the nasal septum bilaterally, the nasal floor bilaterally, the inferior turbinates bilaterally, and the middle turbinates bilaterally. The cocaine pledgets were then once again inserted, and the face was prepped and draped in the usual sterile fashion. After removing the cocaine packs, a right hemitransfixion incision was made. Paparella knife was used to confirm the adequate level of dissection through the mucoperichondrium on the right. Using a Cottle elevator, the mucoperichondrium was elevated off the underlying quadrilateral cartilage to the level of the bony cartilaginous junction, which was then dislocated with the Cottle elevator. The mucoperiosteum was elevated off the bony septum bilaterally with the Cottle elevator. Using scissors, a superior cut was made in the bony septum. Using Takahashi forceps, the deviated portion of the bony septum was then removed. Minimally deviated superior bony nasal septum was removed with double action Jansen-Middleton rongeurs.[2] Inspection at this time demonstrated an inferior spur of the quadrilateral cartilage. This was removed using a septal D-knife and Takahashi forceps. Examination subsequent to this demonstrated excellent bilateral nasal area. A plain gut suture with a Keith needle was used for septal quilting stitch. The hemitransfixion incision was then closed with interrupted 4-0 chromic sutures. Attention was then turned toward the inferior turbinates. Using a Sayre elevator each inferior turbinate was infractured and then outfractured. Using a spinal needle the inferior turbinates were then cauterized superiorly and inferiorly and posteromedially. The endoscopic sinus equipment was then brought in, and using a 0-degree telescope, the middle turbinate was easily visualized. This was infractured using a Freer elevator. Using a sickle knife the uncinate process was entered.

This was subsequently removed with Takahashi forceps. The anterior ethmoidectomy was then performed using Takahashi forceps. See above for findings. At no time was there evidence of herniation of orbital fat, nor did any of the specimens float in water. Next, attention was turned toward the natural ostium of the maxillary sinus, which was easily identified and probed with a curved sucker. This was extremely small. Therefore, using a backbiter, the natural ostium was enlarged. The middle meatus was then packed with Surgicel impregnated with bacitracin ointment. Bilaterally, Doyle splints were placed, with Telfa impregnated with bacitracin also placed in the nares bilaterally lateral to the Doyle splints. The Doyle splints were secured anteriorly with a transcolumellar suture using a chromic stitch. The Telfa pads were anteriorly tied together with a chromic stitch to prevent slippage back into the nasopharynx. The columella was protected with a piece of Telfa impregnated with bacitracin. The patient was then awakened from anesthesia, having tolerated the procedure extremely well. There were no intraoperative complications. Condition of patient to recovery is stable postoperatively. Fluids: 1100 cc of crystalloid. Estimated blood loss: Less than 50 cc. Please note in the PACU,[3] the patient had full range of extraocular motion, and no clinical evidence of an orbital hemorrhage.

Footnotes:

1. 1.It might seem that this should be diagnoses instead of diagnosis (since there are more than one listed), but there are a number of reasons diagnosis works as well: 1) the heading *diagnosis* can be used for a group of diagnoses, 2) it may be the "preferred heading" by the client, and 3) the headings may be preformatted in this report and changing them is not an option.
2. 2.This report is full of uniquely named surgical equipment. A surgical word book would go a long way in verifying the accurate spelling of these dictated equipment terms.
3. 3.PACU = post-anesthesia care unit.

SPELLING.
Determine if the following words are spelled correctly. If the spelling is correct, leave the word as it has already been entered. If the spelling is incorrect, provide the correct spelling.

1. eustasian _____
2. antrotomy _____
3. cautery _____
4. cotonoid _____
5. Paparella _____
6. Cauttle _____
7. Jansen-Middleton _____
8. rongers _____
9. quadrilateral _____
10. Doyle _____

Fill in the Blank.
Using the word(s) in the box, fill in the blanks.

1. _____ elevator
2. _____ splints
3. _____ pads
4. _____ forceps
5. _____ rongeur
6. _____ knife
7. _____ needle

Cottle
Doyle
Jansen-Middleton
Keith
Paparella
Takahashi
Telfa

OTORHINOLARYNGOLOGY REPORT 4 – OPERATIVE NOTE

PREOPERATIVE DIAGNOSIS: Laryngeal mass, rule out malignancy.

POSTOPERATIVE DIAGNOSIS: Laryngeal mass, rule out malignancy.

PROCEDURE PERFORMED: Direct laryngoscopy with biopsies.

INDICATIONS: The patient is a 38-year-old man who recently underwent an esophagogastroduodenoscopy for reflux. Incidentally during this exam, an exophytic mass of the larynx was noted. He was referred to ENT. On fiberoptic laryngoscopy he had an exophytic mass at the base of his epiglottis that extended to the false vocal cord on the left side. He is being taken to the operating room for biopsy of this mass for diagnosis and for staging.

DESCRIPTION OF PROCEDURE: After informed consent was obtained from the patient, he was taken to the operating room and placed in the supine position. General endotracheal anesthesia was administered. A shoulder roll was placed under his shoulder. The head was extended as far as possible. However, this extension was limited by the patient's cervical arthritis. This arthritis prevented rigid esophagoscopy and/or bronchoscopy. Thorough inspection of the oral cavity was first performed. No mucosal lesions were noted, and no submucosal lesions were palpated. An anterior commissure laryngoscope was then inserted into the larynx without difficulty. The patient was noted to have a benign appearing vallecular cyst. Further examination of the larynx was hindered by this cyst. Therefore this cyst was unroofed and was evacuated. A portion of the cyst wall was sent to the pathology department for permanent section. The remainder of the cyst was aspirated, and the cyst was marsupialized. The laryngoscope was then inserted further and immediately an exophytic mass was noted at the base of the epiglottis. This extended from the base of the epiglottis in about the midline to the left false vocal cord. The false vocal cord appeared to be involved. However, the true vocal cord appeared to be free of tumor. The piriform sinuses on either side appeared to be free of tumor. The anterior commissure of the vocal cords appeared to be free of tumor. Several biopsies were taken from this exophytic mass and were sent to the pathology department for frozen section. This resulted in only minimal bleeding. The laryngoscope was then withdrawn carefully. No injury to the teeth or lips was noted. The patient was awakened and extubated in the operating room and was taken to the recovery room in good condition. He tolerated the procedure well. Estimated blood loss: Minimal. Fluids: 1 L of crystalloid. Complications: None.

TNM Cancer Staging

T tumor size or involvement

N regional lymph node involvement

M extent of metastasis

Letters and numerals following TNM

X means assessment cannot be done

0 (zero) indicates no evidence found

Arabic numerals indicate increasing evidence of the characteristics represented by those letters

FINDINGS

1. Benign appearing vallecular cyst.
2. Exophytic lesion extending from the midline of the base of the epiglottis to the left false vocal cord.
3. The true vocal cords appeared to be free of tumor and were freely mobile. No neck nodes were palpated under general anesthesia.

DIAGNOSIS: The final diagnosis is pending the permanent pathology report. However, at this point, this is being staged as a T2 N0 MX[1] squamous cell carcinoma of the larynx pending final pathology.

Footnotes:

1. 1. TNM staging is presented with Arabic numerals after the letter and a space after each number (no commas).

Spelling.

Determine if the following words are spelled correctly. If the spelling is correct, leave the word as it has already been entered. If the spelling is incorrect, retype the word with the correct spelling.

1. _____   2. _____

3. _____   4. _____

5. _____

Multiple Choice.

Choose the best answer.

1. The patient is being seen to rule out (○ malignency, ○ malignancy).

2. The true vocal (○ cords, ○ chords) appeared to be free of tumor.

3. The cyst was unroofed and was (○ valleculated, ○ evacuated).

4. Pending diagnosis is (○ squamus, ○ squamous) carcinoma of the larynx.

5. The patient recently underwent an (○ EKG, ○ EGD) for reflux.

OTORHINOLARYNGOLOGY REPORT 5 – OPERATIVE NOTE

PREOPERATIVE DIAGNOSIS: Recurrent tonsillitis and upper airway obstruction.

ANESTHESIA: General endotracheal.

POSTOPERATIVE DIAGNOSIS: Recurrent tonsillitis and upper airway obstruction.

OPERATION PERFORMED: Tonsillectomy and adenoidectomy.

INDICATIONS: The patient is a 25-year-old male who has a long history of recurrent sore throats. He reports that almost monthly he gets recurrent sore throats that sometimes are positive for strep.[1] This has resulted in significant loss of his work time. In addition, he reports that at night he is a very loud snorer and suffers from persistent nasal congestion that has been unresponsive to medical therapy. He is being taken to the operating room for tonsillectomy and adenoidectomy for treatment of his recurrent sore throats and upper airway obstruction.

DESCRIPTION OF PROCEDURE: After informed consent was obtained from the patient, he was taken to the operating room and placed in the supine position. General endotracheal anesthesia was administered. The face was prepped and draped in the usual sterile fashion. A McIvor mouth gag was placed into position, and the patient was suspended from the stand. A rubber catheter was inserted through the nose and withdrawn through the mouth in order to retract the soft palate. Adenoidectomy was addressed first. Inspection of the adenoid bed using a nasopharyngeal mirror revealed moderate hypertrophy. Several cuts using a large adenoid curet were made, resulting in a modest amount of adenoid tissue being obtained. This was sent for permanent section. A tonsil sponge was then placed in the area for hemostasis. The left tonsil was then addressed. Using a curved Allis to retract the tonsil medially, an incision was made in the superior pole using electrocautery. The plane between the tonsil and underlying musculature was identified using the cautery. Dissection along this plane was carried inferiorly until the tonsil was removed. Only minimal bleeding resulted at this time. This was controlled easily with suction cautery. The right tonsil was addressed in a similar fashion. Similarly, only suction cautery was required for hemostasis. Reinspection of the left side revealed a small amount of residual tonsil tissue at the inferior pole. This was removed sharply. Additional hemostasis was achieved with suction cautery, and a single figure-of-eight 3-0 chromic stitch was placed in the inferior pole on this side. No further bleeding was noted from the right side. Inspection of the adenoid bed revealed only minimal bleeding that was easily controlled with suction cautery. The nasopharynx and oropharynx were then copiously irrigated with normal saline. The mouth gag was then let down for several seconds. Upon reopening, no further bleeding was noted. The mouth gag and the catheter through the nose were then withdrawn. The patient was awakened and extubated in the operating room and was taken to the recovery room in good condition. He tolerated the procedure well. Estimated blood loss: 50 cc. Fluids: Approximately 1200 cc of crystalloid. Complications: None.

FINDINGS: Hypertrophic tonsils and adenoids.

Footnotes:

1. 1. Genus names, such as strep or streptococcus, should be edited lowercase when they stand alone (without a species name).

Multiple Choice.
Choose the correct spelling for the term defined.

1. Abnormal enlargement of organ or body part.

   ○ hypotrophic

   ○ hypertrophic

   ○ hypratrophic

   ○ hypatrofic

2. The diffuse lymphoid tissue and follicles in the roof and posterior wall of the nasopharynx.

   ○ adinoid

   ○ adenod

   ○ adenoid

   ○ edanoid

3. The muscular part of the roof of the mouth.

   ○ soft palate

   ○ soft pallate

   ○ soft palite

   ○ soft pallite

4. Inflammation of the tonsils.

   ○ tonsilitis

   ○ tonsiloatrophy

   ○ tonsillitis

   ○ tonsilloatrophy

5. A shortened and commonly used form of the bacteria that are gram-positive cocci.

   ○ strep

   ○ strept

   ○ Strept

   ○ Strep

Multiple Choice.
Choose the best answer.

1. The patient reports that almost monthly he gets (○ reocurrent, ○ recurrent) sore throats.

2. The (○ sinus, ○ oropharynx) was copiously irrigated with normal saline.

3. (○ Dissection, ○ Disection) along this plane was carried inferiorly until the tonsil was removed.

4. Only suction (○ cautery, ○ ligature) was required for hemostasis.

5. The patient was awakened and (○ exibated, ○ extubated) in the operating room.

OTORHINOLARYNGOLOGY REPORT 6 – DISCHARGE SUMMARY

CHIEF COMPLAINT: The patient is a 31-year-old female who has a long history of nasal congestion and snoring.

HISTORY OF PRESENT ILLNESS: The patient has a long history of nasal congestion and snoring along with facial pain and pressure. She underwent sinus surgery and a septoplasty in February, but received no benefit in her nasal breathing or her snoring. She did not have a sleep study; however, she does not have any signs or symptoms of obstructive sleep apnea. She was admitted to the hospital for surgery to attempt correction of her snoring and nasal obstruction.

PHYSICAL EXAMINATION: At the time of admission, the patient's physical exam was significant for very hypertrophic inferior turbinates as well as a rather redundant soft palate. The remainder of her physical exam was benign.

HOSPITAL COURSE: The patient was admitted to the hospital on July 2, 2006. She underwent a surgery along with a submucous resection of the inferior turbinates on July 3, 2006. The surgery was uncomplicated. Her postoperative course was routine. She was started on a clear liquid diet and advanced to a soft diet. She was tolerating oral intake adequate to discontinue her IV by the 1st postoperative day. She then remained in the hospital until July 5, 2006. Her pain is well controlled with oral analgesics, and she remains on oral antibiotics.

DISCHARGE DIAGNOSES

1. Snoring.
2. Hypertrophic inferior turbinates.

OPERATION: The patient underwent uvulopalatopharyngoplasty and a submucous resection of the inferior turbinates on July 3, 2006.

DISCHARGE MEDICATIONS: The patient was discharged with Percocet and Tylenol with Codeine[1] for pain. She was also discharged to finish a course of amoxicillin. She was given viscous lidocaine for the symptomatic relief of her throat pain.

DISCHARGE ACTIVITY: The patient was instructed to avoid any strenuous physical activity for at least 3 weeks. It is recommended that she be on leave from work for 3 weeks. In addition, the patient was counseled regarding the risk of bleeding postoperatively. Should bleeding occur within the next week to 10 days, the patient will seek medical attention at her local medical center, and will notify the ENT service at Princeton-Plainsboro Teaching Hospital.

DIET: The patient was instructed to follow a soft diet for approximately 1 week. She is then to advance her diet to her regular diet as tolerated.

COMPLICATIONS: None.

Footnotes:

1. 1.While codeine is typically not capped (it is generic), Tylenol with Codeine is a trade name.

SPELLING.
Determine if the following words are spelled correctly. If the spelling is correct, leave the word as it has already been entered. If the spelling is incorrect, provide the correct spelling.

1. submucus _____

2. apnea _____

3. lidocane _____

4. uvulopalatopharyngoplasty _____

5. Percicet _____

TRUE/FALSE.
Mark the following true or false.

1. The patient has received only conservative treatment for snoring in the past.

   ○ true

   ○ false

2. The patient has no signs or symptoms of obstructive sleep apnea.

   ○ true

   ○ false

3. The patient was sent home on no antibiotics.

   ○ true

   ○ false

4. The patient is to follow a soft diet for 3 weeks.

   ○ true

   ○ false

5. The patient was discharged on restricted activity for 3 weeks.

   ○ true

   ○ false

OTORHINOLARYNGOLOGY REPORT 7 – OPERATIVE NOTE

PREOPERATIVE DIAGNOSIS: Chronic tympanic membrane perforation.

POSTOPERATIVE DIAGNOSIS: Chronic tympanic membrane perforation.

OPERATION PERFORMED: Left tympanoplasty, type 1,[1] with a postauricular approach.

INDICATIONS: The patient is a 4-year-old female with a several year history of recurrent otorrhea on the left side. She eventually presented to the ENT service with a draining left ear. This was treated for several weeks with antibiotic drops and oral antibiotics. Eventually this otorrhea resolved, and the patient was left with a large, approximately 40%, anteriorly located tympanic membrane perforation on the left side. This has remained clean and dry for several weeks. The patient is thus being taken to the operating room for definitive care of a chronic perforation.

DESCRIPTION OF PROCEDURE: After informed consent was obtained from the patient, she was taken to the operating room and placed in a supine position. General endotracheal anesthesia was administered. The table was turned 180 degrees from the anesthesiologist, and the endotracheal tube placement and other monitoring devices were confirmed in their proper position. The head was then turned to the left, and the left shoulder was lowered as much as was possible. The hair, approximately 3 cm behind the left ear, was then shaved. The hair was held out of place using a 10 x 10 drape. The left ear was then prepped and draped in the usual sterile fashion. Care was taken to cover the face only with see-through drapes to monitor the face during the procedure. The postauricular area was then infiltrated with 2% lidocaine with 1:100,000 epinephrine. The operating microscope was then brought into position, and the external auditory canal was also infiltrated with 2% lidocaine with 1:100,000 epinephrine.

A vascular strip incision was first made in the external auditory canal. This was accomplished using a sickle knife and round knife, and the flap was elevated laterally to expose the bone of the external auditory canal. The operating microscope was then removed from the immediate field. A postauricular incision was made approximately 2 fingerbreadths behind the auricle from the level of the mastoid to the temporalis muscle. This was carried down sharply to the periosteum inferiorly and to the superficial layer of the temporalis fascia superiorly. An inverted 7 incision was made in the periosteum immediately behind the external auditory canal. A Lempert elevator was used to elevate the periosteum anteriorly to expose the external auditory canal. The operating microscope was then brought back into the field, and dissection was carried further down the external auditory canal until the vascular strip incision made earlier was identified. A tympanic membrane flap was then elevated from approximately 12 o'clock to 6 o'clock. The chorda tympani nerve was identified and preserved. Prior to elevating the flap, the perforation was inspected in its entirety, and the rim of tympanic membrane around the perforation was removed using a sharp needle and microcup forceps. Gelfoam soaked in 1:1,000 epinephrine was placed in the middle ear to achieve hemostasis. Meanwhile, a graft of superficial temporal fascia was harvested from the superior part of the incision. This was cleaned of overlying debris and muscle and was pressed and dried. In addition, it was dyed blue with several drops of methylene blue. The operating microscope was then brought back into position, and the Gelfoam was removed from the middle ear. Small pieces of pressed Gelfoam were then stuffed into the middle ear space. The graft was then trimmed to an appropriate size and was placed under the tympanic membrane flap and over the Gelfoam in the middle ear. The flap was then placed in its anatomic position, and the graft was positioned appropriately, such that the entire portion of the perforation was covered medially with the graft. Several more pieces of pressed Gelfoam were placed lateral to the graft to hold it in place. The external canal was then stuffed with additional pieces of pressed Gelfoam. The periosteum was then closed with interrupted 4-0 Vicryl sutures. The postauricular incision was then closed in 2 layers, closing the subcutaneous layer with interrupted 4-0 Vicryl and closing the skin with a running, locking 4-0 nylon suture. A 1/4-inch Penrose drain was placed prior to the closure and was brought out the inferior portion of the wound. With the auricle in its normal anatomic position, the operating microscope was brought back into position and the vascular strip flap was placed back into its anatomic position. Additional pieces of pressed Gelfoam were stuffed into the external auditory canal to hold the vascular strip flap into its proper position. Finally, a piece of cotton was placed into the meatus of the external auditory canal. A mastoid dressing was applied.

The patient was awakened and extubated in the operating room and was taken to the recovery room in good condition. She tolerated the procedure well. Estimated blood loss was approximately 50 cc. Fluids were approximately 2000 cc of crystalloid. Complications were none.

FINDINGS: A large, approximately 40%, anterior perforation of the tympanic membrane was noted. The ossicular chain was inspected and was tested to ensure that it was intact. No signs of chronic infection or cholesteatoma were noted.

Footnotes:

1. 1.A type 1 tympanoplasty (also acceptably edited as type I) is called myringoplasty and only involves the restoration of the perforated eardrum by grafting.

SPELLING.

Determine if the following words are spelled correctly. If the spelling is correct, leave the word as it has already been entered. If the spelling is incorrect, provide the correct spelling.

1. otorhea _____

2. methilene _____

3. mastoid _____

4. ossiculer _____

5. cholesteatoma _____

True/False.

Mark the following true or false.

1. A postauricular incision was made approximately 1 fingerbreadth behind the auricle.

   ○ true

   ○ false

2. The preoperative and postoperative diagnoses turned out to be different.

   ○ true

   ○ false

3. The vascular strip incision was made with 2 knives.

   ○ true

   ○ false

4. Gelfoam soaked in 1:100,000 epinephrine was placed in the middle ear for hemostasis.

   ○ true

   ○ false

5. There were no complications during the surgery.

   ○ true

   ○ false

OTORHINOLARYNGOLOGY REPORT 8 – OPERATIVE NOTE

PREOPERATIVE DIAGNOSIS: Chronic sinusitis.

POSTOPERATIVE DIAGNOSIS: Chronic sinusitis.

PROCEDURE PERFORMED

1. Bilateral intranasal endoscopic ethmoidectomy.
2. Bilateral endoscopic intranasal nasal antral windows.
3. Bilateral endoscopic partial middle turbinectomies.

INDICATIONS: The patient is a 16-year-old female who has a long history of recurrent and chronic sinusitis. Despite maximum medical therapy, including long courses of antibiotics, she continues to have problems with nasal obstruction, postnasal drip, headache, and facial pain. A CT scan of the sinuses revealed thickened mucosa in the ethmoid air cells and in the area of the ostiomeatal complex. She is being taken to the operating room for definitive care of chronic sinusitis.

DESCRIPTION OF PROCEDURE: After informed consent was obtained, the patient was taken to the operating room and placed in the supine position. General endotracheal anesthesia was administered. The face was prepped and draped in the usual sterile fashion. Cocaine pledgets were first placed into the nose bilaterally. These were withdrawn, and the middle turbinates and ethmoid bullae were injected bilaterally with 1% lidocaine with 1:100,000 epinephrine. The cocaine pledgets were then replaced into the nose. Bilateral endoscopic intranasal ethmoidectomies were performed first. On the left side, using a 0-degree telescope for visualization, the medial turbinate was medially infractured. A sickle knife was then used to make an incision in the ethmoid bulla. The ethmoid cavity was then opened with a Freer elevator, and the ethmoid air cells were exenterated using Takahashi forceps. This exenteration was continued anteriorly and superiorly using an upbiting forceps. An ethmoid curet was then used to remove the remaining bony spicules.[1] A curved sucker tip was placed anteriorly into the nasal frontal duct, which was confirmed to be patent. This procedure was repeated on the right side. On both sides chronically inflamed, thickened mucosa was encountered along with a large amount of very thick mucoid material.

Bilateral intranasal endoscopic partial middle turbinectomies were then performed. Right-biting turbinate scissors were used on the left side to trim the inferior portion of the middle turbinate. This was removed in its entirety using the Takahashi forceps. This opened up the ethmoid labyrinth quite well. This procedure was repeated on the right side.

Bilateral endoscopic intranasal nasal antral windows were then performed. On the left side a right angle sucker tip was used to locate the natural ostium of the maxillary sinus. Once this was located, a backbiting forceps was inserted into the ostium, and the ostium was opened anteriorly. The ostium was opened posteriorly using a Takahashi forceps. The right angle sucker tip was then reinserted into the new ostium, which was confirmed to be approximately 2 cm in an anterior/posterior dimension and 1 cm in a superior/inferior dimension. Chronically inflamed mucosa was noted in the maxillary sinus. This procedure was repeated on the right side. Small pieces of Surgicel were then inserted into the marsupialized ethmoid cavities bilaterally, and the ethmoid cavities were filled with bacitracin ointment. The nose was then packed bilaterally using bacitracin-impregnated Vaseline gauze. This resulted in excellent hemostasis.

The patient was awakened and extubated in the operating room and taken to the recovery room in good condition. The patient tolerated the procedure well. Estimated blood loss was approximately 150 cc. Fluids: Approximately 1200 cc crystalloid.

FINDINGS: Chronically thickened mucosa was encountered in the ethmoid and maxillary sinuses. In addition, very thick mucoid material was noted in the ethmoid cavities.

Footnotes:

1. 1.If you are unsure just what bony spicules are, be sure to look them up.

Spelling.
Determine if the following words are spelled correctly. If the spelling is correct, leave the word as it has already been entered. If the spelling is incorrect, retype the word with the correct spelling.

1. _____   2. _____

3. _____   4. _____

5. _____

Multiple Choice.
Choose the best answer.

1. Despite long (○ courses, ○ coarses) of antibiotics, the patient continued to suffer from sinusitis.

2. The patient was placed in the (○ dorsal lithotomy, ○ supine) position.

3. A trimmed portion of the middle turbinate was removed using (○ Takahashi, ○ Takehashi) forceps.

4. The nose was then packed bilaterally using (○ bacitracin, ○ Vaseline) -impregnated gauze.

5. A CT scan of the sinuses revealed thickened mucosa in the (○ postauricular, ○ ostiomeatal) complex.

HISTORY OF PRESENT ILLNESS: The patient is a 53-year-old white male with a 6- to 8-month history of dysphagia to solids. He is also complaining of halitosis and occasionally has to swallow his food several times in order to get it down. Upper gastrointestinal series showed a moderately large Zenker diverticulum with a widened mouth.

PAST MEDICAL HISTORY: Significant for depression over approximately the last 4 years, for which he takes Wellbutrin XL 150 mg p.o. q.d. He had a questionable episode of angina in June 2007, with subsequent graded exercise tolerance test times 2 being normal. His most recent graded exercise tolerance test was in January 2008.

PAST SURGICAL HISTORY: Left and right inguinal hernia repairs times 2 each.

PHYSICAL EXAMINATION: The patient was a well-developed, well-nourished white male in no acute distress. Head, eyes, ears, nose, and throat exam: Unremarkable. The neck was supple and nontender, without any palpable mass or lymphadenopathy. Thyroid exam was unremarkable. There were no bruits noted. The lungs were clear to auscultation bilaterally. The heart was regular rate and rhythm without murmur. The abdomen was soft and nontender without masses or hepatosplenomegaly. Genitourinary exam: Normal circumcised male with bilaterally descended testes, which were without masses. Rectal exam: Normal prostate, Hemoccult negative stool. Extremity and neurology exams were grossly intact.

HOSPITAL COURSE: The patient was admitted on January 28, and taken to the operating room for an elective excision of his Zenker diverticulum. He tolerated the procedure well, and was started on a clear liquid diet on postoperative day #2. He was discharged on January 31, 2008, on a soft diet. The patient was experiencing very little tenderness over the area of the incision and no difficulty with swallowing.

OPERATIONS: Excision of Zenker diverticulum, January 28, 2008.

LABORATORY: Complete blood count, PT/PTT, urinalysis, and comprehensive metabolic panel were unremarkable.

FINAL DIAGNOSES

1. Zenker diverticulum.
2. History of depression.

DISPOSITION: The patient was discharged to home with followup in the general surgery clinic on February 11. The patient is to keep the wound clean and dry until followup appointment.

DIET: Diet is to be soft foods only, with strict avoidance of coarse foods.

ACTIVITY: No driving for 2 weeks and no strenuous activity for 2 to 4 weeks.

DISCHARGE MEDICATIONS: Wellbutrin XL 150 mg p.o. q.d.

Multiple Choice.
Choose the correct spelling of the term.

1. A pulsion diverticulum developing between the inferior pharyngeal constrictor and the cricopharyngeus muscle.

   ○ zenker

   ○ Zenker

   ○ zencker

   ○ Zencker

2. Guaiac test for occult blood.

   ○ hemocult

   ○ hemoccult

   ○ Hemocult

   ○ Hemoccult

3. Enlargement of the liver and spleen.

   ○ splenomegaly

   ○ hepatosplenomegaly

   ○ hepetomegaly

   ○ hepetosplenomegaly

4. Offensive breath.

   ○ halitosis

   ○ haletosis

   ○ halatosis

   ○ halletosis

5. Difficulty in swallowing.

   ○ dysphasia

   ○ disphasia

   ○ desphagia

   ○ dysphagia

TRUE/FALSE.

Mark the following true or false.

1. The patient has no past surgical history.

   ○ true

   ○ false

2. On exam, the patient's thyroid was enlarged.

   ○ true

   ○ false

3. The patient is on Wellbutrin XL 150 mg daily.

   ○ true

   ○ false

4. The patient's heart was regular rate and rhythm without murmur.

   ○ true

   ○ false

5. The patient stayed in the hospital for 5 days.

   ○ true

   ○ false

ORAL SURGERY

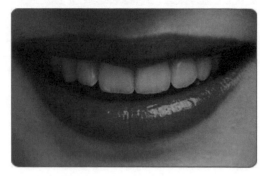

Dental is a term denoting teeth and is one with which you are probably familiar. It is possible that you could work for a dentist or oral surgeon as a transcription editor, in which case you would primarily deal with dental reports. However, as a hospital transcription editor, you will find that dental reports are quite rare. These would include the removal of teeth, root canals, assistance for severe facial trauma, and capping, and occasionally some reports related to TMJ (temporomandibular joint) problems. It is rarely necessary to hospitalize a patient primarily for a dental consideration, and therefore, a discharge summary with a D.D.S. as the primary physician is unlikely. In hospital transcription editing, you will almost exclusively do operative reports related to dentistry. In an effort to be comprehensive, we have included a few oral surgery reports in this ENT unit.

ORAL SURGERY REPORT 1 – OPERATIVE NOTE

PREOPERATIVE DIAGNOSIS: Impacted teeth #1, #16, #17 and #32.[1]

POSTOPERATIVE DIAGNOSIS: Impacted teeth #1, #16, #17 and #32.

OPERATION PERFORMED: Surgical removal of impacted #1, #16, #17 and #32.

DESCRIPTION OF PROCEDURE: The patient was placed on the operating table in a supine semi-reclining position. After adequate oral endotracheal anesthesia was administered, the patient was prepped and draped in the usual fashion for a surgical approach to the third molars. The oropharynx was suctioned free of all secretions, and an oropharyngeal pack was placed. 0.5% Marcaine with 1:200,000 epinephrine was injected for the administration of bilateral inferior alveolar, long buccal, posterior/superior alveolar, and greater palatine nerve blocks. Attention was directed to the mucosa overlying tooth #17. Utilizing a Bard-Parker #15 blade, an incision was carried through the mucosa beginning at the inferior aspect of the left mandibular ramus and continued anteriorly to the distal aspect of tooth #18. A full-thickness mucoperiosteal flap was reflected from the superior and buccal aspect of the alveolar bone overlying tooth #17. Utilizing a surgical handpiece and 703 bur, tooth #17 was exposed and suctioned and the tooth delivered from its socket with Cryer dental elevators. The wound was copiously irrigated with normal saline, and the mucosal flap was replaced to its appropriate position. Attention was then directed to tooth #16. Using a Bard-Parker #15 blade an incision was made beginning at the proximal aspect of the left tuberosity and carried anteriorly to the distal aspect of tooth #15. With the utilization of a periosteal elevator, a full-thickness mucoperiosteal flap was reflected superiorly, exposing the bone lateral to tooth #15. Utilizing an osteotome the bone buccal to the crown of #16 was removed, and the tooth was delivered from its socket with the use of dental elevators. The mucosa was then placed back in its anatomic position and secured with a 4-0 chromic suture. Tonsil sponges were placed over the surgical sites, and attention was directed to the areas of teeth #1 and #32, which were removed in like fashion. The surgical sites at the conclusion of the procedure were inspected and found to be clotting well. Large tonsil sponges were then placed in the surgical sites and secured to the cheeks with Steri-Strips. The oropharynx was suctioned free of all irrigants and blood products, and the throat pack was removed. The patient was awakened and extubated in the operating room, with respirations remaining spontaneous and vital signs stable. The patient was transferred to recovery on supplemental oxygen.

Footnotes:

1. 1.Some clients may use platforms that do not recognize the # symbol and may require it be spelled out to "number." (This is just FYI—tuck it away as possible future useful information.)

SPELLING.
Determine if the following words are spelled correctly. If the spelling is correct, leave the word as it has already been entered. If the spelling is incorrect, provide the correct spelling.

1. Marcaine _____

2. oropharenx _____

3. Bard-Barker _____

4. tuberosity _____

5. osteotome _____

True/False.
Mark the following true or false.

1. The patient was seen for impaction of 5 teeth.

    ○ true

    ○ false

2. Marcaine with 1:100,000 epinephrine was injected.

    ○ true

    ○ false

3. Cryer dental elevators were utilized during the surgery.

    ○ true

    ○ false

4. The patient was extubated in the recovery room.

    ○ true

    ○ false

5. Steri-Strips were used to secure the sponges to the cheeks.

    ○ true

    ○ false

ORAL SURGERY REPORT 2 – OPERATIVE NOTE

PREOPERATIVE DIAGNOSIS: Mandibular atrophy.

POSTOPERATIVE DIAGNOSIS: Mandibular atrophy.

PROCEDURE PERFORMED

1. Mandibular vestibuloplasty.
2. Split-thickness skin graft from right leg to mouth.
3. Lowering the floor of the mouth.

ANESTHESIA: Nasoendotracheal general anesthesia.

INDICATIONS FOR PROCEDURE: The patient is a 69-year-old male with a long history of denture wear. Secondary to this, he has atrophy and now is unable to wear his dentures. He now presents for corrective surgery for this.

DETAILS OF OPERATION: The patient was taken to the operating room with IV infusing Solu-Medrol and aqueous penicillin G. He was placed supine on the operating room table. SCDs were placed, and a Foley catheter was also placed. The patient was then given anesthesia and intubated by the anesthesia department orally. This was carried with a 2-0 suture through the membranous portion of the septum. After this was completed, a moistened throat pack was then placed. The face was then prepped and draped in the usual sterile fashion. The thigh was also prepped prior to prepping the face, and a Biodrape[1] dressing was placed to isolate the groin from the operative field. Sterile towels were placed over the right leg at the proposed skin grafting harvest site and at the outer thigh in the nonhair-bearing region. After this was completed, the patient's mouth was injected with a total of 6 cc of 2% lidocaine with 1:100,000 epinephrine locally for hemostasis control. Attention was then turned back towards the leg. Under sterile technique, a dermatome was used to remove approximately 6 cm x 3-cm section of skin at the pre-set depth eleven thousandths of an inch.[2] This was then taken to the back table, and epinephrine 1:10,000-soaked sponge was then placed on the wound for hemostasis control. The patient was then prepped and draped again in the usual sterile fashion. Attention was then turned towards the mouth where intraoral dissection was begun. A 15 blade was used to make an incision from the left retromolar pad lingually to approximately the right canine, just inside the attached mucosa. Sponge sticks were then used to roll this mucosa towards the tongue, thereby exposing underlying mylohyoid muscle. A curved Kelly clamp was then used to place this anteriorly and extending posteriorly to expose the mylohyoid. This was then attached to the tendinous portion of the mandible without complication. A similar procedure was then carried out on the left side. Moistened sponges were then placed to control hemostasis. An incision was then made on the left side, now on the buccal side of the attached mucosa, extending to the right canine. A distal release was also made at approximately the retromolar pad. Superperiosteal dissection was then carried out using small iris scissors. This was done carefully, and the middle nerve was identified from the right, again without complication and with careful dissection. A similar procedure was then carried out for the right and then anteriorly. Care was taken to maintain a large, 0.1 mentalis anteriorly. After this was completed, the Obwegeser mandibular awl was then passed with a single 3-0 stitch to attach the lingual tissue to posterior to the nerve and to anterior to the nerve on the left and then the right. The sutures were then tied, thereby completing the lingual tissues inferiorly and creating a space for the skin graft on the buccal mucosa. A stent which had previously been fabricated was then tried to the mouth and seen to fit satisfactorily. After this was completed, the skin graft was cut into 2 pieces and placed into the mouth and was attached to the mandible with Mersilene sutures. The patient's mouth was then irrigated, and the moistened throat pack was removed. All sponge and needle counts were correct times 2 at the end of the case. There were no apparent complications.

Footnotes:

1. 1.Biodrape is a tradename and should be capped.
2. 2.It is difficult to know with complete certainty how this measurement should be edited. You wouldn't do 0.011 as eleven thousandths because it is generally preferred not to mix metric and English (decimals and inches). You probably don't need the hyphen between eleven and thousandths because inches is not directly following the measurement. It could also be edited accurately as 11/1000 of an inch.

Multiple Choice.
Choose the best answer.

1. A distal release was also made at approximately the (○ retromolar, ○ retromoler) pad.

2. Attention was turned towards the mouth where (○ intraoral, ○ interoral) dissection was begun.

3. An incision was made from the left pad to the right (○ cannine, ○ canine).

4. Moistened sponges were placed to control (○ hemastasis, ○ hemostasis).

5. The underlying (○ mylohyoid, ○ mylohoid) muscle was exposed.

Matching.
Match the correct terms.

1. ____ Obwegeser		A.	sutures
2. ____ Kelly		B.	dressing
3. ____ Mersilene		C.	awl
4. ____ Biodrape		D.	catheter
5. ____ Foley		E.	clamp

UNIT 10
Pediatrics

PEDIATRICS – INTRODUCTION

Pediatrics is that branch of medicine devoted to the care of children. Specifically, this includes the ages of infant through eighteen. There are some medical problems that are unique to smaller bodies and are only dealt with in the pediatric stage. For example:

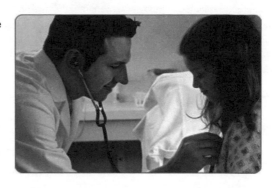

- underdeveloped heart valves
- cleft palates
- myringotomies with tubes
- cancer

Some types of cancer are primarily present and treated in the early stages of life. However, many problems that affect children are the same problems that affect adults. Therefore, you will see many types of illnesses, procedures, diseases, and treatments that are similar in a pediatric setting as in an adult one. For example, tonsillectomies and appendectomies can be performed on adults as well as children since they are caused by the same processes. The reason that they are followed and treated by pediatric specialists is because smaller bodies often need different precautions taken, smaller instruments used, or even different care altogether than adults.

Pediatric illnesses, diagnostics, and treatments are mostly the same as the adult equivalent, and because of this a somewhat generalized language workshop and review is included in this unit. Without further ado, we jump into pediatric reports.

PEDIATRICS LANGUAGE WORKSHOP

Pediatric terminology is similar to general adult medicine terminology, but we felt there were some differences, or even focuses, of medicine that made a language workshop and review a valid and useful tool for this FOMS unit. Childhood is the time of greatest growth, development, and maturation of the body organ systems. Congenital defects, genetic variance, childhood illnesses, and immunological diseases are commonly diagnosed and treated by pediatricians. While the following terms and word parts are not exclusive to Pediatrics, they are terms you will likely be exposed to in this unit.

Common Pediatrics Root Words and Combining Forms

Root Word & Combining Form	Meaning	Example
abdomin/o	abdomen	abdominal
acr/o	extremities	acromegaly
alb/o	white	albino
angi/o	vessel	angiogram
atel/o	imperfect	atelectasis
brachi/o	arm	brachiocephalic
carcin/o	cancer	carcinogenic
cerebr/o	brain	cerebral
chondr/o	cartilage	chondromalacia
cost/o	rib	costovertebral
cyan/o	blue	cyanotic
dactyl/o	finger, toe	hexadactylism
dips/o	thirst	polydipsia
encephal/o	brain	encephalitis
galact/o	milk	galactorrhea
gnath/o	jaw	gnathodynia
hered/o	inherited	heredoimmunity
immun/o	immune	immunodeficiency
leuk/o	white	leukemia
muc/o	mucus	mucoperiosteal
narc/o	sleep, numbness	narcolepsy
ne/o	new	neoblastic
phleb/o	vein	phlebolith
phon/o	sound, voice	phonation
pneum/o	air, breathing	pneumothorax
pseud/o	false	pseudarthrosis
py/o	pus	pyoid
rhin/o	nose	rhinoplasty
somat/o	body	somatization
tox/o	poison	toxemia

Common Pediatrics Prefixes

Prefix	Meaning	Example
a-/an-	no, without	amenorrhea, anechoic
brady-	slow	bradycardia
circum-	around	circumcision
con-	with	congenital
dys-	difficult, abnormal	dysphasia
in-	not	inability
infra-	beneath	infraorbital
intra-	within, inside	intrauterine
micro-	small	microhematuria
para-	near, beside	parahepatic
peri-	around, near	periventricular
tachy-	fast	tachyarrhythmia

Common Pediatrics Suffixes

Suffix	Meaning	Example
-algia	pain	myalgia
-emesis	vomiting	hematemesis
-gram	record	cholangiogram
-graph	instrument for recording	polygraph
-graphy	process of recording	echocardiography
-kinesis	movement	hypokinesis
-meter	instrument to measure	glucometer
-metry	process of measuring	spirometry
-oma	tumor	lymphoma
-plasia	to form, develop	aplasia
-penia	deficiency	osteopenia
-scopy	exam with instrument	colonoscopy
-trophy	nutrition	hypertrophy

Common Pediatrics Abbreviations

Abbreviation	Expansion
NAD	no acute distress
PERRLA	pupils equal, round, and reactive to light and accommodation
EOM	extraocular movements
EOMI	extraocular movements intact
REM	rapid eye movements
TM	tympanic membranes
NSR	normal sinus rhythm
CP	cerebral palsy
CMV	cytomegalovirus
OE	otitis externa
OI	otitis interna
OM	otitis media
PDA	patent ductus arteriosus
PPV	positive/pressure ventilation
RDS	respiratory distress syndrome
RSV	respiratory syncytial virus
ROP	retinopathy of prematurity
SIDS	sudden infant death syndrome
TEF	transesophageal fistula
TPN	total parenteral nutrition

REVIEW: PEDIATRICS LANGUAGE

Multiple Choice.
Choose the best answer.

1. (○ Rhinorrhea, ○ Rhinoplasia) is a term for nasal discharge.

2. (○ Polydipsia, ○ Polykinesis), or excessive thirst, is often a symptom of diabetes.

3. (○ Cytology, ○ Cytomegalovirus) causes circulatory dysfunction and microcephaly in infants.

4. (○ Cerebral, ○ Bell's) palsy is a term encompassing a group of non-progressive, non-contagious diseases that lead to physical disability in childhood development.

5. (○ Random, ○ Rapid) eye movements are normal eye movements that occur during sleep.

6. The abbreviation TPN stands for total (○ parental, ○ parenteral) nutrition.

TRUE/FALSE.
Mark the following true or false.

1. A child experiencing cyanosis usually has a yellowish tint to the skin.

    ○ true

    ○ false

2. Otitis interna is an infection of the outer ear.

    ○ true

    ○ false

3. The term *circumcision* means "to cut around."

    ○ true

    ○ false

4. The abbreviation *NSR* stands for normal sinus rhythm.

    ○ true

    ○ false

Fill in the Blank.
Using the word(s) in the box, fill in the blanks.

patent	
infant	
retinopathy	
syncytial	
immunodeficiency	

1. The term _____ means there is a deficiency in the immune system.

2. _____ ductus arteriosus is a congenital heart defect wherein a child's ductus arteriosus fails to close after birth.

3. Sudden _____ death syndrome is the sudden and unexpected death of a healthy child who is younger than one year old, usually during sleep.

4. _____ of prematurity is a disease of the eye that affects prematurely born babies.

5. Respiratory _____ virus is a highly contagious virus which is quite prevalent during the winter months and can especially cause serious illness in infants under 2 years of age.

PEDIATRICS REPORTS

Pediatricians deal with all types of medical problems, as they relate to minors. Our bodies go through so many changes from birth through adulthood; they are forming, growing, changing, and developing at such rapid rates that they are subject to different types of problems than adult bodies are AND quite similar problems to adult bodies. A pediatrician deals with both types of problems.

In transcription editing of pediatric reports, therefore, you will come across both common and familiar diseases, procedures, and treatments from other specialties, as well as healthcare unique to smaller developing bodies.

PEDIATRICS REPORT 1 – DISCHARGE SUMMARY

DISCHARGE DIAGNOSES

1. Febrile seizure.
2. Otitis media.
3. Sepsis ruled out.

HISTORY OF PRESENT ILLNESS: The patient is an 8-month-old female from Lombard, IL, who was well until the day prior to admission when she developed fevers of greater than 104. She was given Tylenol and sponge baths by her parents. However, the fevers continued, and on the day of admission she was taken to the clinic. At the walk-in clinic, the child was noted to have otitis, and while at the clinic she "started shaking, turned blue, and her eyes rolled back in her head." The shaking episode lasted approximately 5 minutes. At that time, her temperature was 106 degrees. The patient was flown to the County General Hospital for further evaluation by Dr. Archie Morris.

PAST MEDICAL HISTORY: Birth history: The patient was adopted by her aunt. She was reported to be full term with no complications at birth.

CURRENT MEDICATIONS: Amoxicillin prophylaxis for recurrent otitis, Tylenol.

ALLERGIES: The patient has a bad reaction to Pediazole[1] from which she gets bad diarrhea.

FAMILY HISTORY: The patient does have a cousin with a history of seizure disorder. Her biological parents are in good health.

PHYSICAL EXAMINATION: The child was alert upon awakening, although she did fall asleep easily. Head was normocephalic, atraumatic. Eyes: Pupils were equal, round, and reactive to light. Extraocular movements were intact. Fundi were benign. On examination of her ears, her right TM had decreased mobility and increased redness. Nose had crusty rhinorrhea. Throat had no erythema. Her neck was supple with no masses. Lung exam showed good aeration bilaterally. Cardiovascular exam was regular without murmur. Her abdomen was soft, no tenderness to palpation. Extremities had no cyanosis. On examination of her skin, she did have a small rash on her right cheek with some swelling.

LABORATORY DATA: White count 14.2 with 45 segs, 32 bands, 20 lymphs, and 3 monos. Hemoglobin was 11.2, hematocrit 34, and platelet count 286. UA was negative. Sodium was 141, potassium 4.3, chloride 98, bicarb 25, glucose 101, BUN 12, creatinine 0.3. Uric acid 3.9, phosphate 5.1, calcium 9.6, and magnesium 2.3.

HOSPITAL COURSE/PROBLEM LIST[2]

1. Fluids, electrolytes, and nutrition: Initially, the child was started on D5 quarter-normal saline[3] with 20 mEq KCl which was run at 1-1/2 times maintenance. She had had some poor p.o. intake noted the day prior to admission. During her hospital course, her diet was advanced to p.o. ad lib and her IV was maintained at TKO.[4]
2. Seizures: There were no seizures noted during this admission. Therefore, it was felt that the seizure witnessed at the clinic was due to her increased temperature and was therefore classified as a febrile seizure.
3. Infectious diseases: Blood culture and urine cultures were negative. The child was initially started on ceftriaxone, but developed a rash and was therefore changed to chloramphenicol. She responded well to this medication, and 24 hours prior to discharge her IV chloramphenicol was changed over to p.o. chloramphenicol, and she remained afebrile.
4. Otitis: The patient did have a right otitis and this was responding well to the chloramphenicol.

DISCHARGE MEDICATIONS: Chloramphenicol 75 mg/kg per day[5] q.6 hours p.o.

FOLLOWUP: Ear recheck in 2 weeks with the health aide.

DISPOSITION: The patient was discharged to home in good condition.

Footnotes:

1. 1.Pediazole is erythromycin and sulfisoxazole for treatment of susceptible bacterial infections of the upper and lower respiratory tract, otitis media in children caused by susceptible strains of Haemophilus influenzae, and many other infections in patients allergic to penicillin.
2. 2.This is a somewhat atypical way to present the hospital course information. Past reports from this author or a style guide from this client would be helpful in knowing how to present the information.
3. 3."D5 quarter-normal saline" is the proper way to notate this. The D5 indicates the solution contains 5% dextrose.
4. 4.The abbreviation *p.o.*, as you know, stands for per os or by mouth. The phrase *ad lib* is the shortened form of *ad libitum*, meaning freely or as desired. And *TKO* is the abbreviation for To Keep Open. In this use, it means just what it says—her IV was kept open.
5. 5.Typically it is preferred to avoid using more than one virgule per expression, but it would not necessarily be incorrect to edit this as mg/kg/day. There is acceptable variation to how this information is presented.

Multiple Choice.
Choose the correct spelling of the term.

1. The presence of pathogenic microorganisms or other toxins in the blood.

   ○ sepis

   ○ spesis

   ○ sepsis

   ○ sipses

2. Having no fever.

   ○ afebrile

   ○ a febrile

   ○ afebrille

   ○ a febrille

3. Any of various ions, such as sodium or chloride, required by cells to regulate the electric charge and flow of water molecules across the cell membrane.

   ○ electriclytes

   ○ electrolytes

   ○ electrolites

   ○ electrylites

4. Examination with the hands.

   ○ palpitation

   ○ palpetation

   ○ palption

   ○ palpation

5. Prevention of disease, prevention treatment.

   ○ prophelaxis

   ○ prophelaxes

   ○ prophylaxis

   ○ prophelaxys

Multiple Choice.
Choose the best answer.

1. There were no (◯ siezures, ◯ seizures) noted during this admission.

2. Her right (◯ tympanic, ◯ timpanic) membrane had decreased mobility.

3. Pediazole gives the patient (◯ diarrhea, ◯ diarhhea).

4. Ear recheck in 2 weeks with the health (◯ aid, ◯ aide).

5. Cardiovascular exam was regular without (◯ murmur, ◯ murmer).

PEDIATRICS REPORT 2 – DISCHARGE SUMMARY

ADMITTING DIAGNOSIS: Bronchiolitis[1] and hypoxia.

HISTORY OF PRESENT ILLNESS: This is a 5-month-old male with a 4-day history of cough and upper respiratory symptoms. Prior to admission, he was seen on November 22, and said to have an upper respiratory infection by the health aide. He was seen again by the health aide on the day prior to admission and diagnosed with bronchiolitis and otitis media. Ceclor and Metaprel were started on that day, and he had 2 doses of each medicine prior to admission. Mom noted that he had been afebrile and feeding well; however, on the morning of admission, he began to cough and spit up. She also notes that he had urinated 4 to 5 times on the morning of admission. Immunizations appear up to date.

PAST MEDICAL HISTORY: Significant for a term birth at 3629 gm, 52 cm in length, and 35.5 cm head circumference. Birth and prenatal history are without complications. The patient was noted to have preauricular skin tags at birth. The patient was diagnosed with bronchiolitis on November 24, but was not admitted. He was started on oral Metaprel. The patient has had 3 otitis medias since April and has been treated with amoxicillin, Pediazole, and Ceclor for these.

ALLERGIES: The patient has no known allergies.

FAMILY HISTORY: Mom is 33, dad 31, sibs are 6 and 3, respectively; all are healthy. He has an aunt with asthma.

PHYSICAL EXAMINATION: Weight is 21 pounds 7 ounces, which is markedly over the 95th percentile for age. Temperature is 99.7, pulse 158, respiratory rate 72, sat 96% on room air initially. In general, the patient was alert with mild substernal retractions. HEENT: Normocephalic, anterior fontanelle was soft. Extraocular movements were intact. There was a positive red reflex bilaterally. Tympanic membranes were pink and mobile, but mobility may have been somewhat decreased. Nose had positive clear discharge. Throat was clear without exudates. Mucous membranes were moist. Neck was supple, no adenopathy. Lungs: Pretreatment, coarse rhonchi and upper airway sounds; posttreatment were almost clear with some right-sided rhonchi still noted. The patient still had a respiratory rate of 70-80 after the treatments. Heart had regular rate and rhythm, no murmur. Abdomen was soft, bowel sounds present, no hepatosplenomegaly. Extremities showed good pulses and perfusion. Ortolani and Barlow maneuvers were intact. Neurologic exam revealed an alert male patient with good tone and good suck. GU revealed male patient with testes downgoing, uncircumcised. The penis was buried in fat, but was 3- to 4-cm long.

The **red reflex test** is used to screen for abnormalities of the back of the eye (posterior segment) and opacities in the visual axis, such as a cataract or corneal opacity. An ophthalmoscope held close to the examiner's eye and focused on the pupil is used to view the eyes from 12 to 18 inches away from the subject's eyes. To be considered normal, the red reflex of the two eyes should be symmetrical. Dark spots in the red reflex, a blunted red reflex on one side, a lack of a red reflex, or the presence of a white reflex (retinal reflection) are all indications for referral to an ophthalmologist.

HOSPITAL COURSE: Patient's diagnosis on admission was noted to be bronchiolitis. He was placed on high-flow nebulizers q.4 h. and a mist tent. We discontinued the Ceclor because we were not sure about the ear infection initially. However, the night after admission patient spiked a temperature to 103 and was cultured. The next morning, because his respiratory rate was still in the 70s to 80s, it was elected to restart Pediazole for an antibiotic, and over the next 24 hours the patient had continued respiratory rates in the 80s to 90s and began to have an oxygen requirement overnight. He was placed on oxygen, and an ABG was done the next night which revealed a pH of 7.41, pCO2 of 17, and pO2 of over 100.[2] This was consistent with a marked metabolic acidosis, not a respiratory process, and it was felt that the patient may have become dehydrated over the past 24 hours. Multiple, multiple attempts were made to place an IV in this patient. This was very difficult due to his fat, and after multiple attempts at IVs and attempts to feed him p.o., we elected to place an NG tube and feed him via NG to give him liquids. This resulted in a marked improvement in his pCO2, with ABG about 12 hours after this was started of pH 7.41, pCO2 of 31, and pO2 still over 100. Over the next several days, the patient maintained a respiratory rate in the 80s to 90s with what were felt to be "not too many" in the way of lung symptoms. Because he continued his respiratory rates in the 80s to 90s, another chest x-ray was done, and it was noted at this time that he had a right upper lobe atelectasis and some questionable increase in the amount of infiltrate over his initial chest x-ray on admission. The patient had been switched to Augmentin on day 2 of admission, and at this time another IV was attempted. It was felt that if we were not able to get this, we might send him into Children's Hospital just to get a central line and treat him IV.

However, we were successfully able to obtain an IV and placed him on IV cefuroxime and some fluids and continued aggressive chest PT and high-flow nebulizers and oxygen. It took him a while, but over the next several days he calmed down, and his respiratory rates went gradually into the 60s and then into the 40s. He was weaned to room air on December 3, with high saturations and a respiratory rate in the 40s with a good appetite. Repeated chest x-rays, however, showed that his atelectasis persisted, although it looked better than when we first noticed it. He is eating well, afebrile, with clear lungs, and is on albuterol syrup. We will discharge him today, December 5, to continue his syrup and aggressive chest PT centering on the right upper lobe area. The mother has been trained on how to do this. He had a full 10-day course of antibiotics and will be followed up in 2 weeks in the pediatric clinic for repeat chest x-ray. Mother has been given instructions to return if he becomes short of breath, has chest sucking in, or he will not feed because he is too tired. She has also been given albuterol for his bronchodilator therapy syrup. She will give him 2.4 cc q.8 h. and do chest PT 30 minutes afterward. She has also been given nystatin solution and ointment for both an oral and diaper candidiasis, and she was given Eucerin for the dry skin on his face.

Footnotes:

1. <u>1.</u>This refers to inflammation of the bronchioles, usually secondary to viral infection (RSV). If you aren't sure what hypoxia is, look it up!
2. <u>2.</u>It is acceptable to edit blood gases in all caps PCO2/PO2. Reference materials will often show the 2 in subscript. Most platforms will not allow for super- and/or subscripts, so a good old plain numeral 2 is your best option.

Spelling.
Determine if the following words are spelled correctly. If the spelling is correct, leave the word as it has already been entered. If the spelling is incorrect, retype the word with the correct spelling.

1. _____   2. _____

3. _____   4. _____

5. _____

TRUE/FALSE.
Mark the following true or false.

1. The patient was transferred to Children's Hospital to place a central line.

    ○ true

    ○ false

2. The patient's pCO2 was over 100 each time it was tested.

    ○ true

    ○ false

3. The patient is uncircumcised.

    ○ true

    ○ false

4. Repeat x-rays showed the atelectasis cleared.

    ○ true

    ○ false

5. The patient's Ceclor was discontinued soon after admission.

    ○ true

    ○ false

PEDIATRICS REPORT 3 – DISCHARGE SUMMARY

DISCHARGE DIAGNOSIS: Urinary tract infection.

ADMITTING HISTORY: This is a 10-week-old male infant who had been sick for 3 days prior to admission with fever to 103 degrees, fussiness, but good appetite, no vomiting or diarrhea. He had noted a slight cough and runny nose. He had been seen in the emergency room on the evening prior to admission with a normal exam. He did not look particularly ill. He returned on the day of admission for recheck. He had continued to run fevers, but had not otherwise seemed sick. He had been seen 6 days prior to admission in the emergency room with a history of vomiting, diagnosed with an upper respiratory infection. No one else was sick at the time of his admission.

PAST MEDICAL HISTORY: He was born by a vaginal delivery in Scranton at 40 weeks' gestation, birth weight of 3,830 gm,[1] with Apgars of 8 and 9, to a 31-year-old primipara.[2] His newborn exam was normal, and there were no complications. He had no sicknesses prior to this illness. He had HepB at 1 day of age. At 8 weeks he had HepB, DTaP, Hib, IPV, and PCV.[3] His diet was breast milk and Similac, with occasional strained vegetables.

PHYSICAL EXAMINATION: On admission, he was an alert baby, smiling and cooing, not looking ill. His skin was warm with no rashes, good turgor. His temperature on admission was 102.4, pulse 160, respiratory rate 32. HEENT exam showed a slightly depressed anterior fontanelle, normal TMs, normal eye exam, clear nose, normal throat, and no cervical lymphadenopathy. His lungs were clear. He had a 1/6 systolic ejection murmur at the left upper sternal border with a regular heart rhythm. The abdomen was soft and nontender, but slightly distended, no masses. GU exam showed normal male genitalia with no rashes. Testicles were both descended. Extremities showed good range of motion with no deformity.

LABORATORY FINDINGS: A white count was 23.7 with 41 segs and 1 band. Hemoglobin of 8.6, hematocrit of 27.3. A cath UA showed 1+ blood, 30-35 white cells, and 1+ rods.

HOSPITAL COURSE: Blood cultures were obtained, and he was admitted with a diagnosis of a urinary tract infection. He was continued on p.o. feedings and begun on ampicillin at a rate of 200 mg/kg per day and gentamicin 7.5 mg/kg per day. The urine culture grew E. coli, resistant to ampicillin, sensitive to gentamicin, resistant to sulfa and Septra, and only moderately sensitive to Augmentin. When the culture returned, the ampicillin was discontinued, and he was continued on the gentamicin.

His hospital course was unremarkable with continued temperature spikes for the first 3 hospital days. He subsequently remained afebrile. He ate well, good voiding. He did have an ultrasound of the kidneys done during the hospital stay. This was a normal study. The hospitalization was prolonged only because of the absence of any good choices for oral medications to treat his UTI. He was eventually discharged on February 9, to continue on Ceclor for a total of a 10-day course. He was instructed to return to the emergency room for a recheck 2 days after discharge, sooner should his temperature rise above 100.5.

DISPOSITION: He will need a voiding cystourethrogram scheduled at some point in the future once the UTI has cleared. He will be seen in the outpatient clinic in followup with a repeat urine culture, after he has completed his full course of antibiotics.

Footnotes:

1. 1.When presenting a value that contains 4 numerals, a comma is optional (both 3830 and 3,830 are acceptable). When presenting a number containing 5 or more numerals, it is preferred to use a comma (e.g., 35,729 and not 35729). And grams, of course, can also be abbreviated as g.
2. 2.A primipara is a woman who bears a child for the first time.
3. 3.HepB (hepatitis B), DTaP (diphtheria, tetanus, and acellular pertussis), Hib (Haemophilus influenza b), IPV (inactivated polio vaccine), and PCV (pneumococcal conjugate vaccine).

Fill in the Blank.
Using the word(s) in the box, fill in the blanks.

1. UTI – urinary _____ infection

2. VCUG – voiding _____

3. TM – tympanic _____

4. HEENT – head, ears, eyes, _____ and throat

5. DTaP – _____, tetanus, and acellular pertussis

cystourethrogram
Diphtheria
membrane
nose
tract

Multiple Choice.
Choose the best answer.

1. The patient was born by vaginal delivery 40 (◯ week's, ◯ weeks') gestation.

2. The patient will (◯ followup, ◯ follow up) in the outpatient clinic.

3. When the culture returned, the (◯ ampicillin, ◯ ampocillin) was discontinued.

4. The patient was born to a 31-year-old (◯ primepara, ◯ primipara).

5. His skin was warm with no rashes, good (◯ turgor, ◯ turger).

PEDIATRICS REPORT 4 – DISCHARGE SUMMARY

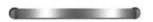

DISCHARGE DIAGNOSES

1. Rule out partially treated meningitis.
2. Impetigo.[1]
3. Immunizations.

PROCEDURES: Lumbar puncture, IV antibiotics.

HISTORY OF PRESENT ILLNESS: This is the 2nd Seattle Grace admission for an 13-month-old who was seen in the emergency room 8 days prior to admission with impetigo, adenitis, URI symptoms, and a father who had clinical strep. The child was treated with erythromycin and bacitracin ointment with good results. He was well until the day prior to admission when he developed fever, irritability, and a stuffy nose, without vomiting, diarrhea, cough, or dyspnea. Physical exam showed marked irritability in contrast to his prior examinations. Therefore, a septic workup was done, and the child was admitted for rule out meningitis.

PAST MEDICAL HISTORY: He was on erythromycin. He has no allergies, is up to date with his immunizations. Negative family history. He had been admitted at 11 months for pneumonia.

PHYSICAL EXAMINATION: Exam shows a furious, robust, fighting infant moving head well, although he did not tolerate neck flexion or other manipulation. Nares were clear. TMs benign. Throat was injected. Neck had shotty nodes[2] with moderate meningismus. Lungs were clear with an occasional cough. Abdomen was benign. There were no skin lesions.

LABORATORY DATA: CBC had a white count of 41,000[3] with 70 neutrophils, 10 bands, and 8 lymphs, hemoglobin of 11.3, and platelet count of 511,000. CSF was colorless, slightly hazy, with 26 red cells and 14 white cells, all of which were lymphs. Protein was 15 and glucose was 86. Gram stain[4] was negative. Chest x-ray showed patchy right middle lobe infiltrates. UA was negative.

HOSPITAL COURSE: In view of his irritability and increased white count, and the lymphocytosis on his CSF, it was felt that this might represent a partially treated meningitis, as he had been on erythromycin, or more likely a viral process although his white count had an extraordinary shift which may have partly been due to his pneumonia. He was placed on IV Rocephin and defervesced over the next 36-48 hours. After 24 hours of hospitalization, he was happy and active. Repeat CBC on the 2nd hospital day showed a white count of 6.3 down from 41. All of his cultures were negative. After 72 hours, his IV antibiotics were discontinued, and he was switched to oral Keflex. He was discharged on the 4th hospital day, cheerful and active, normal tympanic membranes, normal pharynx, supple neck, clear lungs, and normal skin.

DISCHARGE INSTRUCTIONS: Discharge instructions included Keflex 40 mg/kg per day divided t.i.d. for 6 days and an MMR. He is to follow up with Pediatrics in 1 week.

ADDENDUM: Viral cultures done with his CSF returned negative on January 11, 2008.[5]

Footnotes:

1. 1.A contagious infection of the skin caused by staphylococcal and streptococcal bacteria and characterized by blisters that form yellow-brown scabs.
2. 2.Shotty nodes are small nodes that resemble the pellets used in shotgun cartridges (small and round). This is never shoddy nodes.
3. 3.The normal range for a child's white blood count is 5,000 to 10,000. A WBC of 41,000 (also acceptably dictated as 41) is a red flag for infection (among other things).
4. 4.This is occasionally dictated as Gram's stain. The correct presentation is with a capital G—as this method for differential staining of bacteria was developed by Hans Gram. Of note, the results of a Gram stain are presented as gram-negative or gram-positive (lowercase g).
5. 5.An addendum is information which is added to a document after it is initially submitted.

Spelling.
Determine if the following words are spelled correctly. If the spelling is correct, leave the word as it has already been entered. If the spelling is incorrect, retype the word with the correct spelling.

1. _____

2. _____

3. _____

4. _____

5. _____

Multiple Choice.
Choose the best answer.

1. The cerebrospinal (○ fluid, ○ filling) was colorless.

2. The patient presented with an upper (○ respiratory, ○ respirations) infection.

3. The repeat complete (○ bolus, ○ blood) count showed a decreased white count.

4. The child's (○ tubular, ○ tympanic) membranes were benign.

5. The (○ urinalysis, ○ urineanalysis) was negative.

PEDIATRICS REPORT 5 – DISCHARGE SUMMARY

PRIMARY DIAGNOSIS: Newborn female, 34 weeks' gestation.

SECONDARY DIAGNOSIS: Born by primary cesarean section.

HOSPITAL COURSE: This was a 5 pounds 12 ounces female, product of a gravida 8, para 6, abortus 1,[1] African-American female at 34 weeks' gestation with preterm labor and complete cervical dilatation and a transverse lie with a full bag and umbilical cord as presenting part.[2] The mother was taken to cesarean section. There was never any fetal distress. There was a difficult breech extraction at delivery with the child somewhat depressed at birth. She needed some early stimulation and some blow-by O2.[3] However, subsequent to that, the child's neonatal course was unremarkable. The first dextrose stick soon after delivery was 23. However, the child drank 1 oz of formula and the repeat dextrose stick one-half hour later was 63. Her oxygen saturation and exams were always reassuring with no indications of neurologic or musculoskeletal complications from the moderately difficult breech extraction. The young patient continued to do well throughout her hospitalization. She did show some signs of slight jaundice. However, she was feeding well with a good suck and passing stool and urinating well, and clinically was in stable condition. She is expected to have a somewhat higher physiologic jaundice because of her 34 week gestation and because mom is breastfeeding. She did not suffer extensive bruising from the delivery, and so we would not consider this contributory to this potential problem. Mom's blood type is O+ and so is baby's. On the date of discharge her physical exam remained stable without heart murmur, positive red reflexes bilaterally, hips well approximated. She does have a lower central incisor neonatal tooth versus hypertrophied gum which is soft and does not appear to require any immediate attention.

FOLLOWUP: Followup is to be in 10 days with the community health aide. Her birth weight was 2,605 gm. Her discharge weight is 2,420 gm.

Footnotes:

1. 1.Although it wouldn't be edited this way unless dictated, this is the equivalent of G8, P6, A1 (or Ab1).
2. 2.This is a good example of a run-on sentence. Although minor editing would make it easier to read, it is not a "must" unless required by the client.
3. 3.Blow-by oxygen is provided with oxygen tubing, corrugated tubing, or a simple mask held a short distance from the infant's face.

SPELLING.
Determine if the following words are spelled correctly. If the spelling is correct, leave the word as it has already been entered. If the spelling is incorrect, provide the correct spelling.

1. breech _____
2. abortus _____
3. cervicle _____
4. inciser _____
5. musculoskeletal _____

Multiple Choice.
Choose the best answer.

1. A yellowish staining of the skin with bile pigments (○ jaundice, ○ jaundess).

2. The number of the pregnancy that a woman is in would be known as (○ graviduh, ○ gravida).

3. From the time of fertilization of the ovum until birth is known as (○ gestashun, ○ gestation).

4. A surgical procedure that involves the delivery of the fetus through an abdominal incision is a (○ cesarean, ○ caserean) section.

5. The number of live-born children a woman has delivered is known as (○ para, ○ pera).

PEDIATRICS REPORT 6 – DISCHARGE SUMMARY

DIAGNOSES

1. Right peritonsillar abscess this admission.
2. History of recurrent ileocecal intussusception.
3. History of recurrent otitis medias.
4. History of Candida vaginitis.
5. Immunization up-to-date with HepB vaccine.

HISTORY OF PRESENT ILLNESS: The patient is an 8-year-old girl from Denver, Colorado, who reports 4-day history of sore throat, rhinorrhea, and clear discharge. She also reports subjective fevers and right ear pain. The child was treated by her pediatrician on February 19, with amoxicillin 3 times per day. She was advised to come to Denver General by Dr. Jonas Edwards. The mother also treated the patient with chewable Tylenol for fevers and pain. The child was not eating solids or sleeping through the night due to throat pain and was taking less liquids than usual. She denies abdominal pain, cough, nausea, vomiting, change in bowel movements, or headaches. A younger sibling at home is also sick with sore throat and cough.

SOCIAL HISTORY: The patient lives with mom and dad, 2 brothers and 1 sister.

ALLERGIES: No known drug allergies.

FAMILY HISTORY: Heart problems in maternal grandmother, noninsulin-dependent diabetes mellitus in mother, hypertension in paternal grandmother.

PHYSICAL EXAMINATION: The patient is a quiet, well-developed, well-nourished, young girl in no acute distress, but somewhat uncomfortable. Temperature 97.5 axillary, pulse 76, respirations 12, weight 58 lb. HEENT: Right ear slightly erythematous, slightly bulging, good light reflex and landmarks. Left is gray, clear. Eyes: Sclerae clear. Extraocular muscles are intact. Pupils are equal and reactive to light. Fundi: Normal discs[1] and vessels. Nose: Crusty and clear with blood-tinged discharge, erythema, and chafing below the nares. Mouth: Only able to open slightly, mucous membranes moist. Throat: Erythema right tonsillar area, much greater than left, but both erythematous without exudates. Neck is supple with large 3- to 4-cm submandibular nodes, 1- to 2-cm left submandibular node, tender, not stiff, good anterior occipital movement. Chest: Lungs equal movement without retractions, clear to auscultation without rales, rhonchi, or wheezes. Heart: Regular rate and rhythm, S1, S2. Abdomen: Good bowel sounds, soft, nontender, no hepatosplenomegaly or masses. Extremities: Normal muscle strength. Vascular: 2+ pulses. Neurologic: Normal. GU: Deferred.

LABORATORY DATA: White count 40,600, hemoglobin, 13.0, platelet count 429,000.

HOSPITAL COURSE: The patient was treated for a peritonsillar abscess and possible early right OM. She was treated with penicillin G 1 million units IV piggyback q.6 h. for 3 days. She was rehydrated with fluids and was given Tylenol and PediaProfen for pain. She tolerated all of these treatments well and by the 3rd hospital day was feeling ready to go home. She was switched to oral antibiotics and tolerated these without problems. She was discharged to home under the care of her mother.

DISCHARGE MEDICATIONS: Pen-Vee K[2] 250 mg p.o. q.i.d. and Tylenol p.r.n.

FOLLOWUP: She is to follow up with her pediatrician if her condition worsens.

Footnotes:

1. 1. Also acceptably edited as disks.
2. 2. Pen-Vee K has been discontinued. If this were a live report (in real time), the use of this med would be "flag worthy," to bring to the attention or ask for clarification from the client.

Fill in the Blank.
Using the word(s) in the box, fill in the blanks.

1. The patient has a history of recurrent _____ media.

2. Oral exam revealed moist _____ membranes.

3. The patient has a history of nasal discharge, also known as _____ .

4. The patient was treated for a _____ abscess.

5. The patient has a history of _____ , vaginal yeast infections.

Candida vaginitis
mucous
otitis
peritonsillar
rhinorrhea

Multiple Choice.
Choose the correct spelling of the term.

1. Skin that is reddened by congestion of the capillaries.

   ◯ erythematous

   ◯ erethymatus

   ◯ erethymatous

   ◯ erythymatus

2. Of or relating to the armpit.

   ◯ axilary

   ◯ axellary

   ◯ axilery

   ◯ axillary

3. Part of the fibrous layer forming the outer envelope of the eyeball.

   ◯ slcera

   ◯ seclera

   ◯ sclera

   ◯ sclerra

4. Term for an added sound heard on auscultation of breath sounds.

   ◯ rhale

   ◯ rale

   ◯ ralle

   ◯ rail

5. Any fluid that has exuded out of a tissue or its capillaries.

   ◯ exate

   ◯ exudate

   ◯ exxudate

   ◯ excudte

PEDIATRICS REPORT 7 – OPERATIVE NOTE

OPERATION PERFORMED: Right orchiopexy with high ligation of hernia sac.

ANESTHETIC: General mask with augmentation of caudal block.

INDICATIONS: A 16-month-old white male noted to have increased swelling of the right groin area with Valsalva or crying. This would reduce when supine. There was also no palpable testis in the right hemiscrotum. The patient presents at this time for orchiopexy and repair of hernia.

DESCRIPTION OF PROCEDURE: The patient was taken to the operating room after preoperative preparation, counseling, and consent of the parents. He received general mask anesthesia and placement of a caudal block. He was then placed in the supine position, prepped and draped in the usual sterile fashion. An incision was made over the right groin sharply down to the level of the external oblique fascia. The cord structures were noted medially at the external ring. The hernia sac was separated from the surrounding tissue. The right testicle was in the distal portion of the hernia sac and was felt to be normal anatomically. The external oblique fibers were then opened. The ilioinguinal nerve was identified and preserved, and the hernia sac was clear down to the internal ring. This was separated from the cord structures. A high ligation was then performed using stick ties. Excess hernia sac was then removed. The stick tie was performed after replacing the abdominal contents into the peritoneal cavity and entering. No abdominal contents were involved within this tie. At this time, a right dartos scrotal sac was made, and the testicle was brought into the right hemiscrotal dartos sac without twisting or tension. The tunic of the testis was affixed with one single 5-0 chromic suture to the dartos. The scrotal skin incision was then closed using 5-0 chromic in a simple interrupted fashion and covered with collodion.[1] Attention was then turned again to the right inguinal incision. The external oblique fibers were then closed using a 4-0 chromic in a running continuous fashion with care to preserve the ilioinguinal nerve from the fibers of the closure. The Scarpa fascia[2] was then approximated using 4-0 undyed Vicryl in a simple interrupted fashion, and the skin was closed using 5-0 undyed Vicryl in a subcuticular fashion. The wound was then covered with collodion, Steri-Strips, and a dry sterile dressing. After having tolerated this procedure well, the patient was awakened and taken to the recovery room in stable condition. Specimens: Hernia sac. Estimated blood loss: Less than 10 cc. Fluids: 150 cc crystalloid.

Footnotes:

1. 1.A clear syrupy liquid used as a topical protectant, applied to the skin to close small wounds, abrasions, and cuts, to hold surgical dressings in place, and to keep medications in contact with the skin.
2. 2.Scarpa fascia is capped because it is named after Antonio Scarpa. You can find more about eponymous terms by going to www.whonamedit.com.

SPELLING.
Determine if the following words are spelled correctly. If the spelling is correct, leave the word as it has already been entered. If the spelling is incorrect, provide the correct spelling.

1. dartos _____

2. oblicque _____

3. caudle _____

4. Steri-Strips _____

5. tunic _____

6. ilioinguuinal _____

7. crystalloid _____

TRUE/FALSE.
Mark the following true or false.

1. The patient is a 16-year-old male.

   ○ true

   ○ false

2. The patient received a caudal block and general mask anesthesia.

   ○ true

   ○ false

3. Prior to the surgery, the patient had no palpable left testicle.

   ○ true

   ○ false

4. The patient lost a total of 160 cc of blood.

   ○ true

   ○ false

5. The skin was closed with Vicryl.

   ○ true

   ○ false

PEDIATRICS REPORT 8 – DISCHARGE SUMMARY

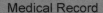

ADMISSION DIAGNOSES

1. Reactive airway disease.
2. Otitis media.

HISTORY OF PRESENT ILLNESS: The patient is 2 years old[1] and presents with a 4-day history of cough and rhinorrhea. He also had some decreased p.o. intake x2 days. The mother of the child reported that he had low-grade fevers, increasing cough, and increasing difficulty with sleeping. The patient was seen in the Bainbridge Island Medical Clinic on the day of admission and was given 2 albuterol nebulizers. However, the patient continued to have increased respiratory distress with nasal flaring and chest retractions. He was seen in the Denny Duquette Memorial Clinic here for respiratory distress and was admitted to Seattle Grace for further management of reactive airway disease.

PAST MEDICAL HISTORY: The patient is a former 1600-gram 32-week premature infant. There was a positive maternal history for alcohol use. The patient is noted to have some developmental delay as well. History also includes recurrent otitis media and septic hip in October 2007.

PAST SURGICAL HISTORY: N/A.[2]

MEDICATIONS: Septra prophylaxis for recurrent otitis.

IMMUNIZATIONS: Up to date.

SOCIAL HISTORY: The patient is currently in foster care.

DEVELOPMENTAL HISTORY: The patient was recently evaluated by the Infant Learning Program. He has approximately a 6-month delay in some areas. His vocabulary consists of about 20-30 words, and he is beginning to put 2 words together. He does help with undressing.

PHYSICAL EXAMINATION: Temperature 101, pulse 132, weight 26 lb. The child was alert, but anxious. Respirations were 62. He was in some mild-to-moderate distress. HEENT: Significant for left TM redness with decreased mobility. The child's throat was red, but had no exudates. Lungs: There were diffuse wheezes bilaterally, again with mild-to-moderate retractions.

HOSPITAL COURSE/PROBLEM LIST

1. Fluids, electrolytes, and nutrition: The patient had no difficulty with fluid intake during this admission, and IV medication was not required.
2. Respiratory: The patient was started out on albuterol nebs 0.5 cc in 2 cc normal saline q.4 hours for 2 days p.r.n. along with prednisone 1 mg/kg per day. Over his 2-day hospitalization, the child's respiratory status improved significantly. He did not require oxygen.
3. Otitis: The patient was started on amoxicillin 15 mg/kg per dose t.i.d. times 10 days, and his temperature decreased.

DISPOSITION: The patient was discharged to home in good condition.

DISCHARGE MEDICATIONS: Albuterol syrup 0.3 mg/kg per day divided t.i.d. and amoxicillin as prescribed during hospitalization.

FOLLOWUP: The patient was to follow up with the clinic in 2 weeks for an ear recheck.

Footnotes:

1. 1.Hyphens are not used here because the age is not adjectival in nature. Had the author said "...is a 2-year-old child," then hyphens would have been required.
2. 2.N/A = not applicable.

SPELLING.

Determine if the following words are spelled correctly. If the spelling is correct, leave the word as it has already been entered. If the spelling is incorrect, provide the correct spelling.

1. Septera _____

2. retractions _____

3. wheaze _____

4. hospitalization _____

5. otitus _____

Multiple Choice.

Choose the best answer.

1. The patient was seen for (○ respiratory, ○ febrile) distress.

2. The child did not require (○ antibiotics, ○ oxygen).

3. The patient was given albuterol (○ nebulizers, ○ nebilizers).

4. He has approximately a 6-month (○ advancement, ○ delay) in some areas.

5. History includes (○ reocurrent, ○ recurrent) otitis media.

PEDIATRICS REPORT 9 – DISCHARGE SUMMARY

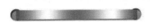

ADMISSION DIAGNOSES

1. Periorbital cellulitis.
2. Sinusitis.
3. Otitis.

HISTORY OF PRESENT ILLNESS: The patient is a 1-year-old female from the Bronx with a 4-day history of redness and swelling around the left eye, worsening, with redness spreading to the cheek over the last 2 days. The patient also has had a history of greenish-yellow discharge from her nose, and low-grade fevers. There has been no history of trauma, insect bite, or pustule in the area of the eye. The patient was sent by Dr. Baker and is admitted for further evaluation and treatment of left eye swelling.

PAST MEDICAL HISTORY: Bronchiolitis at 1 month of age. Birth history: The patient was born at 40 weeks' gestation, Apgar scores of 8 and 9, AGA.[1] Normal spontaneous vaginal delivery with no complications.

PAST SURGICAL HISTORY: None.

ALLERGIES: NO KNOWN DRUG ALLERGIES.

MEDICATIONS: None.

FAMILY HISTORY: The child is the first child in the family. Parents are in good health. Currently the child is still breastfeeding. Immunizations are up to date.

PHYSICAL EXAMINATION: The child was alert and active. HEENT: Significant for red TMs with decreased mobility bilaterally. Left eyelid was swollen and red. The redness spread to the mid-cheek. The remaining physical exam was normal.

HOSPITAL COURSE: The patient had no difficulty with fluid intake on the first day of admission, and her diet was advanced as tolerated. Regarding her periorbital cellulitis, the patient was initially started on Clindamycin and cefuroxime. She responded well to these medications and on the day prior to discharge was switched over to oxacillin 75 mg/kg per day q.i.d. The redness slowly decreased along with the swelling. On the day of discharge, the redness had decreased significantly. There were never any problems with extraocular movements. Vision was intact. With regard to her otitis, the patient's fever decreased significantly during her hospitalization, and the ear had not worsened during her hospitalization.

DISCHARGE DIAGNOSIS

1. Periorbital cellulitis.
2. Sinusitis.
3. Otitis.

DISPOSITION: The patient was discharged to home with her mother.

DISCHARGE MEDICATIONS: Augmentin 5 mg/kg per dose t.i.d. p.o. times 21 days. The mother was informed that the patient may develop diarrhea.

FOLLOWUP: The patient is to follow up with Dr. Baker in 3 weeks for an ear recheck.

Footnotes:

1. 1.AGA = appropriate for gestational age.

SPELLING.

Determine if the following words are spelled correctly. If the spelling is correct, leave the word as it has already been entered. If the spelling is incorrect, provide the correct spelling.

1. Apgar _____

2. cefuroxeime _____

3. Augmenten _____

4. sinusitus _____

5. imunizations _____

Multiple Choice.

Choose the best answer.

1. A visible collection of pus within or beneath the epidermis.

   ○ pustulle

   ○ pustule

   ○ pushtule

   ○ pusstule

2. Situated around the eye socket.

   ○ periorbital

   ○ paraorbital

   ○ perriorbital

   ○ peryorbital

3. Happening or arising without apparent external cause.

   ○ spontaneus

   ○ spontaineus

   ○ spontaneous

   ○ spontanus

4. Inflammation of subcutaneous tissue.

   ○ cellulittis

   ○ celulitis

   ○ sellulitis

   ○ cellulitis

5. Inflammation of the membranes lining the bronchioles.

   ○ bronchiolitis

   ○ bronkiolitis

   ○ broncholitis

   ○ bronchiolitus

UNIT 11

Surgery

SURGERY – INTRODUCTION

As you begin to study this unit on surgery, keep in mind that there are two broad categories of surgery: General Surgery (specific to a specialty) and surgery in general (the hodgepodge of the operating room). They sound similar, a mere rearranging of words, yet they are not the same thing, and it is important to be able to distinguish between the two. While this unit will focus on the surgical specialty of General Surgery, we'll start by discussing surgery in general.

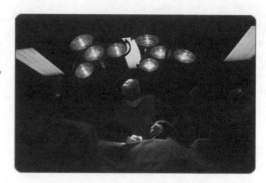

The term **surgery** is somewhat loosely defined as the branch of medical science that treats disease or injury by operative procedures. The majority of surgeons generally concentrate their efforts in a specific area or discipline in medicine. These can be classified along specialty or subspecialty lines. For example, a cardiovascular surgeon, as one might assume, would focus on heart-related surgeries. A neurosurgeon would specialize in brain surgery and certain spinal cord procedures. An orthopedic surgeon might replace a hip, reconstruct a knee, or repair a fracture. The one surgical category that does not follow this "appropriately named" design is general surgery. While general surgeons do handle a variety of body ailments, they are most commonly associated with surgical treatment of diseases or injuries of the abdomen.

General Surgery, as opposed to surgery in general, is a specific department of medicine within a hospital that treats general disorders of the body, typically with surgical intervention. The most common and well-known types of disorders included in this category are appendicitis and cholecystitis (acute inflammation of the appendix and gallbladder, respectively). These are treated by removal of the offending organs— appendectomies and cholecystectomies. In fact, as the name would indicate, most of the treatment rendered by doctors in this category consists of surgery. A general surgeon may perform a laparoscopy to determine the nature of a patient's complaint and then oftentimes remove the offending organ.

Subspecialties in General Surgery include:

- Breast Surgery
- Trauma Surgery
- Colorectal Surgery
- Upper Gastrointestinal Surgery
- Endocrine Surgery
- Transplant Surgery
- Vascular Surgery

In addition to a focus on General Surgery, this unit will conclude with a mini-unit, so to speak, focused on plastic surgery reports. **Plastic Surgery** is a branch of medicine that deals with surgical reconstruction. This type of surgery is often considered "elective" and solely for cosmetic purposes by the general public, which is often the case with face lifts, "nose jobs," or breast augmentations. In fact, it is sometimes also referred to as cosmetic surgery. However, plastic surgery serves both useful and life-saving functions as well. Rhinoplasties (reconstructive nose surgeries) are used to alleviate congestion and sinus problems and open clogged breathing passages. Blepharoplasties tighten up drooping eyelids, increasing the field of vision. These are common types of plastic surgery. Breast augmentations and reconstructions are often performed following mastectomies for breast cancer. Furthermore, burn victims' lives are sometimes only spared by extensive grafting, and they are able to sustain normal living as a result of reconstructive dermal and subdermal surgery.

SURGERY LANGUAGE WORKSHOP

Surgery, in general, has a vocabulary all its own. The MTE who edits surgical reports must know not only the basic medical terminology—the anatomical and physiological terminology required by the discipline or whatever medical specialty the surgery represents—but also know (or know where to find) the names of the surgical instruments, sutures, dressings, incision types, positions, and procedural protocols, among other things. With the advances in medicine and surgical procedures, the required vocabulary and knowledge also grows and changes. Understanding and editing surgical reports can definitely be a challenge for the MTE.

This surgery language workshop will cover both General Surgery terminology and surgical terminology in general.

Common Surgery Root Words and Combining Forms

Root Word & Combining Form	Meaning	Example
acr/o	extremities	acromegaly
adip/o	fat	adipose
aer/o	air	aeration
angi/o	vessel	angiogram
ankyl/o	crooked or fused	ankylosing
bucc/o	cheek	buccal
caud/o	tail	caudate
cephal/o	head	cephalad
chondr/o	cartilage	chondromalacia
colp/o	hollow/vagina	colporrhaphy
cost/o	rib	costovertebral
cry/o	cold	cryogenic
crypt/o	hide, conceal	cryptorchism
cyan/o	blue	cyanotic
dist/o	far/distant from origin	distally
dors/o	toward back/on the back	dorsolateral
enter/o	intestine	enterocolitis
hist/o	tissue	histoplasmosis
lapar/o	flank/abdominal wall	laparotomy
myel/o	marrow/spinal cord	myeloma
ne/o	new	neoblastic
necr/o	dead/corpse	necrosis
odyn/o	pain/distress	odynophagia
pneum/o	air/breathing/lung	pneumoperitoneum
proxim/o	nearest point of origin	proximal
py/o	pus	pyoid
scoli/o	twisted or crooked	scoliosis
spondyl/o	vertebra	spondylosis
thromb/o	clot	thrombosis

Common Surgery Prefixes

Prefix	Meaning	Example
bio-	life	biohazard
circum-	around, circular	circumferential
cry-	cold	cryotherapy
de-	down from, removing	decomposition
dia-	through, between, across	diaphragm
ecto-/ex-/exo-	outside, without, away	exophytic
eu-	good, normal	euthymic
lith-	stone	lithotripsy
meso-	middle, moderate	mesothelial
nulli-	none	nulliparous
primi-	first	primigravida
retro-	behind, backward	retrofit
sub-	beneath, below	subtalar
syn-/sym-	together, union	symphysis
trans-	across, through	transurethral

Common Surgery Suffixes

Suffix	Meaning	Example
-centesis	puncture to withdraw fluid	thoracentesis
-clasis	break, breaking	osteoclasis
-desis	binding, stabilizing, fixation	pleurodesis
-ectomy	excision or removal	tonsillectomy
-esthesia	perception, sensitivity	paresthesia
-lysis	loosening, freeing	adhesiolysis
-meter	instrument to measure	glucometer
-metry	process of measuring	spirometry
-oid	resembling	ovoid
-oma	tumor	lipoma
-opsy	excision or removal of	biopsy
-pexy	fixation, surgical fixation	retinopexy
-plasty	surgical repair	abdominoplasty
-ptosis	to droop or fall	enteroptosis
-rrhaphy	suture	herniorrhaphy
-rrhexis	rupture	capsulorrhexis
-stomy	forming an opening	tracheostomy
-tripsy	surgical crushing	lithotripsy

Common Surgery Abbreviations

Abbreviation	Expansion
AAA	abdominal aortic aneurysm
AVM	arteriovenous malformation
BiPAP	bilevel positive airway pressure
CPAP	continuous positive airway pressure
CPR	cardiopulmonary resuscitation
DNR	DO NOT RESUSCITATE
DOB	date of birth
DT	delirium tremens
ESWL	extracorporeal shock-wave lithotripsy
IMA	internal mammary artery
IOL	intraocular lens
KVO	keep vein open (IV)
LET	lidocaine, epinephrine, tetracaine
NG	nasogastric (tube)
NPO	nothing by mouth (Latin: nil per os)
NS	normal saline
OR	operating room
TKO	to keep open (IV)
TPN	total parenteral nutrition
ICU	intensive care unit
BICU	burn intensive care unit
CCU	coronary care unit
CICU	cardiac intensive care unit, coronary intensive care unit
CMICU	coronary/medical intensive care unit
CSDU	cardiac step-down unit
CSICU	cardiac surgery intensive care unit
CVICU	cardiovascular intensive care unit
ICU	intensive care unit
MICU	medical intensive care unit, mobile intensive care unit
NICU	neonatal intensive care unit
PICU	pediatric intensive care unit
SCICU	spinal cord intensive care unit
SCVICU	surgical cardiovascular intensive care unit
SICU	surgical intensive care unit
STICU	surgical trauma intensive care unit
TICU	trauma intensive care unit

REVIEW: SURGERY LANGUAGE

Fill in the Blank.
Using the word(s) in the box, fill in the blanks.

lithotripsy	
thoracentesis	
cryptorchism	
adhesiolysis	
resuscitate	

1. *DNR* stands for DO NOT _____.

2. The abbreviation *ESWL* stands for extracorporeal shockwave _____.

3. _____ means puncture to withdraw fluid from the thorax.

4. Term that literally means condition of having hidden or concealed testes.

   _____

5. _____ means freeing of adhesions.

Multiple Choice.
Choose the best answer.

1. (◯ Hemoperitoneum, ◯ Pneumoperitoneum) is a term that means having gas or air in the peritoneal cavity.

2. *BiPAP* stands for bilevel (◯ positive, ◯ positional) airway pressure.

3. *TICU* stands for (◯ trauma, ◯ thoracic) intensive care unit.

4. The term *dorsal* refers to the (◯ front, ◯ back).

5. The abbreviation *NPO* is a latin derivative meaning (◯ nothing, ◯ nasal) by mouth.

TRUE/FALSE.
Mark the following true or false.

1. *NICU* means neonavicular intensive care unit.

   ◯ true

   ◯ false

2. *TPN* stands for total parental nutrition.

   ◯ true

   ◯ false

3. When speaking in terms of an IV, *TKO* means to keep open.

   ◯ true

   ◯ false

4. The abbreviation *AAA* stands for abdominal aortic aneuroplasty.

   ◯ true

   ◯ false

5. The abbreviation *NG*, as in *NG tube*, means nasogastric.

   ◯ true

   ◯ false

SURGERY REPORTS

General surgeons are found in every hospital. The types of reports that you will be studying in this unit are quite common. The nature of the problems associated with general surgery are treatable and are rarely life-threatening; they also afflict a large number of people. The terminology found in these reports is fairly general; however, knowledge of surgical instrumentation will be very helpful in the effort for accurate surgical documentation. **Surgical equipment** is a catchall phrase that simply refers to the tools and instruments a surgeon uses to perform procedures. Surgical equipment ranges from simple tweezers used to remove debris from a scratch to complex laser equipment used to perform intracranial surgery.

Listed below is a sampling of the types of surgical equipment used for operations and procedures in general. This is in no way an exhaustive list, and we highly recommend you purchase a good surgical word book, or even two, as you work through the practicum portion of the program—and definitely once employed as an MTE, as the variety and type of instruments used in medicine is vast.

- burs
- compression devices
- drains
- dressings (mesh, gauze, gel, foam, cement, etc.)
- endoscopes
- forceps (atraumatic, hemostatic, splinter, and sponge)
- lasers
- needles, needle holders
- scissors
- retractors
- scalpels, handles and blades
- speculums
- stethoscopes
- suction tubes
- surgical needles
- suture materials
- towel clamps
- trocars and biopsy needles

SURGERY REPORT 1 – OPERATIVE NOTE

PREOPERATIVE DIAGNOSIS: Choledocholithiasis and cholelithiasis.[1]

POSTOPERATIVE DIAGNOSIS: Choledocholithiasis and cholelithiasis.

MATERIAL TO LAB: Gallbladder and stones.

OPERATION PERFORMED: Open cholecystectomy with common bile duct exploration and placement of T-tube drainage.

ESTIMATED BLOOD LOSS: 250 cc.

INDICATIONS: This is a healthy 41-year-old male who presented to the medicine service with jaundice. Ultrasound of the abdomen revealed cholelithiasis and dilated common bile duct and intrahepatic ducts. Preoperative endoscopic retrograde cholangiopancreatography was attempted but failed to remove a large stone impacted in the distal common bile duct. He is now here for open cholecystectomy and common bile duct exploration to remove the impacted stone.

DESCRIPTION OF PROCEDURE: The patient was taken to the operating room where a general anesthesia was attained. His abdomen was prepped and draped in the usual sterile fashion. A scalpel was used to make a right subcostal incision which was deepened with the electrocautery through the abdominal wall until controlled access could be gained to the abdominal cavity. The fundus of the gallbladder was grasped, and electrocautery was used to create a dissection plane through the peritoneal lining over the gallbladder near the junction with the liver. The peritoneal attachments were divided down toward Hartmann pouch.[2] The gallbladder was freed from the liver bed using the electrocautery. Once freed from the liver bed, hemostasis of the liver was verified. The confluence between the cystic duct and the common bile duct was dissected out carefully. Palpation along the distal common bile duct was performed and revealed a large stone distally. The gallbladder was left in place to aid in traction. A scalpel was used to make a small choledochotomy just distal to the location where the cystic duct joined. This was lengthened with Potts scissors for a total length of approximately 1.5 cm. A red Robinson catheter was inserted proximally and distally, and irrigation with saline performed. Small fragments of stone were retrieved with this procedure. An attempt to milk the stone proximally was made and resulted in fragmentation of the stone. Further irrigation was performed and allowed retrieval of several large fragments of stone. Once no further stone was palpable in the duct and irrigation had been completed, the choledochoscope was inserted, and visualization of the right and left hepatic ducts, as well as the distal common bile ducts, was performed. The intrahepatic[3] ducts were clear, as was the proximal common bile duct. Distally, the duct still contained 2 small fragments of stone. A scoop was then used to retrieve these fragments of fractured stone. The choledochoscope was reinserted, and visualization of the ampulla[4] was performed from within the choledochus. The lining of the duct distally looked irritated with what appeared to be frayed epithelium dangling down from the walls of the duct into the lumen. No further fragments were discernible. During retrieval of the stones with the scoop, the scoop could be felt easily within the lumen of the duodenum. This suggested that we had successfully passed the scoop through the ampulla. At one point during the procedure, the cystic artery was avulsed, with resultant loss of a fair amount of blood. With this, the patient became a bit hypotensive, and anesthesia performed successful resuscitation without much difficulty. The cystic artery was ligated with 0 silk sutures and completely divided. The cystic duct, similarly, was doubly ligated with 0 silk and divided. The gallbladder was passed from the field and sent as a specimen. A 20-French T-tube was then brought onto the field. The limbs of the T were shortened and the posterior wall of the T removed. This was placed into the choledochus and the choledochotomy closed, using a running 4-0 chromic gut suture. A 2-shot T-tube cholangiogram was then performed using injections of 20 cc each of one-half strength Angiovist. The cholangiogram returned revealing a normal appearing common duct proximally. The distal common bile duct was not visualized well on the cholangiogram, and it was thought to be in spasm. There was prompt fill of the duodenum with the cholangiogram. Due to the patient's previous hypotensive episode and a desire to finish the case as expeditiously as possible to preclude any further hemodynamic instability, and since the distal duct was visualized with the choledochoscope and found to be stone-free, closure was undertaken. A separate stab incision was made caudal to the main incision, and the T-tube exited through this site. Care was taken to assure that the T-tube maintained a gentle curve through the abdominal cavity. Closure of the abdominal wall was performed with running #1 Prolene suture in 2 separate layers. The first layer approximated the posterior rectus sheath and the transversus abdominis and internal oblique muscle layers laterally. The second layer approximated the anterior rectus sheath and the external oblique muscle layer laterally. The skin was closed with staples. The drain was secured to the skin with a 0 silk suture. All wounds were dressed with Xeroform gauze and 4 x 8 sponges. The patient was awakened and extubated. The patient was then taken to the recovery room awake and with stable vital signs. Estimated blood loss was 250 cc. There were no apparent complications.

Footnotes:

1. 1.Choledocholithiasis = Presence of a stone in the common bile duct. Cholelithiasis = Presence of concretions (gallstones) in the gallbladder or bile ducts.
2. 2.Named after French surgeon Henri Albert Hartmann, the Hartmann pouch is a spheroid or conical out-pouching of the wall of the gallbladder at the junction of the neck of the gallbladder and the cystic duct.
3. 3.Although they sound similar, it will always be "intrahepatic" and never "interhepatic." *Intrahepatic* means within the liver. *Interhepatic* would mean between the liver, which isn't really feasible.
4. 4.Anatomical term designating a flasklike dilatation of a tubular structure.

SPELLING.

Determine if the following words are spelled correctly. If the spelling is correct, leave the word as it has already been entered. If the spelling is incorrect, provide the correct spelling.

1. choledocholithiasis _____
2. jondice _____
3. cholangiopancreatography _____
4. Hartman _____
5. Potts _____
6. ampula _____
7. Angiovist _____
8. prolean _____

TRUE/FALSE.

Mark the following true or false.

1. The patient's gallbladder was removed.

   ○ true

   ○ false

2. The surgery was performed under spinal anesthesia.

   ○ true

   ○ false

3. There were no apparent complications.

   ○ true

   ○ false

4. The skin was closed with 0 silk sutures.

   ○ true

   ○ false

5. During the procedure a cystic artery was torn, and the patient lost a fair amount of blood.

   ○ true

   ○ false

SURGERY REPORT 2 – OPERATIVE NOTE

PREOPERATIVE DIAGNOSIS: Bilateral recurrent inguinal hernias.

POSTOPERATIVE DIAGNOSIS: Bilateral recurrent inguinal hernias.

OPERATION PERFORMED: Preperitoneal hernia repair bilaterally with placement of Marlex mesh.

ESTIMATED BLOOD LOSS: Less than 20 cc.

INDICATIONS: The patient is a healthy 37-year-old male who is status post bilateral inguinal herniorrhaphies in the past. He now relates recurrence[1] of groin bulges bilaterally, and this is confirmed on physical exam. He is scheduled for elective bilateral inguinal herniorrhaphy.

DESCRIPTION OF PROCEDURE: The patient was taken to the operating room where an epidural anesthetic was attained. His groin and lower abdomen were prepped and draped in the usual sterile fashion. A scalpel was used to make a transverse skin incision approximately 1 to 2 fingerbreadths above the pubic bone. Dissection was carried down to the anterior rectus sheath. The midline was then opened and careful dissection performed so as to stay superficial to the peritoneum. Each abdominal wall was then elevated and the peritoneum pushed down as the dissection was continued laterally and inferiorly. As the dissection continued, the spermatic cord could be seen passing up and through the internal ring. The dissection continued until the cord was freed circumferentially. Inferiorly, the peritoneum was pushed away until it was seen falling away down in toward the pelvic bowl. A sheet of Marlex mesh was then fashioned so as to be approximately 4 x 6 cm in size. Laterally, a slit was made in the mesh so as to allow passage of the cord. The mesh was laid[2] down into the pelvic bowl following the normal anatomic curve. The cord was passed through the laterally placed slot in the mesh. The patch was tacked in place at 4 different locations to keep it from migrating. The mesh was reapproximated lateral to the cord so as to create a tight internal ring. Examination within the cord failed to reveal the presence of an indirect hernia sac. The repair on the opposite side was then performed in identical fashion and, again, failed to reveal an indirect hernia sac. At completion of both repairs, both sides were irrigated copiously with antibiotic irrigation. The midline was reapproximated with a running #1 Prolene suture. The skin edges were reapproximated with staples. A dressing of Xeroform gauze and 4 x 8 sponges was placed. The patient was then transported to the recovery room awake and with stable vital signs. Estimated blood loss was less than 20 cc. There were no apparent complications.

Footnotes:

1. 1.Note this is always "recurrence," even if dictated as "reocurrence."
2. 2.The word *laid* is the past tense and past participle of *lay*. In the present tense, if the subject is acting on some other object you use *lay*. If the subject is lying down, then it is *lie*. In a verbatim account, it would be edited as dictated.

Multiple Choice.
Choose the best answer.

1. A transverse skin incision was made approximately 1 to 2 (○ fingersbreadth, ○ fingerbreadths) above the pubic bone.
2. A sheet of (○ Marlex, ○ Marlix) mesh was cut and placed.
3. As the (○ disection, ○ dissection) continued, the spermatic cord was identified.
4. A (○ scalple, ○ scalpel) was used to make a transverse skin incision.
5. He is scheduled for elective bilateral (○ inguinal, ○ ingunal) herniorrhaphy.

Multiple Choice.
Choose the best answer.

1. In a crosswise direction.

   ○ transverce

   ○ transverse

   ○ transferse

   ○ transferce

2. A group of structures which go through the inguinal canal to the testis.

   ○ spermatic cord

   ○ spermadic cord

   ○ spermatic chord

   ○ spermadic cord

3. A rupture in smooth muscle tissue through which a bodily structure protrudes.

   ○ hurnia

   ○ hurnea

   ○ hernea

   ○ hernia

4. Having two sides or parts.

   ○ bilateral

   ○ bilaterall

   ○ billateral

   ○ bylateral

5. Upon or outside the dura mater.

   ○ eppidural

   ○ epedural

   ○ epidural

   ○ epadural

SURGERY REPORT 3 – DISCHARGE SUMMARY

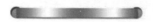

HISTORY OF PRESENT ILLNESS: The patient is a 46-year-old white female who presented to the medicine service in February 2006 secondary to abdominal pain, and was felt to have ovarian cysts with thrombocytopenia. She was noted to have a platelet count of 30,000. At that time, she was diagnosed with idiopathic thrombocytopenic purpura and was started on steroid therapy. Her prednisone was increased to a maximum of 80 mg per day with a good response. Her platelet count increased to 244,000. Over the past few weeks, her platelet count has decreased to 79,000 post[1] stopping the prednisone. She is referred to surgery for an elective splenectomy. She had immunizations against encapsulated bacteria prior to surgery.

PAST MEDICAL HISTORY: Noncontributory.

PAST SURGICAL HISTORY: None.

SOCIAL HISTORY: She denies alcohol or tobacco use.

ALLERGIES: She has no known drug allergies.

MEDICATIONS ON ADMISSION: None.

REVIEW OF SYSTEMS: Noncontributory.

PHYSICAL EXAMINATION: Vital signs are stable. She is afebrile. In general, she is a well-developed, well-nourished, 46-year-old white female, alert and oriented x3, in no apparent distress. She has slightly cushingoid facies.[2] HEENT exam is benign. Heart: Regular rate and rhythm without gallops or murmurs. The lungs are clear to auscultation bilaterally. Her breast exam is all within normal limits. There is no axillary adenopathy. Abdominal exam: Soft and nontender, no hepatosplenomegaly, no masses. She has normoactive bowel sounds. Extremities: No clubbing, cyanosis or edema. Back: There are no noted deformities. The neurological exam is nonfocal. The GU exam is deferred.

LABORATORY DATA ON ADMISSION: Significant for a platelet count of 20,000.

HOSPITAL COURSE: The patient was admitted to surgery. After thorough counseling as to the indications, procedure, and complications of the procedure, the patient was taken to the operating room on February 4, 2006, and a splenectomy was performed. Prior to surgery, she was given Solu-Cortef 100 mg IV piggyback as prophylaxis. In addition she was given Ancef 1 g IV piggyback. The patient tolerated the procedure well, but secondary to the area being notable for a constant ooze, she was administered 6 units of platelets with a postoperative platelet count of greater than 100,000. The patient was subsequently transferred to the ward. The patient's postoperative course was unremarkable with her NG tube removed on postoperative day 3. The patient started on a clear liquid diet after the return of bowel functions, which was tolerated without difficulties. Her diet was subsequently advanced to regular and again tolerated without difficulties. Her platelet count was noted to be increasing over her hospital course, with her platelet count at the time of discharge being greater than 380,000. At the time of the patient's discharge, she was ambulating without assistance and without complaints.

FINAL DIAGNOSIS: Idiopathic thrombocytopenic purpura.

OPERATION PERFORMED: Splenectomy, February 4, 2006.

DISCHARGE MEDICATIONS: Percocet 1-2 tablets p.o. q.4-6 h. p.r.n. for pain.

DISPOSITION AND FOLLOWUP: The patient is to follow up with the general surgery clinic on February 15, 2006 at 1300 hours. She is not to lift greater than 5-10 pounds for the next 4-6 weeks. She should have a CBC performed 2 hours prior to coming to the general surgery clinic on February 15, 2006. She should return to the emergency room as soon as possible if she develops any symptoms of infection. Regular diet. Her activities are otherwise as tolerated.

Footnotes:

1. 1.*Post*, when standing on its own, means after. *Post* is also a prefix. *Post* can also be used as part of a hyphenated compound modifier (post-surgery scar). The phrase *status post* means state or condition after or following.
2. 2.The term *cushingoid facies* is a medical sign for when the face swells up into a rounded shape. This is sometimes called "moon face." It is often associated with Cushing disease. The *c* in cushingoid is not capped because this word means resembling or similar to Cushing disease; it is the adjectival form and not the noun itself.

SPELLING.

Determine if the following words are spelled correctly. If the spelling is correct, leave the word as it has already been entered. If the spelling is incorrect, provide the correct spelling.

1. spleenectomy _____

2. noncontributory _____

3. Solu-Cortif _____

4. ideopathic _____

5. Ancef _____

True/False.

Mark the following true or false.

1. At the time of the patient's discharge, she was ambulating with a cane.

   ○ true

   ○ false

2. Extremities were without clubbing, cyanosis or edema.

   ○ true

   ○ false

3. Lab data on admission showed a platelet count of 30,000.

   ○ true

   ○ false

4. The patient does not have a history of thrombocytopenic purpura.

   ○ true

   ○ false

5. On discharge, the patient was instructed to not lift greater than 5-10 pounds for the next 4-6 weeks.

   ○ true

   ○ false

SURGERY REPORT 4 – OPERATIVE NOTE

PREOPERATIVE DIAGNOSIS: Gastroesophageal reflux disease.

POSTOPERATIVE DIAGNOSIS: Gastroesophageal reflux disease.

OPERATION PERFORMED: Nissen fundoplication and incidental splenectomy.

INDICATIONS: This is a 50-year-old female who complains of reflux symptoms with burning substernal chest pain, with esophagogastroscopy revealing esophagitis with a hiatal hernia. The patient had a positive Bernstein test.[1] She had some relief with the use of omeprazole but not complete resolution of her symptoms, and she now presents for Nissen fundoplication in order to relieve her gastroesophageal reflux from her hiatal hernia.

DESCRIPTION OF PROCEDURE: She was administered a general endotracheal anesthesia in the supine position. The abdomen was prepped and draped in the usual sterile fashion. A midline skin incision was made extending from the xiphoid to the umbilicus, and the abdomen was entered through the linea alba. A Buchwalter self-retaining retractor was placed. The patient was noted to have an extremely elongated left lobe of her liver, which extended back further posterior to the spleen and further inferior than the spleen's attachments. The triangular ligament of the left lobe of the liver was taken down sharply with the electrocautery. Dissection then took place over the esophageal hiatus, with the left lobe of the liver retracted out of the way, and the peritoneum was cleared over the esophagus, being certain to preserve the 2 vagus nerves. Control was then gained circumferentially about the esophagus with a 1-inch Penrose drain. In attempting to divide the short gastric arteries in order to clear the fundus for the planned wrap, a splenic capsular tear was found that was likely made during the dissection of the left lobe of the liver. The anterior and superior aspects of the splenic capsule had been avulsed, and we were not able to control this. Secondary to this, a splenectomy was performed. The hilar vessels in the spleen were divided and ligated with silk ligatures, and the lateral attachments were divided sharply so the specimen could be passed off the field and sent to Pathology. The short gastrics along the greater curvature were then individually ligated and divided with silk ligatures in order to gain enough distance from the fundus for planned wrap. After this was performed, the crural repair was performed after passage of a 40-French bougie and an 18-French nasogastric tube into the stomach. The crural repair was performed with interrupted 0 Nurolon sutures such that a finger could pass into the hiatus freely. The hiatus was known to be greatly patulous prior to this repair. The fundus was then passed posteriorly about the esophagus, and a fundoplication was performed utilizing 4 interrupted 2-0 silk sutures. The inferior and superior sutures were additionally passed through the muscular layer of the esophagus for anchoring. After this was performed, 1 anchoring stitch was placed from the wrap on the fundus of the stomach to the undersurface of the diaphragm to anchor the fundoplication in the abdomen. Hemostasis was then assured. The abdomen was well irrigated. The nasogastric tube was assured to be in good position in the stomach and left in place, and the midline wound was closed with running #1 Prolene suture, begun from either apex. The skin was closed with staples. Sterile dressing was applied. She was awakened from general endotracheal anesthesia, extubated, and returned to the recovery room awake, alert and in stable condition.

Footnotes:

1. 1.A Bernstein test is performed to help establish that substernal pain is due to reflux esophagitis.

Multiple Choice.
Choose the best answer.

1. The (○ hylar, ○ hilar) vessels in the spleen were divided and ligated.

2. The abdomen was well (○ hemostased, ○ irrigated).

3. Esophageal control was gained with a 1-inch (○ Penrose, ○ Buchwalter) drain.

4. The (○ crural, ○ crual) repair was performed with interrupted 0 Nurolon sutures.

5. The patient was administered a general endotracheal anesthesia in the (○ supine, ○ prone) position.

Matching.
Match the correct term to the definition.

1. ____ Bernstein   A. drain

2. ____ Prolene   B. retractor

3. ____ Penrose   C. fundoplication

4. ____ Nissen   D. test

5. ____ Buchwalter   E. suture

SURGERY REPORT 5 – OPERATIVE NOTE

PREOPERATIVE DIAGNOSIS: Appendicitis.

POSTOPERATIVE DIAGNOSIS: Suppurative nonperforated appendicitis.[1]

OPERATION PERFORMED: Appendectomy.

INDICATIONS: The patient is a 29-year-old white female with the clinical evidence of appendicitis during her 24th week of gestation. Preoperative ultrasound earlier in the day demonstrated some periappendiceal fluid with mucosal thickening and luminal dilatation. White blood count was approximately 21,000 with 87% granulocytes, indicating a left shift. The patient was clinically afebrile.

DESCRIPTION OF PROCEDURE: The patient was taken to the operating room and placed on the operating table in the supine position. The patient was sterilely prepped and draped prior to the administration and induction of general anesthesia. Just prior to the incision being made, anesthesia was induced and 2 g of Cefotan antibiotics was[2] administered intravenously. A 3-cm transverse incision was made in the right lateral umbilical region. Dissection through the subcutaneous tissues continued with a combination of scalpel and electrocautery. Scarpa fascia was sharply opened. Each adjacent muscle layer of the abdominal wall was opened, starting with the external oblique, the internal oblique, and transversus. The peritoneum was tented up and sharply divided using the scalpel. Entry into the abdomen was extended with Metzenbaum scissor technique. The cecum was identified and was found to be densely adherent to the retroperitoneum, as well as the pelvis superiorly. Mobilization was continued through a combination of alternating direction traction and blunt dissection. A seropurulent appearing abdominal fluid was obtained, and cultures were sent for Gram stain[3] and sensitivity. The appendix was found to have a purulent fibrinous plaque adherent to it. It was mobilized, and the mesoappendix was taken down sharply and divided by Metzenbaum scissor technique. Each was tied with a 2-0 Vicryl suture. The stalk of the appendix was then identified and crushed with a straight clamp. The clamp was milked distally along the appendiceal stalk. A 0 silk tie was placed in the crush groove. Another tie of 0 silk was placed proximal to the initial tie. The straight clamp was then reapplied to the appendix, and the appendix was sharply divided with a scalpel blade. Specimen, scalpel, and clamp were removed from the field as contaminated. The distal stump of the appendix was fulgurated with electrocautery on scalpel tip. Adequate hemostasis was obtained throughout the procedure at various levels. Pulse sucker was placed into the pelvis, and the abdomen was irrigated with antibiotic containing solution. The cecum[4] was returned to the abdomen. Peritoneal edges were identified with a Crile clamp. A running 3-0 Vicryl suture was placed in the peritoneum. The internal and external oblique muscle fascias were closed with a running PDS 0 suture. Irrigation was performed at each level. Hemostasis was obtained throughout. The abdominal wall and skin were closed with skin staples. Sterile dressing was applied. The patient was awakened from general endotracheal anesthesia. The cultures and appendix were sent to the pathology department as specimens.

Footnotes:

1. 1.When something creates pus it is called suppurative. Therefore, a suppurative nonperforated appendix would be a pus-creating appendix with no holes in it.
2. 2.The correct verb here is "was" and not "were." Units of measurement such as 2 g of Cefotan are treated as a singular entity.
3. 3.As you learned in previous units, Gram stain but also gram-positive or gram-negative.
4. 4.Originally the report said, "the cecum and the appendix were returned to the abdomen." It was flagged for clarification though because this is an appendectomy—which means the appendix was removed. It is important to stay on top of the details.

SPELLING.
Determine if the following words are spelled correctly. If the spelling is correct, leave the word as it has already been entered. If the spelling is incorrect, provide the correct spelling.

1. appendiceal _____

2. mucousal _____

3. adbomen _____

4. oblique _____

5. fulgurated _____

TRUE/FALSE.
Mark the following true or false.

1. The patient is pregnant.

   ○ true

   ○ false

2. The appendix was divided using electrocautery.

   ○ true

   ○ false

3. The abdominal wall and skin were closed with skin staples.

   ○ true

   ○ false

4. The patient's Gram stain came back positive.

   ○ true

   ○ false

5. Only Vicryl suture was used throughout.

   ○ true

   ○ false

SURGERY REPORT 6 – DISCHARGE SUMMARY

HISTORY OF PRESENT ILLNESS: The patient is a 36-year-old white male with a history of peptic ulcer disease and gastritis of longstanding duration that has been stable on his medication of Tagamet 300 mg q.i.d. He complains of increasing epigastric abdominal pain for 4-5 days. He was seen in the ER 2 times in the last several days, and placed on an additional H2 blocker and Carafate without resolution of his symptoms. The last 24 hours the pain has descended to the right midquadrant with radiation. He denies a previous history of similar type pains. He denies nausea and vomiting. He does complain of chills that started yesterday. At the time of presentation to the emergency room, he was noted to have a temperature of 102.2. He indicates that he had a right inguinal hernia repair approximately 6 years ago. He has had no p.o. intake over the last 17 hours. He has had no bowel movements times 3 days. He does complain of anorexia. He has had some upper respiratory and flu-type symptoms. He denies any other complaints. He is admitted to the hospital to rule out acute appendicitis versus ulcer disease.

PAST MEDICAL HISTORY: See HPI.

PAST SURGICAL HISTORY: Right inguinal hernia repair 6 years ago and a polypectomy 1 year ago.

SOCIAL HISTORY: He denies tobacco or alcohol use.

MEDICATIONS ON ADMISSION: Tagamet 300 mg p.o. q.i.d. and Carafate p.r.n.

ALLERGIES: NKDA.[1]

REVIEW OF SYSTEMS: Noncontributory.

PHYSICAL EXAMINATION: Vital signs are significant for a temperature of 102.2, and the rest of his vital signs are within normal limits. In general, he is a young-appearing, 36-year-old Hispanic male in moderate distress with any movement. He is otherwise alert and oriented times 3. Head: Normocephalic and atraumatic. Pupils are equal, round and reactive to light. Extraocular movements are intact. He has positive arcus senilis.[2] His nares are bilaterally patent. There is no icterus. His throat is clear. The neck is supple and nontender without thyromegaly or adenopathy. The back is within normal limits. The chest exam is clear to auscultation bilaterally. The heart has a regular rate and rhythm without gallops or murmurs. Abdominal exam: Normoactive bowel sounds with rushes. He has mild epigastric tenderness to palpation. He has a positive Murphy sign. He is exquisitely tender in the right upper quadrant. In addition he is tender in the right lower quadrant with positive rebound and guarding. There is a positive heel tap, positive psoas and obturator signs. Extremities: No clubbing, cyanosis or edema. Rectal exam: He is slightly tender, but the stool is guaiac negative.

LABORATORY DATA ON ADMISSION: Significant for a white count 19.5. The rest of the laboratories are within normal limits.

HOSPITAL COURSE: The patient was admitted to General Surgery. After discussion with staff and hydration of the patient, it was decided to take the patient to the operating room for exploratory surgery. At operation he was found to have a perforated retrocecal appendix with the cecum being very inflamed. A cecectomy with a side-to-side anastomosis was performed. The patient tolerated the procedure well and was transferred to the recovery room in stable condition. At the time of operation a Jackson-Pratt drain was placed, and subsequent to return of the patient's bowel function this drain was removed. The patient was subsequently started on a clear liquid diet with the return of bowel function. This was advanced to a regular diet which was tolerated without difficulties. The remainder of the patient's postoperative course was unremarkable. The patient was discharged home on July 11, 2004, tolerating a regular diet and without complaints. The patient's final pathology returned consistent with acute ruptured appendicitis with cecitis.

FINAL DIAGNOSES

1. Gangrenous appendicitis, ruptured.
2. Cecitis secondary to #1.
3. History of peptic ulcer disease.

PROCEDURES: None.

OPERATION: Exploratory celiotomy with appendectomy and cecectomy.

DISCHARGE MEDICATIONS

1. Augmentin 500 mg p.o. t.i.d. for 2 weeks.
2. Percocet 1-2 tablets p.o. q.4-6 h. p.r.n. for pain.
3. Colace 100-200 mg p.o. b.i.d. p.r.n. for constipation.
4. Tagamet 300 mg p.o. b.i.d.

DISPOSITION AND FOLLOWUP: The patient is to follow up in the general surgery clinic on July 22, 2004, at 1300 hours for a routine postsurgical check. He is to return to the emergency room as soon as possible if he develops signs of infection. He is to maintain his regular diet and should not lift greater than 5-10 pounds for the next 4-6 weeks. He should not drive for an additional week. His activities are otherwise as tolerated.

Footnotes:

1. 1.NKDA = no known drug allergies.
2. 2.If you aren't sure what this is, look it up.

Multiple Choice.
Choose the correct spelling of the term.

1. Surgical removal of the cecum.

   ○ cecumectomy

   ○ celiotomy

   ○ cecumotomy

   ○ cecectomy

2. An abnormal opening or hole in a hollow organ or viscus.

   ○ preforation

   ○ perforation

   ○ preformation

   ○ performation

3. An operative union of two structures.

   ○ anastimosis

   ○ anastemosis

   ○ anastomosis

   ○ anastemosis

4. An opaque ring at the edges of the cornea.

   ○ arcus senilus

   ○ arcus senilis

   ○ arkus senilus

   ○ arkus senilis

5. An indicator of irritation to the iliopsoas group of hip flexors in the abdomen.

   ○ psoas sign

   ○ psois sign

   ○ psoas sine

   ○ psosa sign

Matching.

Match the drug name to the dosage instructions.

1. ____ Carafate

2. ____ Augmentin

3. ____ Percocet

4. ____ Colace

5. ____ Tagamet

A. 500 mg

B. 300 mg

C. 1-2 tablets

D. p.r.n.

E. 100-200 mg

SURGERY REPORT 7 – OPERATIVE NOTE

PREOPERATIVE DIAGNOSIS: Recurrent gastrointestinal hemorrhage of undetermined etiology.

POSTOPERATIVE DIAGNOSES

1. Recurrent gastrointestinal hemorrhage with jejunal ulcerations.
2. Multiple abdominal wall hernias.

OPERATIONS PERFORMED

1. Exploratory laparotomy.
2. Intraoperative endoscopy.
3. Colonoscopy.
4. Jejunal resection times 2, resection of jejunal ulcer with jejunojejunostomy times 2, and primary closure of resection of jejunal ulcer.
5. Closure, multiple abdominal hernias with Gore-Tex.

INDICATIONS: This is a 68-year-old female with previous history of a right hemicolectomy for ischemic bowel disease and a superior mesenteric artery bypass secondary to ischemia. These procedures were done in 2005 with the bypass having been done at Sacred Heart Hospital by Dr. Cook. The patient now presents with recurrent gastrointestinal hemorrhages of undetermined etiology.

Endoscopy was performed from above and below, failing to elucidate[1] a source for these bleeds. The patient underwent CT of the abdomen, as well as an Indium scan in order to determine if the prior SMA graft was infected or fistulizing, and both of these studies failed to reveal any evidence supporting this. The patient underwent numerous tagged red cell studies, with none revealing any evidence for the source of the bleed until 3 days prior to this procedure, when the patient underwent a heparin challenge prior to doing the tagged cell study with a bolus of 5000 units. This revealed evidence of a bleed in the right upper quadrant, possibly in the area of the ileocolic anastomosis. Secondary to this patient having received numerous blood transfusions in the past for these recurrent bleeds, it is felt that exploration is warranted at this time with plans for intraoperative endoscopy from above and below in order to fully evaluate the small intestine to rule out any small intestine source. It was planned that if no source could be found within the small intestine, likely the anastomosis was the site of the bleed, and the anastomosis would be revised. Additionally, if no source could be identified, it was considered to do a diverting ileostomy and colonic mucus fistula in order to attempt to localize any further bleeding to one of these 2 segments. She now presents for a planned exploratory laparotomy.

DESCRIPTION OF PROCEDURE. She was administered a general endotracheal anesthesia in a lithotomy position. The abdomen was prepped and draped in the usual sterile fashion. A skin incision was made through the previous midline wound. Upon making this incision, it was evident that a prior closure had led to numerous midline hernias with the majority of the small intestine now lying in a rather subcutaneous plane. The adhesions were dissected free in the midline in order to enter the abdomen. There were numerous adhesions involving both the large and small bowel, and tedious dissection resulted in freeing up all of the small bowel and remaining colon. The anastomosis was localized in the right upper quadrant. There was an ileotransverse colonic anastomosis. It appeared to be viable with no evidence of any pathology. The small bowel was cleared from the ligament of Treitz to the terminal ileum such that it could be free for planned intraoperative endoscopy. At this point then, a pediatric colonoscope was passed via the mouth into the esophagus and stomach. It was advanced by the operator around the ligament of Treitz. The scope was then grasped, and the small bowel was telescoped up onto the endoscope. Utilizing this procedure, the majority of the small bowel was able to be examined, with the exception of approximately the last 100 cm of terminal ileum. Upon removing the scope and examining the small intestine, areas of ulceration were found in the jejunum in 4 separate sites. Two of these sites were in such continuity that a primary resection and reanastomosis would remove the ulcers without compromising too much of her jejunum. The other ulcers were too far proximal to consider 1 resection, and therefore it was planned that 2 resections would be necessary, and the fourth ulcerated spot was marked with a stitch such that just an excision could be performed on this site with a primary closure. These ulcers were approximately 3-5 mm in size and appeared to have hemorrhaged at some point prior to this procedure. To examine the remainder of the distal small bowel, a colonoscope was then passed via the anus and was advanced into the terminal ileum, and then it was telescoped through the remainder of the distal ileum. There were no findings of any further ulcerations within the terminal ileum.

The colonoscope was removed. At this point then, the area where the 2 ulcers were located in the jejunum was excised by removing approximately a 10-cm segment of jejunum. The bowel was divided utilizing the GIA stapling device, and a primary anastomosis was performed in a side-to-side or functional end-to-end fashion, again utilizing the GIA stapling device, with the opening through which the device had been passed being closed with TA-55 stapler. Two 3-0 silk sutures were used for reinforcement at the apex of the anastomosis. The third ulcer site was identified, having previously been marked with a stitch, and an approximately 5-cm segment was removed of the jejunum. Again, the anastomosis was performed as previously described, and finally, the most proximal ulcer was marked by placing a stitch right through the base of this ulcer. Therefore an excision was performed in a wedge-like fashion of the small bowel, and primary closure was then performed of the jejunum, utilizing a running 3-0 Vicryl suture, followed by lemberted 3-0 silk sutures to create a 2-layer closure. The segments of resected jejunum were examined to be certain that the ulcerations were contained within the specimens. These were sent to Pathology. Hemostasis was then assured within the abdomen. It was then well irrigated with an antibiotic-containing solution. As previously described, upon entering this abdomen, it was apparent there were numerous very large hernias within the abdominal wall. These resulted in most of the intestine coming to lie in a subcutaneous plane, creating very large hernia sacs. There was very little remaining fascia within the midline, and in order to obtain a closure, it was evident that a prosthetic material would be necessary. First, interrupted 0 Surgilon suture was used, beginning in the inferior and superior aspects of the wound for approximately 10 cm on either end, leaving a gap in the middle that was closed utilizing a Gore-Tex material. This was sutured in place to the fascia utilizing running Prolene sutures 0 in size. Additionally, where the midline was closed with the interrupted sutures, #2 nylon retention sutures were placed. Hemostasis was then assured within the subcuticular layer. Two 10-mm Blake drains were brought into the subcutaneous layer through separate stab incisions, and these were secured to the skin with interrupted silk sutures, and the skin was then closed with staples. Xeroform and a sterile dressing were applied. She was then transported to the surgical intensive care unit, intubated, in stable condition. Estimated blood loss was 300 cc.

Footnotes:

1. 1.*Elucidate* is a fancy word meaning to make clear or comprehensible.

SPELLING.

Determine if the following words are spelled correctly. If the spelling is correct, leave the word as it has already been entered. If the spelling is incorrect, provide the correct spelling.

1. Treitz _____ 2. jejunojejunostomy _____

3. hemicholectomy _____ 4. ileocolic _____

5. anastomosis _____

Matching.

Match the correct term to the definition.

1. ____ GIA   A. ligament
2. ____ Gore-Tex   B. stapling device
3. ____ Treitz   C. suture
4. ____ SMA   D. graft
5. ____ Vicryl   E. material

SURGERY REPORT 8 – DISCHARGE SUMMARY

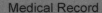

HISTORY OF PRESENT ILLNESS: The patient is a 77-year-old white female who was transferred from Monmouth Junction Hospital secondary to a history of peritonitis status post laparoscopic cholecystectomy, to be administered hyperalimentation. The patient underwent a laparoscopic cholecystectomy on December 8, 2007, which was noted to be uncomplicated. Over the next several days, she complained of periodic abdominal pain, had a period of hypoxia and was subsequently transferred to Princeton-Plainsboro Teaching Hospital. A VQ scan was performed which noted no evidence of pulmonary embolus. A HIDA scan was also performed, which noted good flow through the biliary tree. She was subsequently discharged after 2-1/2 days and was tolerating a regular diet. She presented to the emergency room on December 13, 2007, with complaints of increasing abdominal pain and fever. She was started on IV antibiotics and hydrated, and was subsequently taken to the operating room secondary to abdominal peritonitis. At the time of operation an enterotomy was noted which was closed in 2 layers. At the time of the patient's transfer it was felt that she would need long-term hyperalimentation secondary to her history of peritonitis. She presents here for long-term hyperalimentation and bowel rest.

PAST MEDICAL HISTORY

1. Cholelithiasis.
2. History of a hiatal hernia.
3. History of asthma.
4. See HPI.

PAST SURGICAL HISTORY: TAH/BSO and see HPI.

MEDICATIONS ON ADMISSION: Albuterol nebulizers q.4 h., Timentin 3 g IV piggyback q.6 h., Flagyl 500 mg IV piggyback q.6 h., D5 one-half normal saline with 30 mEq of KCl at 125 cc per hour.

ALLERGIES: ERYTHROMYCIN.

REVIEW OF SYSTEMS: Noncontributory.

PHYSICAL EXAMINATION: In general, the patient is a 77-year-old obese white female who is alert and oriented times 3, in no apparent distress. HEENT is within normal limits. Lungs: Decreased breath sounds bilaterally at the bases with expiratory wheezes. Heart: Rapid rate, normal S1 and S2, no gallops and no murmurs. The abdomen is obese with multiple striae. She has Montgomery straps[1] in place, with the subcutaneous tissue and abdominal fascial layers intact. GU exam: The labia are swollen. There is a Foley catheter in place. The vaginal mucosa is moist. There are no adnexal masses. The rectal exam is without masses, guaiac positive, and there is dark stool in the rectal vault. Extremities: No clubbing, cyanosis or edema. The neurological exam is nonfocal. There is no adenopathy.

LABORATORY DATA ON ADMISSION: Significant for an H&H of 9.6 and 27.9. She is hypokalemic. The remaining labs are within normal limits.

HOSPITAL COURSE: The patient was admitted to General Surgery and was started on hyperalimentation. A chest x-ray was obtained, which noted bilateral pleural effusions. There was also a question of whether the patient was in congestive heart failure. On December 18, 2007, the patient was transferred to the SICU secondary to her SAO2 being in the low 80s. A pulmonary consult was obtained, with recommendations to continue q.4 h. nebulizer therapy and aggressive pulmonary toilet. The remainder of the patient's SICU course was unremarkable. She was subsequently transferred to the ward. She remained on hyperalimentation. A CT scan of the abdomen was obtained on December 25, 2007, which noted bilateral pleural effusions, a right renal cyst, but no evidence of abscess. A fistulogram was performed which noted a fistula between the subcutaneous tissue and a small loop of bowel. After discussion with the staff, it was recommended that the patient be maintained on bowel rest and hyperalimentation, and that the patient be started on somatostatin to decrease flow through the GI tract. This was maintained through her hospital stay, with gradual decrease in her fistula output until it had stopped by January 3, 2008. Somatostatin was continued for the next several days, with her wound always looking good with no evidence of infection. Her dressings were continued to be changed b.i.d. by the nursing staff.

She was subsequently started on a clear liquid diet post discontinuing her somatostatin. The diet was tolerated without difficulties, and subsequently she advanced to a regular diet, again tolerated without difficulties. At the time of the patient's discharge, she was tolerating a regular diet, ambulating without assistance and without complaints.

FINAL DIAGNOSES

1. Enterocutaneous fistula.
2. History of cholelithiasis.
3. History of congestive heart failure, resolved.
4. Right lower lobe pneumonia, resolved.
5. Bilateral pleural effusions, resolving.
6. History of asthma.
7. History of hiatal hernia.

PROCEDURES

1. Fistulogram.
2. CT scan of the abdomen.

OPERATIONS PERFORMED: None.

DISCHARGE MEDICATIONS

1. Colace 100 mg p.o. b.i.d.
2. Metamucil 1 tbsp p.o. b.i.d.
3. Percocet 1-2 tablets p.o. q.6 h. p.r.n. for pain.

DISPOSITION: The patient is to be discharged back home. She is to follow up with her local physician for management of her gastrostomy tube. In addition, she should follow up with her local physician for care of her wound. She should return here p.r.n. She should not lift greater than 5-10 pounds for the next 4-6 weeks. Her activities are otherwise as tolerated. She should maintain her regular diet.

Footnotes:

1. 1.Montgomery straps are medical-grade adhesive tape panels used to secure frequently changed dressings in place.

SPELLING.
Determine if the following words are spelled correctly. If the spelling is correct, leave the word as it has already been entered. If the spelling is incorrect, provide the correct spelling.

1. hyperlimentation _____

2. Timentin _____

3. flagle _____

4. Montgomery _____

5. fistulogram _____

6. Somatostanin _____

7. enterocutaneous _____

Multiple Choice.
Choose the best answer.

1. The patient remained on (○ hyperalimentation, ○ hyperalementation).

2. The patient has a history of a (○ hiatal, ○ hiatle) hernia.

3. Exam revealed no (○ adanexal, ○ adnexal) masses.

4. The patient had a history of (○ peritonitis, ○ peritinitis).

5. The abdomen is obese with multiple (○ striaye, ○ striae).

SURGERY REPORT 9 – OPERATIVE NOTE

OPERATION PERFORMED: Left modified radical mastectomy with axillary lymph node dissection.

INDICATIONS: The patient is a 31-year-old female who felt a lump in her left breast on routine self-breast exam. Biopsy of this revealed infiltrating ductal carcinoma with primary tumor 1.2 cm in greatest dimension in the left upper outer quadrant. She is to undergo modified radical mastectomy. She has been evaluated by the radiation oncology and plastic surgery services, and she opts for modified radical mastectomy.

DESCRIPTION OF PROCEDURE: General endotracheal anesthesia was induced in the supine position, and a sterile prep and drape was then performed in standard fashion. The patient was given 1 g preoperative Ancef prophylactic antibiotic. The margins of resection were outlined with a surgical marking pen on the skin, and incisions were then made and carried down into the subcutaneous tissue utilizing a scalpel. Superior and inferior skin flaps were then raised with the curved Mayo scissors, and hemostasis was obtained and maintained with electrocautery. Following completion of development of the skin flaps, the tissue was then scored at the margins of resection down to the pectoralis muscle through the pectoralis fascia. The breast was then reflected off the pectoralis muscle, taking the fascia and utilizing electrocautery. The fatty tissue in the interpectoral groove was then sharply resected with Metzenbaum scissors, and the dissection then proceeded into the axilla on the chest wall. The axillary vein was identified, and this was the highest extent of the axillary dissection. The fatty tissue was divided from the axillary vein utilizing electrocautery and Metzenbaum scissors. Multiple small vein branches were ligated and divided between 3-0 silk ties. The thoracodorsal nerve was identified and tested with a gentle pinch. On the chest wall, the long thoracic nerve was identified high in the axilla and was tested with gentle pinch. Both of these nerves were functional and were protected from injury throughout the course of the dissection. The fatty tissue between these 2 nerves inferior to the axillary vein and between the chest wall and the anterior edge of the latissimus muscle was then carefully delivered by meticulous blunt and sharp dissection. This was then kept in continuity with the breast specimen. A small surgical clip marked most of highest axillary dissection on the axillary vein, and the highest axillary nodal tissue was marked on the specimen with a 3-0 silk suture ligature. The specimen was then passed off the field. The operative field was irrigated with sterile water, and final hemostasis was achieved with electrocautery and with silk ties. At the completion of the dissection, the nerves were then again tested with gentle pinch and were all seen to be functional. A 7-mm Jackson-Pratt drain was then placed through an inferior flap stab incision and secured with a silk tie. It was then placed in the axilla below the level of the axillary vein. The skin was then reapproximated with interrupted inverted 3-0 undyed Vicryl and skin staples. Bacitracin, followed by dry sterile dressings, was then applied. The patient was awakened and extubated and transported to the recovery room with stable vital signs. Estimated blood loss for the procedure was approximately 300 cc. The patient received no intraoperative blood products.

SPELLING.
Determine if the following words are spelled correctly. If the spelling is correct, leave the word as it has already been entered. If the spelling is incorrect, provide the correct spelling.

1. radical _____

2. biopsy _____

3. Metzenbomb _____

4. fasha _____

5. nodle _____

Multiple Choice.

Choose the correct spelling of the term.

1. The space below the shoulder joint.

   ○ axila

   ○ axillah

   ○ axilla

   ○ axala

2. The cauterization of tissue using electric current to generate heat.

   ○ electricautery

   ○ electrocautery

   ○ cautery

   ○ cateroelectricity

3. Surgical removal of breast.

   ○ mastectomy

   ○ mastetotomy

   ○ breastectomy

   ○ breastotomy

4. Lying face upward.

   ○ prone

   ○ prine

   ○ suppine

   ○ supine

5. A general term denoting a broad structure like a muscle.

   ○ latisimis

   ○ latissimis

   ○ latisimus

   ○ latissimus

PLASTIC SURGERY

Plastic surgery is not one of the more common types of admissions to a hospital. While you will undoubtedly encounter some of these report types, unless you become employed by a plastic surgeon in particular, you will probably not type an abundance of them.

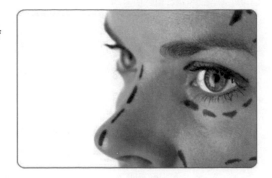

The basic goals of plastic surgery include the following:

- Correction of perceived disfigurement
- Restoration of impaired function
- Improvement of physical appearance

PLASTIC SURGERY REPORT 1 – OPERATIVE NOTE

PREOPERATIVE DIAGNOSIS: Nasal deformity.

POSTOPERATIVE DIAGNOSIS: Nasal deformity.

OPERATION PERFORMED: Open rhinoplasty.

INDICATIONS: The patient is a 21-year-old male who complained of a bulbous[1] tip on his nose. He requested a rhinoplasty for a correction of this cosmetic deformity. He has no breathing problems, and on physical exam his septum is midline. Also on physical exam, he has a rather bulbous tip with an otherwise well-formed nose. There does not appear to be any bony dorsal deformity. The base of the nose appears to be symmetrical with the rest of his face. Essentially, his only deformity is a very bulbous and thick, ill-defined tip region.

PROCEDURE: After informed consent was obtained from the patient, he was taken to the operating room and placed in a supine position. Intravenous sedation was administered. Pledgets soaked in 4 cc of 4% cocaine were placed into the nose for vasoconstriction and topical anesthesia. Lidocaine 2%[2] with 1:100,000 epinephrine was then infiltrated bilaterally into the areas of the infraorbital nerve, ciliary nerve, columella and caudal septum, the vestibular skin of the nose, and along the nasal dorsum.

The nose and face were then prepped and draped in the usual sterile fashion. The cocaine pledgets were then withdrawn. An incision was made in the columella at approximately the midpoint using an inverted V. Dissection through the soft tissue was then accomplished with iris scissors, and the medial crura[3] of the lower lateral cartilages were identified. The incision was then extended along the columella towards the nasal valve and into a rim incision on either side. The lateral crura of the lower lateral cartilages were identified, and dissection above these cartilaginous structures was performed, such that the skin of the nasal tip could be peeled back and the lower lateral cartilages delivered into the operating field. Once this was accomplished, the soft tissue overlying the lateral crura of the lower lateral cartilages was cleaned off. A small amount of apparently fatty and fibrous tissue in the tip of the nose was debulked. The patient had very prominent lateral crura, and this appeared to be contributing to the bulbous nature of his nose. The decision was made to perform a complete strip. The cephalic portions of each lateral crus of the lower lateral cartilages were then trimmed, leaving a remaining strut that was approximately 6 cm in width. The portion of cartilage removed was symmetrical, comparing the right and left. Replacement of the skin of the nose into its anatomic position revealed excellent reduction in the bulbous nature of the tip. To give additional projection of the nasal tip, the domes of the lower lateral cartilages were sewn together using a 4-0 clear nylon suture in a horizontal mattress stitch. Replacement of the nasal skin revealed excellent projection of the nose, along with adequate debulking of the bulbous tip. To give additional support to the tip, the medial crura of the lower lateral cartilages were also sewn together using the clear nylon suture. The nasal skin was then replaced in its anatomic position. The columellar incision was then closed with interrupted 6-0 nylon. The rim incisions were closed with several interrupted 3-0 chromic sutures. Telfa impregnated with bacitracin was placed in either vestibule to supply bolster support to the tip area. Tape was applied over the nasal dorsum to support the tip, and an Aquaplast cast was placed on the dorsum of the nose. This represented the termination of the procedure.

The patient was taken to the recovery room in good condition. He tolerated the procedure well. Estimated blood loss was minimal. Fluids were approximately 700 cc of crystalloid. Complications were none.

FINDINGS: Prominent lateral wings of the lower lateral cartilages were encountered, and a complete strip was performed. Additionally, the domes of the lower lateral cartilages were sewn together to apply additional tip projection.

Footnotes:

1. 1.Bulbous, as in curving outward, like a bulb.
2. 2.It is generally preferred not to begin a sentence with a numeral. Even if dictated as "Two percent lidocaine with..." an MTE might recast this to "Lidocaine 2% with..." so as not to begin the sentence with a numeral. That may or may not have been what happened here (we can't be sure without the accompanying audio).
3. 3.Crura is the plural of crus, which means the leg-like part of something.

Fill in the Blank.
Determine if the following words are spelled correctly. If the spelling is correct, leave the word as it has already been entered. If the spelling is incorrect, provide the correct spelling.

1. columnella _____

2. fibrus _____

3. inverted _____

4. anitomic _____

5. steril _____

True/False.
Mark the following true or false.

1. The operation performed on the patient was a closed rhinoplasty.

   ○ true

   ○ false

2. Bulbous denotes the curving outward, like a bulb.

   ○ true

   ○ false

3. Lidocaine 1% with 1:100,000 epinephrine was infiltrated.

   ○ true

   ○ false

4. Fluids were approximately 700 cc of saline.

   ○ true

   ○ false

5. There were no complications with the surgery.

   ○ true

   ○ false

PLASTIC SURGERY REPORT 2 – OPERATIVE NOTE

PREOPERATIVE DIAGNOSIS: Bilateral silicone gel implant rupture.

POSTOPERATIVE DIAGNOSIS: Bilateral silicone gel implant rupture.

OPERATION PERFORMED: Bilateral implant explantation with capsulectomies.[1]

INDICATIONS: The patient is a 36-year-old female who 10 years ago had bilateral subpectoral gel implants placed for augmentation. Implant size was 205 cc. The patient noticed that approximately 1 year ago there was decrease in size of the implants. A mammogram revealed bilateral rupture of the implants. The patient has had no other significant complaints. However, the left implant has become more cylindrical in shape. She is undergoing the following procedure for removal of the implants with the capsules and possible replacement of textured saline implants if the gel rupture is minimal.

DESCRIPTION OF PROCEDURE: The patient was taken to surgery where general anesthesia by the endotracheal route was performed. After adequate anesthesia was achieved, the patient was prepped and sterilely draped. Utilizing the scars in the inframammary areas, incisions were made. The incision was taken down to the level of the implant capsule using cautery. The capsule was then separated from the surrounding tissue using Bovie cautery. It was noted that there were several ruptures in the implant with several bubbles or extensions of the silicone gel surrounded by fibrous capsule. In one area the capsule was thin and opened, extruding gel. Gel was removed in its entirety. The remaining capsulectomy was completed. It was extended up and separated from the overlying pectoralis muscle. On the right side the extension followed the pectoralis muscle up into the axillary region. The entire capsule was removed. The wound was copiously irrigated with saline solution. Sponge packs were then placed. Next, the left implant was removed. This was done in a similar manner. Again, due to the essentially complete loss of the silicone shell of the gel implant, the implant had several rupture sites with a surrounding capsule. On the left side, the ruptured gel extended up underneath the pectoralis muscle to the axilla and laterally to an area just anterior to the latissimus muscle. Again the entire capsule was removed. There was a small opening and a small amount of gel extruded. This was all removed. Hemostasis was obtained with cautery. Again the implant pocket was copiously irrigated. Due to the extensive dissection up underneath the pectoralis muscle to the axilla and laterally past the anterior axillary line, and due to the extrusion of gel, it was elected not to replace textured saline implants at this time. Therefore, 10-mm Blake drains were placed in the pectoral pockets after again irrigating. The dermis was then closed using 3-0 Vicryl interrupted sutures, and the skin was closed using 5-0 nylon subcuticular running sutures. Sterile dressing of Xeroform, Kling, and Ace wrap was then placed. The patient was extubated in the operating room and taken to the recovery room without difficulty.

Footnotes:

1. 1.Explantation is the removal of an implant. Capsulectomy is removal of a capsule, as around a breast implant.

Spelling.
Determine if the following words are spelled correctly. If the spelling is correct, leave the word as it has already been entered. If the spelling is incorrect, retype the word with the correct spelling.

1. _____   2. _____

3. _____   4. _____

5. _____

Multiple Choice.

Choose the best answer.

1. The entire (○ capsil, ○ capsule) was removed.

2. The patient was prepped and (○ sterilely, ○ sterily) draped.

3. The (○ skin, ○ dermis) was then closed using 3-0 Vicryl interrupted sutures.

4. The wound was copiously irrigated with (○ bacitracin, ○ saline) solution.

5. The patient was (○ extubated, ○ extruded) in the operating room.

ANSWER KEY

Cardiology

REVIEW: CARDIOLOGY LANGUAGE

I. TRUE/FALSE.
false   2. true
false   4. true
false

II. MULTIPLE CHOICE.
coronary   2. rapid
blue   4. bundle
arteries

III. FILL IN THE BLANK.
percutaneous   2. thrombolysis
internal   4. destruction
hypertension

CARDIOLOGY REPORT 1 – DISCHARGE SUMMARY

I. SPELLING.
rheumatic   2. dyspneic
regurgitation   4. reticulocyte
Coombs

II. FILL IN THE BLANK.
congestive heart failure   2. jugular venous distention
BP   4. HJR
central venous pressures   6. subacute bacterial endocarditis
BUN

CARDIOLOGY REPORT 2 – DISCHARGE SUMMARY

I. SPELLING.
nitroglycerin   2. sublingual
Coumadin   4. enalapril
Cardizem   6. Mevacor
Lopressor

II. FILL IN THE BLANK.
A&P   2. LVEDP
CCU   4. percutaneous transluminal coronary angioplasty
LAD   6. paroxysmal nocturnal dyspnea
MI   8. GU
electrocardiogram   10. bid OR b.i.d.

CARDIOLOGY REPORT 3 – OPERATIVE NOTE

I. SPELLING.
hemoclip   2. anastomosis
aortotomies   4. lavage
circuit   6. cannulae OR cannula

II. MATCHING.
B. antegrade   2. C. electrocoagulation
A. Jackson-Pratt   4. D. retrograde
F. cannulation   6. E. hemostasis

CARDIOLOGY REPORT 4 – DISCHARGE SUMMARY

I. SPELLING.

lorazepam
Tegretol
urokinase

2. Benadryl
4. tricyclics
6. Percocet

II. FILL IN THE BLANK.

partial thromboplastin time
RSD
HEENT
twice a day
history of present illness

2. aortofemoral bypass
4. superior mesenteric artery
6. inferior mesenteric artery
8. jugular venous distention
10. PVR

CARDIOLOGY REPORT 5 – OPERATIVE NOTE

I. SPELLING.

Ancef
paraspinous
Bethune
Hespan

2. benzoin
4. Matson
6. Isolyte

II. FILL IN THE BLANK.

carcinoma OR cancer
ET
right upper lobe

2. lactated Ringer's
4. computed tomography

CARDIOLOGY REPORT 6 – DISCHARGE SUMMARY

I. SPELLING.

hilar
mellitus
subcarinal

2. Caucasian
4. tracheal
6. squamous

II. FILL IN THE BLANK.

benign prostatic hypertrophy
operating room
NIDDM

2. UA
4. arterial blood gas
6. CBC

CARDIOLOGY REPORT 7 – OPERATIVE NOTE

I. SPELLING.

Wegener
cavitations
trocar
Satinsky

2. hemoptysis
4. sterilely
6. extubated

II. MATCHING.

D. extubate
A. supine
C. intercostal

2. B. periosteum
4. E. taper

CARDIOLOGY REPORT 8 – DISCHARGE SUMMARY

I. SPELLING.

Klebsiella

anisocoria

cefuroxime

2. Xanax

4. ranitidine

II. FILL IN THE BLANK.

TB

MI

VSD

hemoglobin and hematocrit

2. peptic ulcer disease

4. chronic obstructive pulmonary disease

6. gastrointestinal

CARDIOLOGY REPORT 9 – DISCHARGE SUMMARY

I. SPELLING.

Pediazole

Metaprel

Eucerin

Indocin

2. erythromycin

4. candidiasis

6. dipyridamole

8. Valsalva

II. FILL IN THE BLANK.

ROM

ABI

pulmonary function test

2. pupils equal, round, reactive to light and accommodation OR Pupils equally round and reactive to light and accommodation

4. degenerative joint disease

Gastroenterology

REVIEW: GASTROENTEROLOGY LANGUAGE

I. MULTIPLE CHOICE.
Cholecystectomy
Lithotripsy
hepatojugular

2. rectocele
4. stomach

II. FILL IN THE BLANK.
laparotomy
gastroesophageal
appendectomy

2. oncology
4. lithotomy

III. TRUE/FALSE.
false
false
true

2. true
4. true

GASTROENTEROLOGY REPORT 1 – OPERATIVE NOTE

I. SPELLING.
Kelly
descending
antimesenteric

2. electrocautery
4. terminal
6. spleen

II. MATCHING.
B. omentum
C. colectomy
E. peritoneum

2. F. pubic tubercle
4. A. white line of Toldt
6. D. adenocarcinoma

GASTROENTEROLOGY REPORT 2 – DISCHARGE SUMMARY

I. MULTIPLE CHOICE.
hepatosplenomegaly
aide
vomiting

2. Apgars
4. seizures

II. FILL IN THE BLANK.
tympanic membrane

history of present illness

CNS

2. DTR OR DTRs
4. head, eyes, ears, nose, and throat OR head, eyes, ears, nose and throat

GASTROENTEROLOGY REPORT 3 – OPERATIVE NOTE

I. SPELLING.
imperforate
inspissated
proximal

2. atresia
4. fistula

II. MATCHING.
B. stoma
A. transverse
F. mesentery

2. E. adhesion
4. C. distal
6. D. endotracheal

GASTROENTEROLOGY REPORT 4 – PROCEDURE NOTE

I. SPELLING.

duodenum
pylorus
midazolam

2. reflux
4. sphincter

II. MATCHING.

B. cimetidine
E. omeprazole
C. lidocaine

2. A. ranitidine
4. D. midazolam

GASTROENTEROLOGY REPORT 5 – DISCHARGE SUMMARY

I. SPELLING.

Mylanta
deficiency
guaiac

2. nitrofurantoin
4. Haemophilus

II. FILL IN THE BLANK.

degenerative joint disease
gastrointestinal
PT

2. UTI
4. emergency room
6. IV

GASTROENTEROLOGY REPORT 6 – OPERATIVE NOTE

I. SPELLING.

Zenker
halitosis
bougie
esophagus

2. cricopharyngeal
4. platysma
6. dissection
8. Xeroform

II. MULTIPLE CHOICE.

equipment
anatomical
anatomical
equipment

2. anatomical
4. equipment
6. anatomical
8. equipment

GASTROENTEROLOGY REPORT 7 – OPERATIVE NOTE

I. MATCHING.

C. nocturia
B. herniation
F. fungating

2. E. copious
4. A. suprapubic
6. D. resection

II. MULTIPLE CHOICE.

sigmoid
laparotomy
1300

2. catheter
4. Surgical Intensive Care Unit

GASTROENTEROLOGY REPORT 8 – DISCHARGE SUMMARY

I. FILL IN THE BLANK.

urinary tract infection
gastrointestinal
BUN

2. TB
4. urinalysis
6. NG

II. TRUE/FALSE.

true
true
false

2. false
4. false

GASTROENTEROLOGY REPORT 9 – OPERATIVE NOTE

I. MATCHING.

C. pneumaturia

E. taut

D. musculature

2. A. efflux

4. B. laparotomy

II. MULTIPLE CHOICE.

suprapubic

tract

seepage

2. intermittent

4. peritoneum

Genitourinary

REVIEW: GENITOURINARY LANGUAGE

I. TRUE/FALSE.

false

true

true

2. true

4. false

II. FILL IN THE BLANK.

resection

hydrocele

balanitis

2. extracorporeal

4. anuresis

III. MULTIPLE CHOICE.

Dysuria

Anorchism

enuresis

2. urethrotomy

4. prostate

GENITOURINARY REPORT 1 – OPERATIVE NOTE

I. SPELLING.

torsion

orchiopexy

tunica

DeBakey

mesorchium

2. epididymis

4. hemiscrotum

6. vaginalis

8. raphe

10. albuginea

II. MATCHING.

C. gauze

D. electrocautery

2. A. forceps

4. B. suture

GENITOURINARY REPORT 2 – OPERATIVE NOTE

I. SPELLING.

puboprostatic

devascularization

cystoprostatectomy

conduit

rectourethralis

2. psoas

4. hemodialysis

6. Bricker

8. Storey

10. Babcock

II. TRUE/FALSE.

false

false

true

2. true

4. false

GENITOURINARY REPORT 3 – DISCHARGE SUMMARY

I. SPELLING.

hematuria

nitrites

hyperplasia

2. phallus

4. trabeculations

II. MATCHING.

B. amenable

A. hypertrophy

C. ad lib

2. E. dysuria

4. D. trigone

6. F. anorexia

GENITOURINARY REPORT 4 – OPERATIVE NOTE

I. SPELLING.

prostatic
transurethral
gurney

2. benign
4. verumontanum

II. MATCHING.

D. catheter
F. resectoscope
E. evacuator

2. C. sheath
4. A. sound
6. B. obturator

GENITOURINARY REPORT 5 – PROCEDURE NOTE

I. SPELLING.

circumcision
foreskin
eminence

2. paraphimosis
4. subcutaneously

II. TRUE/FALSE.

true
false
true

2. true
4. false

GENITOURINARY REPORT 6 – OPERATIVE NOTE

I. SPELLING.

varicocele
Veress
quadrant

2. Trendelenburg
4. trocar

II. MATCHING.

B. orogastric
A. ligation
D. fascia

2. C. tympany
4. E. insufflate

GENITOURINARY REPORT 7 – DISCHARGE SUMMARY

I. SPELLING.

recurrence
sessile
tubular

2. tubulovillous
4. transanal

II. TRUE/FALSE.

true
true
false

2. false
4. true

GENITOURINARY REPORT 8 – OPERATIVE NOTE

I. SPELLING.

Ray-Tec
cannulated
endotracheal

2. mucosa
4. transversalis

II. MATCHING.

A. transurethral
B. tenotomy
C. subcutaneous

2. E. perineum
4. D. Scarpa's fascia

GENITOURINARY REPORT 9 – OPERATIVE NOTE

I. SPELLING.

pyelogram

fluoroscopic

dilating

2. lithotripsy

4. ureteral

II. MATCHING.

A. lithotripsy

D. forceps

C. perioperative

2. E. contrast

4. B. edema

Neurology

REVIEW: NEUROLOGY LANGUAGE

I. FILL IN THE BLANK.
emission
computed
encephalitis
neurotome

2. craniomalacia
4. resonance
6. peripheral

II. MULTIPLE CHOICE.
Arthroplasty
Myopathy
ischemic

2. labyrinthitis
4. laminectomy

III. TRUE/FALSE.
false
true
false

2. false
4. true

NEUROLOGY REPORT 1 – OPERATIVE NOTE

I. SPELLING.
paresthesias
myelopathy
Thrombin

2. colli
4. osteophyte

II. MATCHING.
C. rongeur
D. periosteal elevator
E. retractor

2. A. electrocautery
4. B. disk space spreader

NEUROLOGY REPORT 2 – DISCHARGE SUMMARY

I. SPELLING.
encroachment
Azulfidine
hemilaminectomy
pulposus

2. hepatocellular
4. steatohepatitis
6. foraminotomy

II. FILL IN THE BLANK.
DJD
PT
gastrointestinal
cervical spine

2. no known drug allergies
4. LFT
6. HPI
8. twice a day

NEUROLOGY REPORT 3 – OPERATIVE NOTE

I. SPELLING.
dura
schwannoma
craniectomy

2. subocciput
4. Mayfield

II. TRUE/FALSE.
false
true
true

2. false
4. false

NEUROLOGY REPORT 4 – DISCHARGE SUMMARY

I. SPELLING.

pneumocephalus
hemotympanum
psychometrics

2. papilledema
4. ventriculostomy

II. FILL IN THE BLANK.

emergency room
TM
ventriculoperitoneal
loss of consciousness
DC

2. electroencephalogram
4. OT
6. CT
8. deep tendon reflex

NEUROLOGY REPORT 5 – OPERATIVE NOTE

I. SPELLING.

cord
Surgicel
hemostatic

2. platelets
4. pituitary

II. MATCHING.

E. decompression
D. irrigated
B. infiltrated

2. A. paraparesis
4. C. obliteration

NEUROLOGY REPORT 6 – DISCHARGE SUMMARY

I. MULTIPLE CHOICE.

pulposus
dexamethasone
hemilaminectomy

2. antalgic
4. strenuous

II. TRUE/FALSE.

false
false
false

2. true
4. false

NEUROLOGY REPORT 7 – OPERATIVE NOTE

I. SPELLING.

thoracolumbar
cancellous
autologous

2. endplates
4. facets

II. MULTIPLE CHOICE.

decubitus
copious
laminar

2. lordosis
4. periosteum

NEUROLOGY REPORT 8 – DISCHARGE SUMMARY

I. SPELLING.

hepatosplenomegaly

diplopia

meningeal

2. Lyme

4. bioccipital

II. MATCHING.

F. tuberculosis

I. acid-fast bacillus

A. rapid plasma reagin

M. cerebrospinal fluid

G. potassium hydroxide

K. purified protein derivative

J. Epstein-Barr virus

2. C. lumbar puncture

4. H. thyroid stimulating hormone

6. B. fluorescent treponemal antibody absorption

8. L. angiotensin-converting enzyme

10. D. brainstem auditory-evoked response

12. E. cytomegalovirus

NEUROLOGY REPORT 9 – OPERATIVE NOTE

I. MULTIPLE CHOICE.

stenosis

analgesic

herniated

2. scarred

4. annulus

II. MATCHING.

B. recurrent

A. prominence

C. dura

2. D. refractory

4. E. curet

REVIEW: OB/GYN LANGUAGE

I. TRUE/FALSE.

true

false

true

2. true

4. true

6. false

II. FILL IN THE BLANK.

galactorrhea

papilloma

metrorrhagia

2. cephalopelvic

4. bilateral

6. inflammatory

III. MULTIPLE CHOICE.

Menarche

alpha

2. Perineorrhaphy

4. Pseudocyesis

OB/GYN REPORT 1 – OPERATIVE NOTE

I. SPELLING.

endometriosis

Maylard

Metzenbaum

2. fulguration

4. Turner-Warwick

II. MATCHING.

D. scissors

A. retractor

E. drain

2. C. incision

4. B. catheter

OB/GYN REPORT 2 – DISCHARGE SUMMARY

I. SPELLING.

terbutaline

betamethasone

Streptococcus

2. Chlamydia

4. tocolytics

II. MATCHING.

C. gravida

A. terbutaline

B. placenta previa

2. E. para

4. D. magnesium sulfate

OB/GYN REPORT 3 – PROCEDURE NOTE

I. SPELLING.

curettage

Provera

tenaculum

Randall

2. Vabra

4. speculum

6. retroverted

8. uterine cry

II. TRUE/FALSE.

false

true

false

2. true

4. true

OB/GYN REPORT 4 – OPERATIVE NOTE

I. MULTIPLE CHOICE.

pessary

introitus

dissect

2. mucosa

4. colpotomy

II. MATCHING.

B. stitch

E. clamp

D. retractor

A. scissors

2. A. scissors

4. C. tenaculum

6. E. clamp

OB/GYN REPORT 5 – DISCHARGE SUMMARY

I. SPELLING.

uterovaginal

culdoplasty

atrophic

2. McCall

4. hematocrit

II. MATCHING.

C. Minipress

A. Colace

D. cyanosis

2. E. cystocele

4. B. rectocele

OB/GYN REPORT 6 – OPERATIVE NOTE

I. SPELLING.

reanastomosis

scalpel

serosa

2. proximal

4. mesosalpinx

II. MULTIPLE CHOICE.

adhesions

cervix

laparotomy

2. fimbriated

4. Metzenbaum

OB/GYN REPORT 7 – OPERATIVE NOTE

I. SPELLING.

succinylcholine

cul-de-sac

Terbutaline

2. fascial

4. bleeder

II. TRUE/FALSE.

false

false

true

2. true

4. true

OB/GYN REPORT 8 – DISCHARGE SUMMARY

I. SPELLING.

scotomata

Aldomet

preeclampsia

2. clonus

4. oligohydramnios

II. FILL IN THE BLANK.

estimated date of confinement

amniotic fluid index

para

GC

2. history of present illness

4. DTR OR DTRs

6. spontaneous vaginal delivery

8. biophysical profile

OB/GYN REPORT 9 – OPERATIVE NOTE

I. MULTIPLE CHOICE.

infraumbilical

fornix

lithotomy

2. benign

4. cervical

II. MATCHING.

D. squamous

C. agglutination

A. speculum

2. B. tenaculum

4. E. endometriosis

REVIEW: OPHTHALMOLOGY LANGUAGE

I. FILL IN THE BLANK.

sinister
blepharitis
photophobia

2. lacrimal
4. salt

II. MULTIPLE CHOICE.

Phacoemulsification
blepharospasm
iridectomy

2. Ophthalmology
4. conjunctivitis
6. Retinopathy

III. TRUE/FALSE.

false
true
false

2. true
4. false

OPHTHALMOLOGY REPORT 1 – OPERATIVE NOTE

I. SPELLING.

diplopia
Wydase
conjunctiva
bayonet

2. Marcaine
4. palpebral
6. malleable
8. Maxitrol

II. MATCHING.

D. forceps
A. suture
E. retractor

2. B. elevator
4. C. shield

OPHTHALMOLOGY REPORT 2 – OPERATIVE NOTE

I. SPELLING.

McPherson
Lacri-Lube
dexamethasone

2. vitrectomy
4. V-flap
6. Fortaz

II. MULTIPLE CHOICE.

capsulorrhexis
cataract
haptic

2. conjunctiva
4. collagen

OPHTHALMOLOGY REPORT 3 – DISCHARGE SUMMARY

I. SPELLING.

epiphora
Hismanal
cephalosporin
applanation
pinguecula
Schirmer's

2. Premarin
4. Vancenase
6. tonometry
8. puncta
10. macula
12. dacryocystorhinostomy

II. FILL IN THE BLANK.

NAD
millimeters of mercury

right eye

ENT

2. left eye
4. CBC
6. total abdominal hysterectomy/bilateral salpingo-oophorectomy

OPHTHALMOLOGY REPORT 4 – OPERATIVE NOTE

I. FILL IN THE BLANK.

sclerostomy
peritomy
ophthalmoscope

2. vitrectomy
4. epiretinal membrane

II. TRUE/FALSE.

false
true
true

2. false
4. false

OPHTHALMOLOGY REPORT 5 – DISCHARGE SUMMARY

I. SPELLING.

keratopathy
retinopexy
cimetidine
Pred Forte

2. rhegmatogenous
4. diathermy
6. scopolamine

II. FILL IN THE BLANK.

MI
atrioventricular
right eye
OS
ACIOL

2. penetrating keratoplasty
4. IOL
6. dacryocystorhinostomy
8. both eyes
10. mmHg

OPHTHALMOLOGY REPORT 6 – OPERATIVE NOTE

I. SPELLING.

ptosis
pupillary
limbus

2. preaponeurotic
4. orbicularis

II. MATCHING.

E. retractor
A. anesthetic
D. gauze

2. C. scissors
4. B. shields

OPHTHALMOLOGY REPORT 7 – DISCHARGE SUMMARY

I. SPELLING.

Pilogel
Krukenberg's
fluorouracil
Voltaren

2. Neptazane
4. gonioscopy
6. Seidel's

II. MULTIPLE CHOICE.

obstruction
Krukenberg's
OD

2. epithelial
4. bleb

OPHTHALMOLOGY REPORT 8 – OPERATIVE NOTE

I. SPELLING.

dermatochalasis
thermocautery
infraorbital

2. oblique
4. blepharoplasty

II. MULTIPLE CHOICE.

Ice
electrocautery
Tylenol

2. local
4. tetracaine

OPHTHALMOLOGY REPORT 9 – PROCEDURE NOTE

I. SPELLING.

retrobulbar
scleral
Miostat

2. akinesia
4. capsulorrhexis

II. TRUE/FALSE.

true
false
false

2. false
4. true

Orthopedics

REVIEW: ORTHOPEDICS LANGUAGE

I. MULTIPLE CHOICE.
osteotome
inflammation
osteopenia

2. cartilage
4. cruciate

II. TRUE/FALSE.
true
true
true

2. true
4. false

III. FILL IN THE BLANK.
myotomy
metacarpophalangeal
arthroplasty

2. costochondritis
4. carpal

ORTHOPEDICS REPORT 1 – OPERATIVE NOTE

I. SPELLING.
fungal
compressive
Hemovac

2. quiescent
4. anaerobic

II. MULTIPLE CHOICE.
fungal
copious
subcutaneous

2. osteomyelitis
4. purulent

ORTHOPEDICS REPORT 2 – OPERATIVE NOTE

I. TRUE/FALSE.
false
false
true

2. true
4. false

II. MATCHING.
E. gauze
D. drain
C. saw

2. B. wrap
4. A. screw

ORTHOPEDICS REPORT 3 – DISCHARGE SUMMARY

I. FILL IN THE BLANK.
cruciate
hematocrit
degenerative

2. occupational OR Occupational
4. medial
6. bowel

II. TRUE/FALSE.
false
true
true

2. false
4. false

ORTHOPEDICS REPORT 4 – OPERATIVE NOTE

I. SPELLING.

varus

cruciate

Kerlix

2. intercondylar

4. patellar

II. TRUE/FALSE.

true

false

false

2. false

4. true

ORTHOPEDICS REPORT 5 – OPERATIVE NOTE

I. SPELLING.

debridement

gelatinous

cloaca

2. cellulitis

4. loculation

6. lavage

II. MULTIPLE CHOICE.

cloaca

curet

decubitus

2. lavage

4. plane

ORTHOPEDICS REPORT 6 – OPERATIVE NOTE

I. SPELLING.

anesthesia

urokinase

prosthesis

2. Gigli

4. ligation

II. MULTIPLE CHOICE.

left

oscillating

supine

2. Hemostasis

4. prosthesis

ORTHOPEDICS REPORT 7 – DISCHARGE SUMMARY

I. MULTIPLE CHOICE.

pseudolaxity

autologous

meniscectomy

2. prophylaxis

4. suprapatellar

II. FILL IN THE BLANK.

compression

continuous

function

2. embolic OR thromboembolic

4. thrombosis

ORTHOPEDICS REPORT 8 – OPERATIVE NOTE

I. FILL IN THE BLANK.

chondromalacia OR chondromalacial

cyclops lesion

periosteal

2. exsanguinate

4. impingement

II. MATCHING.

D. guide

A. pin

C. cannula

2. E. bur

4. F. suture

6. B. brace

ORTHOPEDICS REPORT 9 – OPERATIVE NOTE

I. MULTIPLE CHOICE.
bursal

activities

epinephrine

2. extubated

4. sterilely

II. MULTIPLE CHOICE.
decubitus

subacromial

glenohumeral

2. posterolateral

4. anterolateral

Otorhinolaryngology

REVIEW: OTORHINOLARYNGOLOGY LANGUAGE

I. FILL IN THE BLANK.
anesthesia

laryngitis

nose

2. suppurative

4. otoscopy

II. MULTIPLE CHOICE.
dysphasia

larynx

bronchospasm

2. hematemesis

4. equalization

III. TRUE/FALSE.
false

true

false

2. true

4. true

OTORHINOLARYNGOLOGY REPORT 1 – OPERATIVE NOTE

I. SPELLING.
turbinates

McIvor

velopharyngeal

Vicryl

epinephrine

pledgets

Sayre

Telfa

crystalloid

2. uvulopalatopharyngoplasty

4. Bovie

6. DeBakey

8. palate

10. vasoconstriction

12. mucoperiosteum

14. bacitracin

16. columella

II. MATCHING.
C. elevator

B. mouth gag

D. cautery

2. E. forceps

4. A. dressing

OTORHINOLARYNGOLOGY REPORT 2 – OPERATIVE NOTE

I. SPELLING.
fingerbreadths

Shiley

elliptical

2. scalpel

4. fenestrated

II. TRUE/FALSE.
false

false

false

2. true

4. true

OTORHINOLARYNGOLOGY REPORT 3 – OPERATIVE NOTE

I. SPELLING.

eustachian
cautery
Paparella
Jansen-Middleton
quadrilateral

2. antrotomy
4. cottonoid
6. Cottle
8. rongeurs
10. Doyle

II. FILL IN THE BLANK.

Cottle
Telfa
Jansen-Middleton
Keith

2. Doyle
4. Takahashi
6. Paparella

OTORHINOLARYNGOLOGY REPORT 4 – OPERATIVE NOTE

I. SPELLING.

epiglottis
marsupialize
vallecula

2. exophytic
4. piriform

II. MULTIPLE CHOICE.

malignancy
evacuated
EGD

2. cords
4. squamous

OTORHINOLARYNGOLOGY REPORT 5 – OPERATIVE NOTE

I. MULTIPLE CHOICE.

hypertrophic
soft palate
strep

2. adenoid
4. tonsillitis

II. MULTIPLE CHOICE.

recurrent
Dissection
extubated

2. oropharynx
4. cautery

OTORHINOLARYNGOLOGY REPORT 6 – DISCHARGE SUMMARY

I. SPELLING.

submucous
lidocaine
Percocet

2. apnea
4. uvulopalatopharyngoplasty

II. TRUE/FALSE.

false
false
true

2. true
4. false

OTORHINOLARYNGOLOGY REPORT 7 – OPERATIVE NOTE

I. SPELLING.

otorrhea
mastoid
cholesteatoma

2. methylene
4. ossicular

II. TRUE/FALSE.

false
true
true

2. false
4. false

OTORHINOLARYNGOLOGY REPORT 8 – OPERATIVE NOTE

I. SPELLING.
patent
ostium
mucosa

2. labyrinth
4. antrum

II. MULTIPLE CHOICE.
courses
Takahashi
ostiomeatal

2. supine
4. bacitracin

OTORHINOLARYNGOLOGY REPORT 9 – DISCHARGE SUMMARY

I. MULTIPLE CHOICE.
Zenker
hepatosplenomegaly
dysphagia

2. Hemoccult
4. halitosis

II. TRUE/FALSE.
false
true
false

2. false
4. true

ORAL SURGERY REPORT 1 – OPERATIVE NOTE

I. SPELLING.
Marcaine
Bard-Parker
osteotome

2. oropharynx
4. tuberosity

II. FILL IN THE BLANK.
false
true
true

2. false
4. false

ORAL SURGERY REPORT 2 – OPERATIVE NOTE

I. MULTIPLE CHOICE.
retromolar
canine
mylohyoid

2. intraoral
4. hemostasis

II. MATCHING.
C. awl
A. sutures
D. catheter

2. E. clamp
4. B. dressing

REVIEW: PEDIATRICS LANGUAGE

I. MULTIPLE CHOICE.

Rhinorrhea

Cytomegalovirus

Rapid

2. Polydipsia

4. Cerebral

6. parenteral

II. TRUE/FALSE.

false

true

2. false

4. true

III. FILL IN THE BLANK.

immunodeficiency

infant

syncytial

2. patent

4. retinopathy

PEDIATRICS REPORT 1 – DISCHARGE SUMMARY

I. MULTIPLE CHOICE.

sepsis

electrolytes

prophylaxis

2. afebrile

4. palpation

II. MULTIPLE CHOICE.

seizures

diarrhea

murmur

2. tympanic

4. aide

PEDIATRICS REPORT 2 – DISCHARGE SUMMARY

I. SPELLING.

albuterol

infiltration

rhonchi

2. atelectasis

4. normocephalic

II. TRUE/FALSE.

false

true

true

2. false

4. false

PEDIATRICS REPORT 3 – DISCHARGE SUMMARY

I. FILL IN THE BLANK.

tract

membrane

Diphtheria OR diphtheria

2. cystourethrogram

4. nose

II. MULTIPLE CHOICE.

weeks'

ampicillin

turgor

2. follow up

4. primipara

PEDIATRICS REPORT 4 – DISCHARGE SUMMARY

I. SPELLING.
adenitis
dyspnea
meningitis

2. defervesced
4. lymphocytosis

II. MULTIPLE CHOICE.
fluid
blood
urinalysis

2. respiratory
4. tympanic

PEDIATRICS REPORT 5 – DISCHARGE SUMMARY

I. SPELLING.
breech
cervical
musculoskeletal

2. abortus
4. incisor

II. MULTIPLE CHOICE.
jaundice
gestation
para

2. gravida
4. cesarean

PEDIATRICS REPORT 6 – DISCHARGE SUMMARY

I. FILL IN THE BLANK.
otitis
rhinorrhea
Candida vaginitis

2. mucous
4. peritonsillar

II. MULTIPLE CHOICE.
erythematous
sclera
exudate

2. axillary
4. rale

PEDIATRICS REPORT 7 – OPERATIVE NOTE

I. SPELLING.
dartos
caudal
tunic
crystalloid

2. oblique
4. Steri-Strips
6. ilioinguinal

II. TRUE/FALSE.
false
false
true

2. true
4. false

PEDIATRICS REPORT 8 – DISCHARGE SUMMARY

I. SPELLING.
Septra
wheeze
otitis

2. retractions
4. hospitalization

II. MULTIPLE CHOICE.
respiratory
nebulizers
recurrent

2. oxygen
4. delay

PEDIATRICS REPORT 9 – DISCHARGE SUMMARY

I. SPELLING.

Apgar
Augmentin
immunizations

2. cefuroxime
4. sinusitis

II. MULTIPLE CHOICE.

pustule
spontaneous
bronchiolitis

2. periorbital
4. cellulitis

REVIEW: SURGERY LANGUAGE

I. FILL IN THE BLANK.

resuscitate OR RESUSCITATE

thoracentesis

adhesiolysis

2. lithotripsy

4. cryptorchism

II. MULTIPLE CHOICE.

Pneumoperitoneum

trauma

nothing

2. positive

4. back

III. TRUE/FALSE.

false

true

true

2. false

4. false

SURGERY REPORT 1 – OPERATIVE NOTE

I. SPELLING.

choledocholithiasis

cholangiopancreatography

Potts

Angiovist

2. jaundice

4. Hartmann

6. ampulla

8. Prolene

II. TRUE/FALSE.

true

true

true

2. false

4. false

SURGERY REPORT 2 – OPERATIVE NOTE

I. MULTIPLE CHOICE.

fingerbreadths

dissection

inguinal

2. Marlex

4. scalpel

II. MULTIPLE CHOICE.

transverse

hernia

epidural

2. spermatic cord

4. bilateral

SURGERY REPORT 3 – DISCHARGE SUMMARY

I. SPELLING.

splenectomy

Solu-Cortef

Ancef

2. noncontributory

4. idiopathic

II. TRUE/FALSE.

false

false

true

2. true

4. false

SURGERY REPORT 4 – OPERATIVE NOTE

I. MULTIPLE CHOICE.
hilar
Penrose
supine

2. irrigated
4. crural

II. MATCHING.
D. test
A. drain
B. retractor

2. E. suture
4. C. fundoplication

SURGERY REPORT 5 – OPERATIVE NOTE

I. SPELLING.
appendiceal
abdomen
fulgurated

2. mucosal
4. oblique

II. TRUE/FALSE.
true
true
false

2. false
4. false

SURGERY REPORT 6 – DISCHARGE SUMMARY

I. MULTIPLE CHOICE.
cecectomy
anastomosis
psoas sign

2. perforation
4. arcus senilis

II. MATCHING.
D. p.r.n.
C. 1-2 tablets
B. 300 mg

2. A. 500 mg
4. E. 100-200 mg

SURGERY REPORT 7 – OPERATIVE NOTE

I. SPELLING.
Treitz
hemicolectomy
anastomosis

2. jejunojejunostomy
4. ileocolic

II. MATCHING.
B. stapling device
A. ligament
C. suture

2. E. material
4. D. graft

SURGERY REPORT 8 – DISCHARGE SUMMARY

I. SPELLING.
hyperalimentation
Flagyl
fistulogram
enterocutaneous

2. Timentin
4. Montgomery
6. somatostatin

II. MULTIPLE CHOICE.
hyperalimentation
adnexal
striae

2. hiatal
4. peritonitis

SURGERY REPORT 9 – OPERATIVE NOTE

I. SPELLING.

radical

Metzenbaum

nodal

2. biopsy

4. fascia

II. MULTIPLE CHOICE.

axilla

mastectomy

latissimus

2. electrocautery

4. supine

PLASTIC SURGERY REPORT 1 – OPERATIVE NOTE

I. FILL IN THE BLANK.

columella

inverted

sterile

2. fibrous

4. anatomic

II. TRUE/False.

false

false

true

2. true

4. false

PLASTIC SURGERY REPORT 2 – OPERATIVE NOTE

I. SPELLING.

augment

implants

pectoralis

2. endotracheal

4. inframammary

II. MULTIPLE CHOICE.

capsule

dermis

extubated

2. sterilely

4. saline